Neuroinflammation

New Insights into Beneficial and Detrimental Functions

Neuroinflammation
New Insights into Beneficial and Detrimental Functions

Edited by

SAMUEL DAVID, PhD

WILEY Blackwell

Published by John Wiley & Sons, Inc., Hoboken, New Jersey
Published simultaneously in Canada

Library of Congress Cataloging-in-Publication Data:

Neuroinflammation (David)
  Neuroinflammation : new insights into beneficial and detrimental functions / edited by Samuel David.
    p. ; cm.
  Includes bibliographical references and index.
  ISBN 978-1-118-73282-3 (cloth)
  I. David, Samuel, editor. II. Title.
  [DNLM: 1. Central Nervous System Diseases–immunology. 2. Central Nervous System Diseases–physiopathology. 3. Autoimmune Diseases–physiopathology. 4. Inflammation–physiopathology. 5. Neurodegenerative Diseases–physiopathology. WL 301]
  RC346.5
  616.8′0479–dc23

                                                                                    2014047521

Cover images: Headache © Ingram_Publishing/iStockphoto
Printed and bound in Malaysia by Vivar Printing Sdn Bhd

1 2015

Contents

Contributors

Stanley H. Appel

Department of Neurology
Methodist Neurological Institute
The Methodist Hospital
Weill Cornell Medical College
Houston, TX, USA

Nathalie Arbour

Department of Neurosciences
Université de Montréal
Centre de Recherche du Centre Hospitalier de l'Université de
Montréal
Montreal, QC, Canada

Lukas Andereggen

Laboratories for Neuroscience Research in Neurosurgery and
F.M. Kirby Neurobiology Center
Boston Children's Hospital
Boston, MA, USA

Department of Neurosurgery
Harvard Medical School
Boston, MA, USA

Ivan Ballesteros

Department of Pharmacology (Medical School)
Universidad Complutense de Madrid
Instituto de Investigación Hospital 12 de Octubre (i+12)
Madrid, Spain

David R. Beers

Department of Neurology
Methodist Neurological Institute
The Methodist Hospital
Weill Cornell Medical College
Houston, TX, USA

Larry I. Benowitz   Laboratories for Neuroscience Research in Neurosurgery and
                               F.M. Kirby Neurobiology Center
                               Boston Children's Hospital
                               Boston, MA, USA

                               Departments of Neurosurgery and Ophthalmology
                               Program in Neuroscience
                               Harvard Medical School
                               Boston, MA, USA

Bibiana Bielekova   Neuroimmunology Branch
                               National Institute of Neurological Disorders and Stroke
                               National Institutes of Health
                               Bethesda, MD, USA

Nathalie Castanon   Laboratory of Nutrition and Integrative Neurobiology
                               INRA UMR 1286
                               Bordeaux, France

                               University of Bordeaux
                               Bordeaux, France

María Isabel Cuartero   Department of Pharmacology (Medical School)
                               Universidad Complutense de Madrid
                               Instituto de Investigación Hospital 12 de Octubre (i+12)
                               Madrid, Spain

James C. Cronk   Center for Brain Immunology and Glia and Department of
                               Neuroscience
                               University of Virginia School of Medicine
                               Charlottesville, VA, USA

Samuel David   Department of Neurology and Neurosurgery
                               Faculty of Medicine
                               Centre for Research in Neuroscience
                               The Research Institute of the McGill University Health Centre
                               Montreal, QC, Canada

Noël C. Derecki   Center for Brain Immunology and Glia and Department of
                               Neuroscience
                               University of Virginia School of Medicine
                               Charlottesville, VA, USA

Ashley M. Fenn   Department of Neuroscience
                               The Ohio State University
                               Columbus, OH, USA

Robin J.M. Franklin
Department of Clinical Neurosciences
Wellcome Trust-MRC Cambridge Stem Cell Institute
University of Cambridge
Cambridge, UK

Andrew D. Greenhalgh
Department of Neurology and Neurosurgery
Faculty of Medicine
Centre for Research in Neuroscience
The Research Institute of the McGill University Health Centre
Montreal, QC, Canada

Jonathan P. Godbout
Department of Neuroscience and Institute for Behavioral
Medicine Research
The Ohio State University
Columbus, OH, USA

Janos Groh
Department of Neurology and Developmental Neurobiology
University of Wuerzburg
Wuerzburg, Germany

Renu Heir
Department of Neurology and Neurosurgery
Centre for Research in Neuroscience
The Research Institute of the McGill University Health Center
Montreal, QC, Canada

Kristopher G. Hooten
Department of Neurological Surgery
University of Florida
Gainesville, FL, USA

Dennis Klein
Department of Neurology and Developmental Neurobiology
University of Wuerzburg
Wuerzburg, Germany

Jonathan Kipnis
Center for Brain Immunology and Glia and Department of
Neuroscience
University of Virginia School of Medicine
Charlottesville, VA, USA

Graduate Program in Neuroscience and Medical Scientist
Training Program
University of Virginia School of Medicine
Charlottesville, VA, USA

Antje Kroner
Department of Neurology and Developmental Neurobiology
University of Wuerzburg
Wuerzburg, Germany

Department of Neurology and Neurosurgery
Faculty of Medicine
Centre for Research in Neuroscience
The Research Institute of the McGill University Health Centre
Montreal, QC, Canada

Steve Lacroix
Centre de Recherche du Centre Hospitalier Universitaire (CHU) de Québec –CHUL
Québec, QC, Canada

Département de Médecine Moléculaire
Faculté de médecine
Université Laval
Québec, QC, Canada

Hans Lassman
Division of Neuroimmunology
Center for Brain Research
Medical University of Vienna
Vienna, Austria

Sophie Layé
Laboratory of Nutrition and Integrative Neurobiology
INRA UMR 1286
Bordeaux, France

University of Bordeaux
Bordeaux, France

Ignacio Lizasoain
Department of Pharmacology (Medical School)
Universidad Complutense de Madrid
Instituto de Investigación Hospital 12 de Octubre (i+12)
Madrid, Spain

Giamal Luheshi
Department of Psychiatry
Douglas Mental Health University Institute
McGill University
Montreal, QC, Canada

Rudolf Martini
Department of Neurology and Developmental Neurobiology
University of Wuerzburg
Wuerzburg, Germany

María Ángeles Moro
Department of Pharmacology (Medical School)
Universidad Complutense de Madrid
Instituto de Investigación Hospital 12 de Octubre (i+12)
Madrid, Spain

Muktha Natrajan
Department of Clinical Neurosciences
Wellcome Trust-MRC Cambridge Stem Cell Institute
University of Cambridge
Cambridge, UK

Diana M. Norden   Department of Neuroscience
                             The Ohio State University
                             Columbus, OH, USA

Alexandre Paré   Centre de Recherche du Centre Hospitalier Universitaire (CHU)
                             de Québec - CHUL
                             Québec, QC, Canada

Alexandre Prat   Department of Neurosciences
                             Université de Montréal
                             Centre de Recherche du Centre Hospitalier de l'Université de
                             Montréal
                             Montreal, QC, Canada

Christopher Power   Department of Medicine (Neurology)
                             University of Alberta
                             Edmonton, AB, Canada

Harald Prüss   Department of Neurology and Experimental Neurology
                             Clinical and Experimental Spinal Cord Injury Research
                             (Neuroparaplegiology)
                             Charite
                             Universitatsmedizin Berlin
                             Berlin, Germany

                             German Center for Neurodegenerative Diseases (DZNE)
                             Berlin, Germany

Catarina Raposo   Department of Neurobiology
                             Weizmann Institute of Science
                             Rehovot, Israel

Jan M. Schwab   Department of Neurology and Experimental Neurology
                             Clinical and Experimental Spinal Cord Injury Research
                             (Neuroparaplegiology)
                             Charite - Universitatsmedizin Berlin
                             Berlin, Germany

                             Spinal Cord Injury Center
                             Trauma Hospital Berlin
                             Berlin, Germany

                             Department of Neurology and Neuroscience
                             Center for Brain and Spinal Cord Repair
                             The Ohio State University Medical Center
                             Columbus, OH, USA

Michal Schwartz   Department of Neurobiology
                             Weizmann Institute of Science
                             Rehovot, Israel

Charles N. Serhan
Department of Anesthesiology
Perioperative and Pain Medicine
Center for Experimental Therapeutics and Reperfusion Injury
Harvard Institutes of Medicine
Brigham and Women's Hospital and Harvard Medical School
Boston, MA, USA

David Stellwagen
Department of Neurology and Neurosurgery
Centre for Research in Neuroscience
The Research Institute of the McGill University Health Center
Montreal, QC, Canada

Ephraim F. Trakhtenberg
Laboratories for Neuroscience Research in Neurosurgery and
F.M. Kirby Neurobiology Center
Boston Children's Hospital
Boston, MA, USA

Department of Neurosurgery
Harvard Medical School
Boston, MA, USA

John G. Walsh
Department of Medicine (Neurology)
University of Alberta
Edmonton, AL, Canada

Yuqin Yin
Laboratories for Neuroscience Research in Neurosurgery and
F.M. Kirby Neurobiology Center
Boston Children's Hospital
Boston, MA, USA

Department of Neurosurgery
Harvard Medical School
Boston, MA, USA

Ji Zhang
The Alan Edwards Centre for Research on Pain and Department
of Neurology and Neurosurgery
Faculty of Dentistry and Medicine
McGill University
Montreal, QC, Canada

Weihua Zhao
Department of Neurology
Houston Methodist Neurological Institute
Houston Methodist Hospital Research Institute
Houston Methodist Hospital
Houston, TX, USA

Preface

When I was approached by the publisher, Wiley, to edit a book on neuroinflammation I felt it was a timely project and one that would have a wide appeal. As a researcher whose work focuses on inflammation in spinal cord injury (SCI), central nervous system (CNS) autoimmune disease, peripheral nerve injury, and stroke, I have a broad perspective on the role of neuroinflammation. Moreover, as someone who has run a graduate level course on neuroinflammation for the past 10 years at McGill University, I have had a close-up view of the wide ranging impact of inflammation in neurology.

This book is divided into three sections. The first part begins with two general chapters, the first chapter provides a broad overview of neuroinflammation and immune pathology in patients with multiple sclerosis (MS) and stroke. It discusses the concept of neuroinflammation and the basic principles of immune surveillance and inflammation by adaptive immune responses. The second chapter provides an overview of *in vivo* imaging of immune and glial cell responses in animal models of CNS injury and disease. The use of intravital microscopy to study CNS inflammation is providing new insights into cell-to-cell interactions and behavior of immune and CNS cells *in situ*. The second part of the book focuses mainly on the detrimental aspects of inflammation, although discussions in many chapters also note some of the beneficial aspects of inflammation that one could modulate to improve outcomes. This section consists of eight chapters ranging from MS and experimental autoimmune encephalomyelitis, SCI, stroke, aging, obesity, neuropathic pain subsequent to peripheral nerve injury, inherited peripheral neuropathies, and CNS viral infections such as human immunodeficiency virus (HIV) and West Nile virus. The third part of the book focuses on areas in which the beneficial aspects of neuroinflammation are seen more prominently. This section consists of seven chapters ranging from CNS injury, remyelination in the CNS, Rett syndrome, amyotrophic lateral sclerosis (ALS), and the role of tumor necrosis factor (TNF) in synaptic plasticity and neuronal function. The book ends with a chapter on the mechanisms underlying resolution of inflammation in CNS. The key reasons for choosing these topics are summarized in the subsequent text and will give the reader an idea of the main objectives of this book.

It is becoming increasingly evident that inflammation plays a role in many if not most neurological disorders. Certain conditions such as MS have long been recognized as a neuroinflammatory condition involving a prominent autoimmune response to CNS myelin antigens. In the case of traumatic SCI and stroke, inflammation triggered locally at the site of injury or stroke has also been recognized as contributing to secondary tissue damage and evolving pathology. Studies on neuroinflammation in MS, SCI, and stroke have a long history, but several recent advances have begun to shed new light that is worth taking note of. In contrast, the involvement of neuroinflammation has not been widely appreciated in aging and obesity. In these areas, neuroinflammation can impact on learning and memory, as well as on mood and cognitive function. With the increase in wealth in formerly developing countries, obesity is increasing worldwide at a shocking rate in children and adults and has an impact not only on cardiovascular health and the development of type 2 diabetes but also on the brain. In HIV/acquired immunodeficiency syndrome (AIDS), despite the effectiveness of combined antiretroviral therapy to markedly improve survival of people with HIV/AIDS, the CNS remains a major reservoir of the virus. About a third of patients on antiretroviral therapy have a spectrum of neurocognitive disorders that contributes significantly to morbidity and mortality and remains an important therapeutic target. Inflammation in peripheral nerves also contributes to pathology as seen in its involvement in neuropathic pain. Interestingly, this involves not only macrophage and cytokine responses locally in the injured nerve but also injury-induced microglia/macrophage and cytokine responses in the spinal cord, which provides multiple novel therapeutic targets for the management of pain. Recent work on inherited peripheral neuropathies, such as Charcot-Marie-Tooth disease, has also shown the involvement of the innate and adaptive immune response in the pathogenesis. Such work has led to the identification of immune cells as mediators and amplifiers of the demyelinating and axonal pathology.

Not too long ago there were long and heated debates on whether inflammation in conditions such as CNS injury is good or bad. One exciting development in other fields of immunology in the past decade that has now trickled into neuroscience, shows that the immune response can be good or bad depending on the state of activation of macrophages and microglia, which is influenced by the tissue environment. The idea that macrophages and microglia are very plastic cells that change their phenotype or polarization state along a continuum from proinflammatory, cytotoxic M1 phenotype at one extreme to an anti-inflammatory, pro-repair M2 phenotype at the other extreme with stages in-between is an important conceptual model with increasing supportive evidence. These cells can be polarized differently in different conditions and can also change their polarization state at different times during the evolving pathology. Macrophage and microglial polarization therefore has wide-ranging implications for neurological conditions. This includes neuroinflammation in SCI and stroke, as well as diverse phenomenon such as remyelination in the CNS, and neuronal survival in neurodegenerative diseases such as ALS. A characteristic feature of the adult mammalian CNS is that axons damaged by injury or disease fail to regenerate in situ. Work done on the optic nerve show that induction of an inflammatory response in the eye triggers long-distance axon regeneration of retinal ganglion cells through the optic nerve, showing how some aspects of neuroinflammation can indeed be beneficial to recovery. In another striking discovery, the transplantation of wild type microglia-like cells into the brains of *Mecp2*-null mice (a model of Rett syndrome) improved survival and motor function. Genetic targeting of microglia to express wild type Mecp2 in *Mecp2* null mice also improved outcome, showing that CNS resident immune cells can be selectively targeted to improve neuronal survival in certain conditions. Another surprising recent discovery is the finding that the proinflammatory cytokine TNF can have profound effects on synaptic plasticity and neuronal function, in particular, the compensatory synaptic adaption in response to prolonged changes in neuronal activity. This has implications for neuronal function in CNS injury and disease in which increases in TNF occur. Finally, no discussion on inflammation would be complete without a section on the active resolution of inflammation and the pro-resolution bioactive lipid mediators such as resolvins and protectins that attenuate inflammation and improve outcome. There is excitement and hope that these pro-resolution mediators will become important therapeutics to treat a variety of neuroinflammatory conditions.

The reader will find differences but also many commonalities in the inflammatory responses in the various neurological conditions covered in this book. This implies that development of treatments against particular neuroinflammation targets for one neurological condition is likely to also be useful for other conditions. Many of us focus our work in our own particular areas of interest and tend to keep to our own silos. My aim is to bring such diverse areas together in one book and to break down these barriers and foster cross-talk and understanding of neuroinflammation in various fields. There is much we can learn from each other.

I want to thank all the authors for taking the time to contribute to this book. I know how much demand there is on their time and am truly appreciative of their efforts. I am indebted to Dr. Antje Kroner, a senior postdoctoral fellow in my laboratory for so generously helping me in editing the chapters and for her keen attention to detail. I could not have done it as easily without her help. I also want to thank Justin Jeffryes, Editorial Director at Wiley for seeking me out for this project. I thank him for his help, advice, and encouragement in taking this project through to completion. I am also grateful to Stephanie Dollan, Senior Editorial Assistant, for making sure I kept on track, for corresponding with the authors, and for making it all so easy.

Samuel David, PhD
Montreal, Canada

PART I
Introduction

1 Immune Response in the Human Central Nervous System in Multiple Sclerosis and Stroke

Hans Lassmann

Division of Neuroimmunology, Center for Brain Research, Medical University of Vienna, Wien, Austria

Introduction

Traditional pathology provides a clear distinction between inflammatory and neurodegenerative disorders. Inflammatory diseases comprise a large spectrum of infectious and autoimmune diseases. In these conditions, a specific immune response against autoantigens or infectious agents is present, which induces inflammation and specific destruction of cells, which contain the inciting agent or autoantigen. In addition, cells and tissue components, which are present in the vicinity of the specific targets of the immune response, also get injured or destroyed by toxic products or mediators of the immune response, a process termed "bystander damage" (Wisniewski and Bloom, 1975). In contrast, in conditions of neurodegeneration or brain ischemia, the primary cause of cell and tissue injury is due to primary metabolic changes. Also, in these conditions, immune mediators, such as cytokines or activated cells of the immune system, as for instance granulocytes or activated macrophages and microglia, are involved in cell and tissue degeneration. This lead to the broad concept of "neuroinflammation" playing a major role in the pathogenesis of a wide spectrum of brain diseases and being a potential target for neuroprotective treatments (Craft *et al.*, 2005, Ransohoff and Liu, 2007).

The Concept of Neuroinflammation

Any type of tissue injury in the central nervous system (CNS) is associated with local changes in the microenvironment, which are in part similar to those seen in inflammatory conditions. Cell injury in the CNS results in activation of microglia and astrocytes (Ransohoff and Brown, 2012). Furthermore, a similar activation of microglia can be induced even by functional changes in neuronal networks, such as for instance sustained overactivation of neuronal circuits in epileptic seizures (Xanthos and Sandkühler, 2013). Activation of glia is induced by different signals, including release of adenosine triphosphate (ATP) and its signaling through G-protein-coupled

Neuroinflammation: New Insights into Beneficial and Detrimental Functions, First Edition. Edited by Samuel David.
© 2015 John Wiley & Sons, Inc. Published 2015 by John Wiley & Sons, Inc.

receptors, by direct neurotransmitter signaling or by the liberation of intracellular components from damaged cells, resulting in the activation of pattern recognition receptors (Iadecola and Anrather, 2011). An important consequence of astrocyte and microglia activation is the production of a wide spectrum of pro- and anti-inflammatory cytokines and growth factors. Thus, microglia and astroglia activation as a reflection of an inflammatory response to tissue injury may have beneficial as well as detrimental consequences for adjacent neurons and glia, depending on the type of the primary tissue injury and on the properties of the environment where it takes place (Griffiths *et al.*, 2007).

In addition, tissue injury and the induction of proinflammatory cytokines and chemokines may lead to disturbance of vascular integrity at the blood–brain barrier, resulting in brain edema and the penetration of serum components into the CNS (Takeshita and Ransohoff, 2012; Erickson *et al.*, 2012). Besides leakage of various additional proinflammatory factors such as complement components, the leakage of fibrin and its coagulation within the perivascular compartment plays an important role in this process. It has been shown in experimental studies that fibrin deposition in the brain augments the inflammatory process and/or the subsequent tissue injury. Thus, inflammatory processes in the brain are much milder in fibrinogen-deficient animals or in conditions of fibrin depletion in the plasma. Fibrin can activate microglia and macrophages through toll-like receptor signaling. In addition, fibrin interacts with microglia through specific binding to the integrin receptor CD11b/CD18, which amplifies the inflammatory process and its associated tissue damage (Davalos *et al.*, 2012). Such a vascular inflammatory process may also recruit inflammatory cells from the circulation. Depending on the type of tissue injury and its local induction of different spectra of adhesion molecules and chemokines, different leukocyte populations will be recruited, such as granulocytes and monocytes, but also different subpopulations of T- and B-lymphocytes (Gorina *et al.*, 2014; Ransohoff and Engelhardt, 2012). This vascular injury is an important component of the inflammatory reaction, giving rise to the cardinal features of an inflammatory response, which have been defined as tissue swelling due to edema (tumor), vasodilatation, and hyperemia (rubor and calor) and activation of sensory receptors (dolor). In the CNS, edema and tissue swelling are the most important consequence, as the brain can swell only to a limited degree due to restrains by the bony skull. Thus, edema results in increased intracranial pressure leading to disturbance of microcirculation and amplification of tissue damage by ischemia (Bor Seng Shu *et al.*, 2013).

Finally, inflammation may also be induced or augmented by specific mechanisms of adaptive immune responses. The prerequisite for such a scenario is that the organism has earlier mounted a specific response of T-lymphocytes or antibodies, which are directed against an antigen that is present within the CNS (Wekerle *et al.*, 1986; Flügel *et al.*, 2001). Inflammation, which is mediated by adaptive immune responses, is especially important in infectious and autoimmune diseases of the nervous system. The diverse patterns of neuroinflammation are summarized in Fig. 1.1.

Basic Principles of Immune Surveillance and Inflammation by Adaptive Immune Responses

The CNS has for long been viewed as an immune-privileged organ, which is shielded from the peripheral immune system by the blood–brain barrier and which does not express major histocompatibility complex (MHC) antigens required for antigen recognition by T-lymphocytes. This

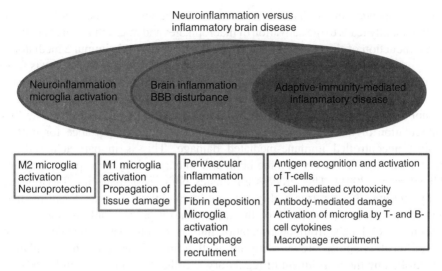

Figure 1.1 Inflammation of the CNS comprises a broad spectrum of tissue alterations including microglia activation, vascular inflammation with blood–brain barrier damage, and inflammation mediated by adaptive immunity. (*See insert for color representation of this figure.*)

concept, however, has been modified during recent years. T-lymphocytes can enter the normal brain through an intact blood–brain barrier in the course of immune surveillance (Wekerle *et al.*, 1986). However, it is only the activated T-cell population, which is able to enter the normal CNS tissue. This implies that a small fraction of T-cells, when activated in the course of an infection, migrates into the brain or spinal cord in search for their specific antigen. When they do not find their cognate antigen, they quickly disappear from the brain tissue due to local destruction by programmed cell death (apoptosis; Bauer *et al.*, 1998). Whether some of these T-cells can also migrate back into the blood stream or into the lymphatic system is currently unresolved. However, when the specific antigen is present in the CNS and is presented in the perivascular or meningeal space by a macrophage population with features of dendritic cells, T-cells receive a further activation signal (Flügel *et al.*, 2001, Mues *et al.*, 2013). They then proliferate and expand clonally and produce additional proinflammatory cytokines and chemokines, which act on endothelia and promote the secondary recruitment of other leukocytes from the bloodstream, such as other T-cells, B-cells, and monocytes (Ransohoff and Engelhardt, 2012). This results in a first stage of perivascular and meningeal inflammation. Proinflammatory cytokines in this condition also activate local microglia and astrocytes, which amplify the inflammatory response through additional production of cytokines, chemokines, and proteases. This further amplifies the perivascular inflammatory response and allows the inflammatory cells to pass the subpial and perivascular astrocytic glia limitans and spread into the CNS parenchyme. Tissue injury can be induced directly by cytotoxic MHC Class I antigen-dependent cytotoxic T-cells (Saxena *et al.*, 2008). These cells can recognize their specific antigen on all cells of the CNS, such as astrocytes, oligodendrocytes, and neurons, as all these cells express MHC Class I antigens in an inflammatory environment (Höftberger *et al.*, 2004). The expression of MHC Class II antigens, which are necessary for antigen recognition by CD4 positive T-cells, is more restricted, being mainly present on macrophages, microglia, and occasionally on astrocytes. Thus, CD4[+] T-cell-mediated inflammation mainly leads to the activation of macrophages and microglia, which are then responsible for the induction of tissue injury through the liberation of toxic immune mediators, such as reactive oxygen or nitrogen species, of cytotoxic cytokines, such as tumor necrosis factor alpha (TNF-α), or of proteases and lipases (Jack *et al.*, 2005). However, direct cytotoxicity can even be mediated by CD4[+] T-cells. When highly activated, they may mediate cytotoxicity in a manner that does not depend on specific antigen recognition on the target cell (Nitsch *et al.*, 2004).

Downregulation of the inflammatory response is of critical importance for protecting the CNS against uncontrolled immune-mediated damage. This is in part achieved by highly efficient destruction of T-cells within the brain and spinal cord through apoptosis (Bauer *et al.*, 1998, Flügel *et al.*, 2001). This process eliminates both antigen-specific T-lymphocytes and secondarily recruited T-cells. It is highly efficient in conditions of acute T-cell-mediated brain inflammation and allows persistence of the inflammatory process only as long as there is a continuous influx of T-cells from the circulation into the lesions. The molecules involved in the induction of T-cell apoptosis are currently not well defined. In addition, brain inflammation is further controlled by the recruitment of regulatory T-cells (Tregs) into the inflamed CNS tissue (O'Connor and Anderton, 2008; Fransson *et al.*, 2012) as well as by downregulation of immune response due to activation of the pituitary/adrenal axis (MacPhee *et al.*, 1989). Clearance of the inciting trigger, such as the infectious agent, also terminates inflammation by the lack of further antigen presentation and T-cell activation. Taken together, these mechanisms grant that the brain is controlled by a strictly regulated immune response, which keeps collateral damage as small as possible.

Immune-mediated damage of the brain by specific antibodies in general is low or absent, as they penetrate the normal blood–brain barrier only to a very limited degree. In addition, antibodies require interaction with complement or activated effector cells such as granulocytes or macrophages to induce tissue damage, factors that are not present in the normal CNS (Vass *et al.*, 1992). However, circulating autoantibodies, directed against foreign or self-antigens, which are present on the extracellular surface of cells, may become pathogenic, when they reach the brain in an inflammatory environment, for instance induced by a T-cell-mediated inflammatory response (Linington *et al.*, 1988). T-cell-mediated inflammation not only opens the blood–brain barrier, but also activates local macrophages and microglia and induces granulocyte and macrophage recruitment from the circulation by inducing local chemokine secretion. It further stimulates the production of complement and inhibits the production of complement-inhibitory proteins. These additional factors allow efficient antibody-mediated cell destruction (Pohl *et al.*, 2013).

Data obtained in diseases, which are mediated by autoantibodies against neurotransmitter receptors or cell surface channels, suggest that even antibodies alone may induce disease and damage in the CNS. In this case, high titers of autoantibodies are present in the circulation, and the antibodies exert their pathogenic role by direct binding to the channels or receptors, thus acting more analogous to a pharmacological agonist or antagonist than as an immunological tool (Hughes *et al.*, 2010). In this situation, massive functional disturbances are seen despite only sparse or absent inflammation and structural tissue damage (Bien *et al.*, 2012).

As mentioned previously, recruitment of T- and B-lymphocytes into the CNS may also occur secondarily to tissue injury, for instance in ischemia or in neurodegenerative diseases

(Gelderblom *et al.*, 2009). However, the mere presence of lymphocytes within a brain lesion does not necessarily imply that they are pathogenic. When there is no activation signal within the CNS tissue, such cells are inert bystanders. Such T-cell infiltrates in brain lesions are potentially pathogenic when they are locally activated, for instance by recognizing specific autoantigens. This is indicated, when the respective T-cells locally proliferate, show clonal expansion, or express activation markers (Liesz *et al.*, 2013a).

Inflammation in the Central Nervous System of Patients with Multiple Sclerosis

Multiple sclerosis (MS) has originally been defined as an inflammatory demyelinating disease, suggesting that the formation of brain and spinal cord lesions in this disease is driven by the inflammatory process (Lassmann *et al.*, 2007). Focal plaques of primary demyelination, reflected by complete loss of myelin, but partial preservation of axons and neurons, are the hallmark of MS pathology. Demyelinated plaques are present in the white matter as well as in the grey matter, such as the cerebral and cerebellar cortex (Peterson *et al.*, 2001) and the deep grey matter nuclei (Vercellino *et al.*, 2009), including the basal ganglia, the thalamus, and hypothalamus (Huitinga *et al.*, 2004). In addition to the focal pathology, reflected by demyelinated plaques, there are also diffuse changes in the brain, consistent of small perivascular demyelinated lesions, diffuse axonal injury and neurodegeneration, generalized microglia activation, and diffuse astrocytic scar formation in the entire white and grey matter of the brain and spinal cord (Kutzelnigg *et al.*, 2005). This finally leads to profound tissue loss and atrophy in the entire CNS. While focal demyelinated lesions in the white matter dominate the pathology of patients with early stages of relapsing remitting MS, cortical demyelination and diffuse damage of the white and grey matter are most prominent in patients during the later progressive stage of the disease (Kutzelnigg *et al.*, 2005).

Active demyelination and neurodegeneration in the MS brain are invariably associated with inflammation, consistent of infiltrates of the tissue by T- and B-lymphocytes and by macrophages (Fig. 1.2; Frischer *et al.*, 2009). Most prominent, however, is the profound

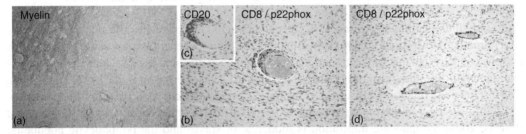

Figure 1.2 Inflammation in multiple sclerosis. (a) Inflammation in active multiple sclerosis lesions is associated with demyelination, reflected by the loss of blue myelin staining in the lesion. (b, c) Infiltration of the tissue with CD8+ T-lymphocytes (b) and CD20+ B-lymphocytes (c) (black cells) in the active lesion edge. The zone of initial demyelination at the lesions edge shows profound microglia activation with intense expression of NADPH oxidase (brown cells; p22phox). (d) CD8+ T-lymphocytes are also present in the lesion center (black cells). Most inflammatory cells are macrophages with low expression of NADPH oxidase (brown cells). (*See insert for color representation of this figure.*)

activation of the local microglia population (Jack *et al.*, 2005). Several arguments speak in favor for a pathogenic role of this inflammatory response. T- and B-cells in the lesions show an activated phenotype and clonal expansion (Babbe *et al.*, 2000; Obermeier *et al.*, 2011), most likely due to proliferation following the encounter with their cognate antigen in the lesions. Furthermore, active lesions in the white matter of patients with MS show contrast enhancement as a consequence of inflammation-induced blood–brain barrier damage (Miller *et al.*, 1988; Gaitan *et al.*, 2011). Most importantly, anti-inflammatory or immunomodulatory treatments have a beneficial effect, in particular in patients in the early relapsing stage of their disease (Wiendl and Hohlfeld, 2009).

There is still some debate, whether inflammation also drives neurodegeneration in the progressive stage of the disease, because in such patients, lesions with contrast enhancement are rare and current anti-inflammatory treatments are no longer effective. Thus, a widely proposed concept for the pathogenesis of the progressive stage of MS is that inflammation in early relapsing disease initiates a cascade of events, which leads to demyelination and neurodegeneration in the progressive stage and becomes independent of the original inflammatory response (Trapp and Nave, 2008). However, detailed pathological studies showed that active tissue injury in the progressive stage is associated with T- and B-cell infiltrates in the CNS and that in patients in whom lymphocyte infiltration in the brain has declined to levels seen in age-matched controls, no active demyelination is found and neurodegeneration also is reduced to levels seen in the respective controls (Frischer *et al.*, 2009). Yet, the nature of the inflammatory response appears to be different between early and late stages of MS. While in new active lesions in acute and relapsing/remitting MS, inflammation is associated with massive blood–brain barrier damage, inflammation in the progressive stages occurs at least in part behind a closed or repaired blood–brain barrier (Hochmeister *et al.*, 2006). Furthermore, aggregates of inflammatory infiltrates, which consist of T-cells, B-cells, and plasma cells and may even form lymph follicle-like structures, are present in the meninges and perivascular spaces (Serafini *et al.*, 2004). The extent of meningeal inflammation and the formation of inflammatory aggregates correlate well with the extent of active cortical demyelination and neurodegeneration (Magliozzi *et al.*, 2007).

The Nature of the Inflammatory Response in Actively Demyelinating Lesions in MS

Profound inflammation, consisting of T-cells and B-cells, is a characteristic feature of actively demyelinating MS lesions. Active demyelination and neurodegeneration are associated with the presence of activated macrophages and microglia, which are present in close contact with degenerating myelin sheaths and axons (Prineas and Graham, 1981; Ferguson *et al.*, 1997; Trapp *et al.*, 1998). However, inflammation in active lesions appears to occur as a two-step phenomenon. In the initial stage, termed initial (Marik *et al.*, 2007) or pre-phagocytic lesions (Barnett and Prineas, 2004), lymphocyte infiltration is moderate or sparse and the lymphocytic population mainly consists of MHC Class-I-restricted CD8$^+$ T-cells. In contrast, when myelin sheaths have been destroyed and taken up by microglia and macrophages, inflammatory infiltration is much higher and a wide spectrum of different leukocyte populations is found, including CD4$^+$ and CD8$^+$ positive T-cells, B-cells, hematogeneous macrophages, and a variable number of plasma cells (Marik *et al.*, 2007; Henderson *et al.*, 2009). Thus, a small number of T-cells (mainly CD8$^+$

cells) appear to enter the brain in the course of immune surveillance, encounter their specific antigen, and start the lesions through microglia activation. However, when myelin and oligodendrocytes get destroyed, intracellular and myelin components are liberated into the extracellular space and provide an additional proinflammatory stimulus. This, then, leads to secondary amplification of the inflammatory process in the lesions.

It has, however, been questioned, whether the mild T-cell infiltration in initial lesions is sufficient to drive the demyelinating process. The alternative interpretation of these findings is that initial demyelination occurs independently from adaptive T- and B-cell responses and that inflammatory cells are secondarily recruited into sites of pre-existing tissue injury, where they then may amplify demyelination and neurodegeneration (Barnett and Prineas, 2004; Henderson *et al.*, 2009).

Both T- and B-cells show clonal expansion in the MS brain, and for B-cells, this is reflected by the presence of oligoclonal intrathecal antibody synthesis (Skulina *et al.*, 2004; Obermeier *et al.*, 2008). Regarding T-cells, the most pronounced clonal expansion is seen for MHC Class-I-restricted CD8$^+$ cells, which also dominate in initial lesions stages. Genome-wide association studies in patients with MS versus controls identified a large number of different genes to be associated with MS susceptibility (Sawcer *et al.*, 2011). Most of them have putative functions in the immune system. Finally, anti-inflammatory or immunomodulatory treatments are beneficial at least in early disease stages (Wiendl and Hohlfeld, 2009).

Studies on local cytokine and chemokine expression in MS lesions are limited but consistent with an inflammatory response, which is driven by T- and possibly B-lymphocytes. Active lesions show the expression of various adhesion molecules (Washington *et al.*, 1994; Allavena *et al.*, 2010; Cavrol *et al.*, 2008; Ifergan *et al.*, 2011; Larochelle *et al.*, 2012) and chemokines (Trebst *et al.*, 2001; Kivisakk *et al.*, 2004), which are instrumental for leukocyte migration through the blood–brain barrier (Steiner *et al.*, 2010). Antigen-specific activation of T-cells in MS lesions is also indicated by the expression of activation antigens (Pohl *et al.*, 2013; Annibali *et al.*, 2010), the presence of costimulatory molecules (Windhagen *et al.*, 1995; Gerritse *et al.*, 1996) or autoantigen and MHC complexes (Krogsgaard *et al.*, 2000), and by the local expression of various pro- and anti-inflammatory cytokines (Mycko *et al.*, 2003; Tzartos *et al.*, 2008, 2011). This has so far been mainly described in classical active lesions. Detailed studies on the phenotype of lymphocytes in different stages of the disease and in relation to the activity of inflammation and neurodegeneration are still missing.

Macrophages and Microglia in MS Lesions

Much of our knowledge on the role of microglia and macrophages comes from experimental studies performed in rodents. However, there are species-related functional differences between rodent and human microglia, which involve cytokine signaling, response to innate immunity stimuli, and effector functions (Smith and Dragunow, 2014). Thus, to understand microglia function in brain disease, analysis of their function in human disorders is important.

There is good agreement that active demyelination and axonal injury in MS occurs in close apposition with activated microglia and macrophages (Prineas *et al.*, 2001; Lassmann, 2011). In the normal-appearing white matter around actively demyelinating lesions, microglia nodules are seen, which are in close contact with myelinated nerve fibers. In initial lesions, massive microglia activation is associated with oligodendrocyte apoptosis and initial changes of myelin disintegration. Myelin is then taken up by phagocytic cells. Toward the lesion center, there is a continuous transition between cells with microglia and macrophage phenotype, suggesting that most of the phagocytic cells in the lesions come from the microglia cell pool. Furthermore, dystrophic axons within and around active MS lesions are seen in close contact with microglia or macrophages (Ferguson et al., 1997). Activated microglia and macrophages in initial and active MS lesions express a variety of markers, including MHC class I and Class II molecules (Höftberger et al., 2004), Fc-receptors (Ulvestad et al., 1994), and markers associated with phagocytosis, such as CD68 (Brück et al., 1995). Most importantly, they highly express components of the nicotinamide adenine dinucleotide phosphate (NADPH) oxidase (NOX1 and NOX2) complexes, suggesting high oxidative burst activation. In contrast, expression of inducible nitric oxide synthase (iNOS) is sparse or absent in initial lesions, but it is upregulated on a subset of macrophages in established lesions. When myelin has been taken up in macrophage-like cells, they lose their expression of NADPH oxidase but retain the expression of phagocytosis-related molecules, such as CD68 or CD163 (Fig. 1.2; Fischer et al., 2012, 2013). As, however, shown in spinal cord injury, this conversion from an M1 to an M2 phenotype of macrophages in response to myelin phagocytosis can be counteracted by the presence of TNF and by iron loading of macrophages in the lesions (Kroner et al., 2014).

Unrelated to the presence of demyelinated lesions, there is also a general activation of microglia in the normal-appearing white matter in patients with MS and to a lower extent also in the white matter of age-matched controls (Lassmann, 2011). Recent studies suggest that microglia in the normal-appearing white matter of patients with MS are in an alerted state, which may be transformed into a cytotoxic state by the additional presence of proinflammatory cytokines (Vogel et al., 2013). Global microglia activation may in part reflect anterograde and retrograde neuronal and axonal degeneration due to lesions in other brain areas. This may explain why new MS lesions are more frequently seen in areas, which receive axonal input from distant regions, affected by other MS-related pathology (Kolasinski et al., 2012). In addition, global microglia activation in the MS brain also reflects diffuse neurodegeneration in the normal-appearing white and grey matter.

From all these data, it is assumed that activated microglia and macrophages play a major role in the induction of demyelination and tissue degeneration in the brain of patients with MS. However, astrocytes take part in this process as well. As reviewed recently, they are involved in propagating and controlling inflammation. Furthermore, functional impairment of astrocytes in active lesions augments demyelination, oligodendrocyte death, and axonal injury (Brosnan and Raine, 2013). Reactive astrocytes in MS lesions lose their cell polarity, which results in the loss of connexins, the excitatory amino acid transporter EAAT2, and the water channel aquaporin 4 (Masaki et al., 2013). This impairs energy supply to oligodendrocytes and axons and increased excitotoxicity and may also propagate brain edema.

Mechanisms of Demyelination and Neurodegeneration in MS

There are many different acute and chronic inflammatory diseases of the CNS, but the widespread primary demyelination leading to large plaques of myelin destruction with axonal preservation and reactive gliosis is a specific feature of MS pathology. This is best illustrated by the presence of cortical demyelinated lesions, which besides in MS are only seen in conditions of virus infection of oligodendrocytes (Fischer et al., 2013; Moll et al., 2008). Thus, in MS, there must be a specific trigger responsible for the induction of demyelination.

Experimental studies show that immune-mediated tissue injury in inflammatory demyelinating diseases can be mediated by several different mechanisms, involving T-lymphocytes, B-cells, and antibodies, as well as activated macrophages or microglia. This is also reflected by heterogeneous patterns of demyelination seen in active plaques of different patients with MS (Lucchinetti et al., 2000). Applying organotypic tissue culture, it was found that serum and in part also cerebrospinal fluid contains demyelinating activity (Bornstein and Appel, 1965). Experimental data indicate that this demyelinating factor may be an autoantibody response directed against antigens expressed on the surface of myelin or oligodendrocytes (Linington et al., 1988). However, this may not be the case in MS. Depletion of immunoglobulins from MS sera did not abolish demyelinating activity in most tested MS sera (Grundke Iqbal and Bornstein, 1980). Recently, it was shown that supernatants from activated B-cells may contain a demyelinating activity, which could not be ascribed to immunoglobulins (Lisak et al., 2012). Thus, these data indicate that a soluble factor produced by inflammatory cells may be involved in the induction of demyelination in the MS brain, but the nature of this factor remains unknown.

All these different patterns of demyelination in MS lesions, however, have in common the close association between activated macrophages and microglia with active cell and tissue injury. However, microglia and macrophage activation alone does not explain the selectivity of demyelination seen in MS lesions in the cortex and white matter. Active tissue injury in the MS brain is associated with profound oxidative injury, reflected by the presence of oxidized lipids, proteins, and DNA (Bizzozero et al., 2005; van Horssen et al., 2008). Most profound evidence for oxidative injury has been found in oligodendrocytes and myelin, as well as in axons and degenerating neurons. In fact, massive accumulation of oxidized phospholipids was seen in apoptotic oligodendrocytes and in neurons and in fragmented axons and dendrites, and this was associated with DNA oxidation and fragmentation (Haider et al., 2011; Fischer et al., 2013). Oxidative injury appears to be driven by oxidative burst in activated microglia and amplified by mitochondrial injury (Mahad et al., 2008) and liberation of iron from damaged myelin and oligodendrocytes (Hametner et al., 2013; Lassmann et al., 2012).

Inflammation in Stroke Lesions

The primary cause of tissue injury in stroke lesions is hypoxia and ischemia. However, a number of data suggest that an inflammatory reaction within the lesions may amplify functional disturbance and structural damage (Gelderblom et al., 2009). This assumption is mainly based on evidence from experimental models, in which various different anti-inflammatory treatment strategies have been shown to reduce clinical deficit and lesion size. However, in contrast to the situation in MS, anti-inflammatory or immunomodulatory treatments have failed the test in clinical stroke trials so far (Amanthea et al., 2013). Several potential explanations have been forwarded for this unsatisfactory situation. Firstly, experimental research has shown that inflammation in the brain not only is detrimental, but also is beneficial depending on the exact timing of the treatment and the nature of the initiating event (e.g., permanent or transient vessel occlusion, ischemic vs hemorrhagic stroke vs intracerebral hemorrhage). Exact timing of treatment can easily be achieved in experimental models but is very difficult to accomplish in the setting of a complex human trial. Secondly, patients with stroke or with traumatic brain injury go through a phase of generalized immunodepression, which reaches a peak during the first days after CNS injury and is also responsible for an increased susceptibility for systemic infections during this phase. Additional immunosuppression during this phase may increase systemic side effects and dangers (Dirnagl *et al.*, 2007). Finally, information regarding the exact nature of the inflammatory response in human stroke lesions currently is limited and in part controversial.

Microglia Activation and Macrophage Response

Microglia activation mediates the first neuroinflammatory response in cerebral ischemia and intracerebral hemorrhage. The microglia response in experimental stroke lesions has been summarized in detail in a recent review (Taylor and Sansing, 2013); this will be covered in Chapter 5 and will, thus, only be shortly summarized in this chapter. First activation occurs as a result of ischemic cell destruction, mediated besides other mechanisms by the release of ATP and HMGB1 (high-mobility group box 1) into the extracellular space. Importantly, the patterns of microglia activation are different in the ischemic core and the peri-infarct zone (penumbra). In the infarct core, primary microglia activation results in an anti-inflammatory or neuroprotective phenotype during the first hours, but a substantial number of these cells die within the next days due to ischemia (Fig. 1.3). The remaining cells together with macrophages, recruited from the circulation are instrumental in phagocytosis of tissue debris. With increasing time after the acute ischemic event, however, the phenotype of microglia in part changes into a proinflammatory (M1) phenotype. This is associated with the production of different cytokines, such as interleukin (IL)-1ß, TNF-α, IL-6, transforming growth factor ß, and IL-10 (for detailed review see Lambertson *et al.*, 2012). In contrast, in the peri-infarct zone, proinflammatory inflammatory microglia activation dominates (Taylor and Sansing, 2013). The expression of enzymes involved in the production of reactive oxygen and nitric oxide species, such as NADPH oxidase or iNOS together with free radical production through damaged mitochondria results in profound oxidative injury in the lesions, which in the penumbra leads to patterns of demyelination and neurodegeneration, which are in part similar to those seen in MS lesions (Aboul-Enein *et al.*, 2003) and which may also be amplified by similar age-dependent mechanisms. When there is an additional hemorrhagic component or extensive vasogenic brain edema, proinflammatory microglia activation is further enhanced (Taylor and Sansing, 2013).

Granulocyte Infiltration

Granulocyte infiltration into stroke lesions is an early event, and the products secreted by activated granulocytes are toxic for the CNS tissue *in vitro* (Mena *et al.*, 2004; Gronberg *et al.*, 2013). However, the importance of granulocyte infiltration in stroke lesions has been challenged in a recent systematic study on experimental models and human tissue. The study showed that

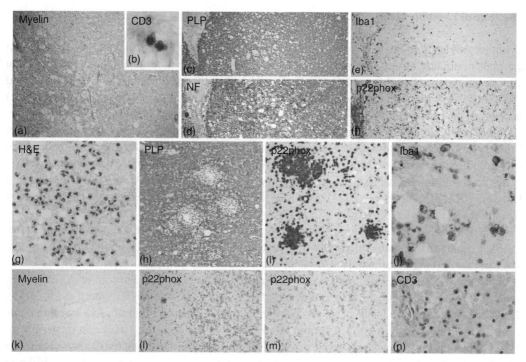

Figure 1.3 Inflammation in stroke. (a–f) Initial white matter stroke lesions (24 h after disease onset) with reduced intensity of staining for conventional myelin markers (a), but preservation of immune reactivity for the (c) myelin protein proteolipid protein (PLP) and (d) neurofilament (NF); such lesions contain single T-cells (b), microglia, which express the pan microglia marker Iba1 (e); NADPH oxidase (brown; p22phox; f) is expressed in microglia at the lesion edge but largely lost from the lesion center. (g–j) Some initial/early stroke lesions (in this example 48 h after disease onset), in which PLP (h) is still preserved, show profound infiltration with granulocytes (g), which intensely express NADPH oxidase (brown cells; p22phox; i), but they reveal very little infiltration of macrophages or microglia activation stained for the microglia and macrophage marker Iba1 (j). (k–n) Advanced stroke lesions, in which myelin and other tissue components are already destroyed (k), reveal profound macrophage activation at the edge (l), macrophages with little NADPH oxidase expression in the lesion center (m), and perivascular or diffuse T-cell infiltrates (n). (*See insert for color representation of this figure.*)

in conditions of pure ischemia, granulocyte infiltration is sparse and that granulocytes mainly remain in the meninges and perivascular spaces. In human stroke as well as in experimental stroke models, the perivascular glia limiting membrane was suggested to be a tight barrier, impeding granulocyte movement from the perivascular space into the brain parenchyma (Enzmann *et al.*, 2013). However, when there is an additional hemorrhagic component, more pronounced granulocyte recruitment and their dispersion into the damaged brain parenchyme are seen (Kalimo *et al.*, 2013). Thus, therapies blocking infiltration and activation of granulocytes in human patients with stroke may only be applicable to a subset of the total patient population (Fig. 1.3). However, augmentation of tissue injury by neutrophils not necessarily means that these cells have had to enter the CNS through the blood–brain barrier. When they adhere to cerebral endothelial cells, the latter may be damaged by the secretion of reactive oxygen species and neutrophil-derived proteases. This may lead to disturbance of microcirculation and brain edema, which by itself may augment tissue injury (Segel *et al.*, 2011).

The Role of Lymphocytes

Lymphocytes accumulate with time in stroke lesions. In experimental stroke lesions, few of them are present already at very early stages and gradually increase in numbers, reaching a plateau after about 5 days (Gronberg et al., 2013). T-cells within the lesions consist of both $CD4^+$ and $CD8^+$ cells. Furthermore, a substantial number of these cells show clonal expansion. This is seen not only in the brain and lesions, but also in draining lymph nodes and spleen (Liesz et al., 2013a, 2013b, 2013c). Interestingly, clonal expansion of T-cells is a late event, occurring mainly between 7 and 14 days after induction of the lesions. Whether proliferation and clonal expansion is driven by recognition of a cognate antigen or by a nonspecific stimulus is currently unknown. However, systemic autoimmune reactions can be triggered as a consequence of stroke (Vogelgesang and Dressel, 2011; Becker et al., 2011), possibly through leakage of brain antigens into draining lymph nodes (Planas et al., 2012).

For a potential design of immunosuppressive or immune-regulatory treatment strategies, it has to be remembered that many different lymphocyte population infiltrate the brain in stroke lesions, some of them having detrimental and others beneficial actions. Thus, this includes $CD4^+$ or $CD8^+$ effector T-cells, Tregs, as well as B-cells and natural killer cells (Gelderblom et al., 2009). In general, $CD4^+$ T-cells appear first followed by $CD8^+$ cells and B-cells (Gronberg et al., 2013). Transfer of autoreactive $CD4^+$ Th1- or Th17-cells at the time of cerebral ischemia augments clinical disease (Zierath et al., 2013), and blockade of T-cell entry into the brain or peripheral T-cell depletion during early stages of reperfusion reduces infarct size in experimental animals (Kraft et al., 2013; Xiong et al., 2013), although the beneficial effect is different between different models (Xiong et al., 2013). However, stroke lesions are also infiltrated by Tregs (Stubbe et al., 2013), and experimental studies have shown a beneficial effect of different regulatory T- and B-cell populations in clinical outcome or lesion size (Engelbertsen et al., 2013; Li et al., 2013; Offner and Hurn, 2012; Liesz et al., 2013b). These studies argue that recruitment of Tregs or B-cells into the lesions reduces neuroinflammation and subsequent tissue damage. This view is contradicted by another study, which showed reduced infarct size after peripheral Treg depletion. Tregs interacted with cerebral endothelial cells in the process of transmigration through the vessel wall, and this interaction caused microvascular dysfunction and thrombosis (Kleinschnitz et al., 2013).

Dynamics of Inflammation in Human Stroke Lesions

Information on the inflammatory response in human stroke lesions is currently limited (Mena et al., 2004, Kalimo et al., 2013). Overall, the response appears to be similar to that seen in experimental models, but the stage-dependent changes in inflammation are less distinct. Four different stages have been defined (Mena et al., 2004). The first, which occurs 1–2 days after disease onset, is characterized by acute neuronal injury and shows a low but variable infiltration by polymorphonuclear leukocytes and some microglia activation (Fig. 1.3a–1.3j). This is followed by a stage of acute inflammation (3–37 days after disease onset), reflected by infiltration of the tissue by granulocytes, lymphocytes, and macrophages, and a phase of chronic inflammation (10–53 days) with dominance of lymphocyte and macrophage infiltrates (Fig. 1.3k–1.3n). Finally, in the resorption phase (26 days to years after disease onset), only macrophages are seen within the lesion in variable numbers. There are several possible reasons for the profound overlap in the dynamics of inflammation in human stroke lesions. Owing to the severe vascular pathology in aged patients with stroke, lesions may not occur as a single event but may progressively or recurrently enlarge with time. In addition, human stroke lesions are rarely purely ischemic but may have in different patients a hemorrhagic component of variable intensity. Finally, human stroke lesions may be complicated by additional comorbidities, such as for instance systemic infections or sepsis.

Conclusions

Neuroinflammation is an important pathophysiological process involved not only in classical inflammatory diseases of the nervous system such as MS, but also in other neurodegenerative conditions such as stroke. In MS, anti-inflammatory treatments have shown clear beneficial effects, when applied during the early stage of the disease. However, in patients with stroke and even in patients with MS who have entered the progressive phase of the disease, such therapeutic strategies have failed so far. One of the reasons for this unsatisfactory situation is that neuroinflammation has both detrimental and beneficial effects, depending on the nature of the primary insult, the nature of the immune response, and the microenvironment within the lesions. Currently, most of our knowledge on brain inflammation in disease comes from experimental studies, while information on the nature and time course of the inflammatory response as well as on the composition, activation state, phenotype, and function of inflammatory cells in brain lesions of patients is very limited. Only when these processes are well defined in human brain diseases and when proper paraclinical markers are developed, which allow to monitor these processes *in vivo*, anti-inflammatory treatment of patients will have a realistic chance of success.

References

Aboul-Enein, F., Rauschka, H., Kornek, B. *et al.* (2003) Preferential loss of myelin associated glycoprotein reflects hypoxia-like white matter damage in stroke and inflammatory brain diseases. *Journal of Neuropathology and Experimental Neurology*, **62**, 25–33.

Allavena, R., Noy, S., Andrews, M. & Pullen, N. (2010) CNS elevation of vascular and not mucosal addressin cell adhesion molecules in patients with multiple sclerosis. *American Journal of Pathology*, **176** (2), 556–562.

Amanthea, D., Tassorelli, C., Petrelli, F. *et al.* (2013) Understanding the multifaceted role of inflammatory mediators in ischemic stroke. *Current Medicinal Chemistry*, **21** (18), 2098–2117.

Annibali, V., Ristori, G., Angelini, D.F. *et al.* (2010) CD161(high)CD8+T cells bear pathogenetic potential in multiple sclerosis. *Brain*, **134**, 542–554.

Babbe, H., Roers, A., Waisman, A. *et al.* (2000) Clonal expansion of CD8$^+$ T cells dominate the T cell infiltrate in active multiple sclerosis lesions as shown by micromanipulation and single cell polymerase chain reaction. *Journal of Experimental Medicine*, **192**, 393–404.

Barnett, M.H. & Prineas, J.W. (2004) Relapsing and remitting multiple sclerosis: pathology of the newly forming lesion. *Annals of Neurology*, **55**, 458–468.

Bauer, J., Bradl, M., Hickey, W.F. *et al.* (1998) T cell apoptosis in inflammatory brain lesions: Destruction of T-cells does not depend on antigen recognition. *American Journal of Pathology*, **153**, 715–724.

Becker, K.J., Kalil, A.J., Tanzi, P. *et al.* (2011) Autoimmune responses to brain after stroke are associated with worse outcome. *Stroke*, **42** (10), 2763–2769.

Bien, C.G., Vincent, A., Barnett, M.H. *et al.* (2012) Immunopathology of autoantibody-associated encephalitides: Clues for pathogenesis. *Brain*, **135** (5), 1622–1638.

Bizzozero, O.A., Dejesus, G., Callaha, K. & Pastuszyn, A. (2005) Elevated protein carbonylation in the brain white matter and grey matter of patients with multiple sclerosis. *Journal of Neuroscience Research*, **81**, 687–695.

Bor Seng Shu, E., Figueiredo, E.G., Fonoff, E.T., Fujimoto, Y., Panerai, R.B. & Texeira, M.J. (2013) Decompressive craniectomy and head injury: Brain morphometry, ICP, cerebral hemodynamics, cerebral microvascular reactivity and neurochemistry. *Neurosurgical Review*, **36** (3), 361–370.

Bornstein, M.B. & Appel, S.H. (1965) Tissue culture studies of demyelination. *Annals of the New York Academy of Sciences*, **122**, 280–286.

Brosnan, C.F. & Raine, C.S. (2013) The astrocyte in multiple sclerosis revisited. *Glia*, **61**, 453–465.

Brück, W., Porada, P., Poser, S. *et al.* (1995) Monocyte/macrophage differentiation in early multiple sclerosis lesions. *Annals of Neurology*, **38**, 788–796.

Cavrol, R., Wosik, K., Berard, J.L. *et al.* (2008) Activated leukocyte cell adhesion molecule promotes leukocyte trafficking into the central nervous system. *Nature Immunology*, **9**, 137–145.

Craft, J.M., Watterson, D.M. & Van Eldick, L.J. (2005) Neuroinflammation: A potential therapeutic target. *Expert Opinion on Therapeutic Targets*, **9** (5), 887–900.

Davalos, D., Ryu, J.K., Merlini, M. *et al.* (2012) Fibrinogen-induced perivascular microglial clustering is required for the development of axonal damage in neuroinflammation. *Nature Communications*, **3**, 1227.

Dirnagl, U., Klehment, J., Braun, J.S. *et al.* (2007) Stroke-induced immunodepression: Experimental evidence and clinical relevance. *Stroke*, **38** (2 Suppl), 770–773.

Engelbertsen, D., Andersson, L., Ljungcrantz, I. *et al.* (2013) T-helper 2 immunity is associated with reduced risk of myocardial infarction and stroke. *Arteriosclerosis, Thrombosis, and Vascular Biology*, **33** (3), 637–644.

Enzmann, G., Mysiorek, C., Gorina, R. *et al.* (2013) The neurovascular unit as a selective barrier to polymorphonuclear granulocyte (PMN) infiltration into the brain after ischemic injury. *Acta Neuropathologica*, **125**, 395–412.

Erickson, M.A., Dohi, K. & Banks, W.A. (2012) Neuroinflammation: A common pathway in CNS diseases mediated at the blood–brain barrier. *Neuroimmunomodulation*, **19** (2), 121–130.

Ferguson, B., Matyszak, M.K., Esiri, M.M. & Perry, V.H. (1997) Axonal damage in acute multiple sclerosis lesions. *Brain*, **120**, 393–399.

Fischer, M.T., Sharma, R., Lim, J. *et al.* (2012) NADPH oxidase expression in active multiple sclerosis lesions in relation to oxidative tissue damage and mitochondrial injury. *Brain*, **135**, 886–899.

Fischer, M.T., Wimmer, I., Höftberger, R. *et al.* (2013) Disease-specific molecular events in cortical multiple sclerosis lesions. *Brain*, **136**, 1799–1815.

Flügel, A., Berkowicz, T., Ritter, T. *et al.* (2001) Migratory activity and functional changes of green fluorescent effector cells before and during experimental autoimmune encephalomyelitis. *Immunity*, **14**, 547–560.

Fransson, M., Piras, E., Burman, J. *et al.* (2012) CAR/FoxP3-engineered T regulatory cells target the CNS and suppress EAE upon intranasal delivery. *Journal of Neuroinflammation*, **9**, 112.

Frischer, J.M., Bramow, S., Dal Bianco, A. *et al.* (2009) The relation between inflammation and neurodegeneration in multiple sclerosis brains. *Brain*, **132**, 1175–1189.

Gaitan, M.I., Shea, C.D., Evangelou, I.E. *et al.* (2011) Evolution of the blood brain barrier in newly forming multiple sclerosis lesions. *Annals of Neurology*, **70**, 22–29.

Gelderblom, M., Leypoldt, F., Steinbach, K. *et al.* (2009) Temporal and spatial dynamics of cerebral immune cell accumulation in stroke. *Stroke*, **40**, 1849–1857.

Gerritse, K., Laman, J.D., Noelle, R.J. *et al.* (1996) CD40-CD40 ligand interactions in experimental allergic encephalomyelitis and multiple sclerosis. *Proceedings of the National Academy of Sciences of the United States of America*, **93**, 2499–2504.

Gorina, R., Lyck, R., Vestweber, D. & Engelhardt, B. (2014) ß2 integrin mediated crawling on endothelial ICAM-1 and ICAM-2 is a prerequisite for transcellular neutrophil diapedesis across the inflamed blood–brain barrier. *Journal of Immunology*, **192** (1), 324–337.

Griffiths, M., Neal, J.W. & Gasque, P. (2007) Innate immunity and protective neuroinflammation: New emphasis on the role of neuroimmune regulation proteins. *International Review of Neurobiology*, **82**, 29–55.

Gronberg, N.V., Johansen, F.F., Kristiansen, U. & Hasseldam, H. (2013) Leukocyte infiltration in experimental stroke. *Journal of Neuroinflammation*, **10**, 115.

Grundke Iqbal, I. & Bornstein, M.B. (1980) Multiple sclerosis: Serum gamma globulin and demyelination in culture. *Neurology*, **30**, 749–754.

Haider, L., Fischer, M.T., Frischer, J.M. *et al.* (2011) Oxidative damage and neurodegeneration in multiple sclerosis lesions. *Brain*, **134**, 1914–1924.

Hametner, S., Wimmer, I., Haider, L., Pfeiffenbring, S., Brück, W. & Lassmann, H. (2013) Iron and neurodegeneration in the multiple sclerosis brain. *Annals of Neurology*, **74** (6), 848–861.

Henderson, A.P.D., Barnett, M.H., Parratt, J.D.E. & Prineas, J.W. (2009) Multiple sclerosis: Distribution of inflammatory cells in newly forming lesions. *Annals of Neurology*, **66**, 739–753.

Hochmeister, S., Grundtner, R., Bauer, J. *et al.* (2006) Dysferlin is a new marker for leaky brain blood vessels in multiple sclerosis. *Journal of Neuropathology and Experimental Neurology*, **65**, 855–865.

Höftberger, R., Aboul-Enein, F., Brueck, W. *et al.* (2004) Expression of major histocompatibility complex class I molecules on the different cell types in multiple sclerosis lesions. *Brain Pathology*, **14** (1), 43–50.

Hughes, E.G., Peng, X., Gleichman, A.J. *et al.* (2010) Cellular and synaptic mechanisms of anti-NMDA receptor encephalitis. *Journal of Neuroscience*, **30** (17), 5866–5875.

Huitinga, I., Erkut, Z.A., van Beurden, D. & Swab, D.F. (2004) Impaired hypothalamus-pituitary-adrenal axis activity and more severe multiple sclerosis with hypothalamic lesions. *Annals of Neurology*, **55**, 37–45.

Iadecola, C. & Anrather, J. (2011) The immunology of stroke: From mechanisms to translation. *Nature Medicine*, **17** (7), 796–808.

Ifergan, I., Kebir, H., Terouz, S. *et al.* (2011) Role of ninjurin-1 in the migration of myeloid cells to central nervous system inflammatory lesions. *Annals of Neurology*, **79**, 751–763.

Jack, C., Ruffini, F., Bar-Or, A. & Antel, J. (2005) Microglia in multiple sclerosis. *Journal of Neuroscience Research*, **81** (3), 363–373.

Kalimo, H., del Zoppo, G.J., Paetau, A. & Lindsberg, P.J. (2013) Polymorphonuclear neutrophil infiltration into ischemic infarctions: Myth or truth? *Acta Neuropathologica*, **125**, 313–316.

Kivisakk, P., Mahad, D.J., Callahan, M.K. *et al.* (2004) Expression of CCR7 in multiple sclerosis: Implications for CNS immunity. *Annals of Neurology*, **55** (5), 627–638.

Kleinschnitz, C., Kraft, P., Dreykluft, A. *et al.* (2013) Regulatory T cells are strong promoters of acute ischemic stroke in mice by inducing dysfunction of the cerebral microvasculature. *Blood*, **121** (4), 679–691.

Kolasinski, J., Stagg, C.J., Chance, S.A. *et al.* (2012) A combined post-mortem MRI and quantitative histological study of multiple sclerosis pathology. *Brain*, **135**, 2938–2951.

Kraft, P., Göb, E., Schuhmann, M.K. *et al.* (2013) FTY720 ameliorates acute ischemic stroke in mice by reducing thrombo-inflammation but not by direct neuroprotection. *Stroke*, **44**, 3202–10.

Krogsgaard, M., Wucherpfennig, K.W., Cannella, B. *et al.* (2000) Visualization of myelin basic protein (MBP) T cell epitopes in multiple sclerosis lesions using a monoclonal antibody specific for the human histocompatibility leukocate antigen (HLA)-DR2-MBP 85–99 complex. *Journal of Experimental Medicine*, **191**, 1395–1412.

Kroner, A., Greenhalgh, A.D., Zarruck, J.G., Passos dos Santos, R., Gaestel, M. & David, S. (2014) TNF and increased intracellular iron alter macrophage polarization to a detrimental M1 phenotype in the injured spinal cord. *Neuron*, **83**, 1–19.

Kutzelnigg, A., Lucchinetti, C.F., Stadelmann, C. *et al.* (2005) Cortical demyelination and diffuse white matter injury in multiple sclerosis. *Brain*, **128**, 2705–2712.

Lambertson, K.L., Biber, K. & Finsen, B. (2012) Inflammatory cytokines in experimental and human stroke. *Journal of Cerebral Blood Flow & Metabolism*, **32**, 1677–98.

Larochelle, C., Cayrol, R., Kebir, H. *et al.* (2012) Melanoma cell adhesion molecule identifies encephalitogenic T lymphocytes and promotes their recruitment to the central nervous system. *Brain*, **135** (Pt 10), 2906–24.

Lassmann, H. (2011) The architecture of active multiple sclerosis lesions. *Neuropathology and Applied Neurobiology*, **37**, 698–710.

Lassmann, H., Brück, W. & Lucchinetti, C. (2007) The immunopathology of multiple sclerosis: An overview. *Brain Pathology*, **17**, 210–8.

Lassmann, H., van Horssen, J. & Mahad, D. (2012) Progressive multiple sclerosis: Pathology and pathogenesis. *Nature Reviews Neurology*, **8**, 647–56.

Li, P., Gan, Y., Sun, B.L. *et al.* (2013) Adoptive regulatory T-cell therapy protects against cerebral ischemia. *Annals of Neurology*, **74** (3), 458–71.

Liesz, A., Karcher, S. & Veltkamp, R. (2013a) Spectratype analysis of clonal T cell expansion in murine experimental stroke. *Journal of Neuroimmunology*, **257**, 46–52.

Liesz, A., Zhou, W., Na, S.Y. *et al.* (2013b) Boosting regulatory T cells limits neuroinflammation in permanent cortical stroke. *Journal of Neuroscience*, **33** (44), 17350–62.

Linington, C., Bradl, M., Lassmann, H., Brunner, C. & Vass, K. (1988) Augmentation of demyelination in rat acute allergic encephalomyelitis by circulating mouse monoclonal antibodies directed against a myelin/oligodendrocyte glycoprotein. *American Journal of Pathology*, **130**, 443–454.

Lisak, R.P., Benjamins, J.A., Nedelkoska, L. *et al.* (2012) Secretry products of multiple sclerosis B-cells are cytotoxic to oligodendrocytes in vitro. *Journal of Neuroimmunology.*, **246**, 85–95.

Lucchinetti, C., Bruck, W., Parisi, J., Scheithauer, B., Rodriguez, M. & Lassmann, H. (2000) Heterogeneity of multiple sclerosis lesions: Implications for the pathogenesis of demyelination. *Annals of Neurology*, **47**, 707–717.

MacPhee, I.A., Antoni, F.A. & Mason, D.W. (1989) Spontaneous recovery of rats from experimental allergic encephalomyelitis is dependent on regulation of the immune system by endogeneous adrenal corticosteroids. *Journal of Experimental Medicine*, **169** (2), 431–445.

Magliozzi, R., Howell, O., Vora, A. *et al.* (2007) Meningeal B-cell follicles in secondary progressive multiple sclerosis associate with early onset of disease and severe cortical pathology. *Brain*, **130**, 1089–1104.

Mahad, D., Ziabreva, I., Lassmann, H. & Turnbull, D. (2008) Mitochondrial defects in acute multiple sclerosis lesions. *Brain*, **131**, 1722–1735.

Marik, C., Felts, P., Bauer, J., Lassmann, H. & Smith, K.J. (2007) Lesion genesis in a subset of patients with multiple sclerosis: A role for innate immunity? *Brain.*, **130**, 2800–2815.

Masaki, K., Suzuki, S.O., Matsushita, T. *et al.* (2013) Connexin 43 anstrocytopathy linked to rapidly progressive multiple sclerosis and neuromyelitis optica. *PLoS One*, **8** (8), e72919.

Mena, H., Cadavid, D. & Rushing, E.J. (2004) Human cerebral infract: A proposed histopathologic classification based on 137 cases. *Acta Neuropathologica*, **108**, 524–530.

Miller, D.H., Rudge, P., Johnson, G. *et al.* (1988) Serial gadolinium enhanced magnetic resonance imaging in multiple sclerosis. *Brain*, **111**, 927–939.

Moll, N.M., Rietsch, A.M., Ransohoff, A.J. *et al.* (2008) Cortical demyelination in PML and MS: Similarities and differences. *Neurology*, **70**, 336–343.

Mues, M., Bartolomäus, I., Thestrup, T. *et al.* (2013) Real-time in vivo analysis of T cell activation in the central nervous system using a genetically encoded calcium indicator. *Nature Medicine*, **19** (6), 778–783.

Mycko, M.P., Papoian, R., Boschert, U., Raine, C.S. & Selmaj, K.W. (2003) cDNA microarray analysis in multiple sclerosis lesions: Detection of genes associated with disease activity. *Brain*, **126**, 1048–1057.

Nitsch, R., Pohl, E.E., Smorodchenko, A., Infante-Duarte, C., Atkas, O. & Zipp, F. (2004) Direct impact on T-cells on neurons revealed by two-photon microscopy in living brain tissue. *Journal of Neuroscience*, **24**, 2458–2464.

O'Connor, R.A. & Anderton, S.M. (2008) Foxp3+ regulatory T cells in the control of experimental CNS autoimmune disease. *Journal of Neuroimmunology*, **193** (1–2), 1–11.

Obermeier, B., Mentele, R., Malotka, J. (2008) Matching of oligoclonal immunoglobulin transcriptomes and proteomes of cerebrospinal fluid in multiple sclerosis. *Nature Medicine*, **14**, 688–93.

Obermeier, B., Lovato, L., Mentele, R. *et al.* (2011) Related B-cell clones that populate the CSF and CNS of patients with multiple sclerosis produce CSF immunoglobulin. *Journal of Neuroimmunology*, **233** (1–2), 245–248.

Offner, H. & Hurn, P.D. (2012) A novel hypothesis: Regulatory B lymphocytes shape outcome from experimental stroke. *Translational stroke research*, **3** (3), 324–330.

Peterson, J.W., Bo, L., Mork, S., Chang, A. & Trapp, B.D. (2001) Transected neurites, apoptotic neurons and reduced inflammation in cortical multiple sclerosis lesions. *Annals of Neurology*, **50**, 389–400.

Planas, A.M., Gomez-Choco, M., Urra, X., Gorina, R., Caballero, M. & Chamorri, A. (2012) Brain-derived antigens in lymphoid tissue of patients with acute stroke. *Journal of Immunology*, **188** (5), 2156–2163.

Pohl, M., Kawakami, N., Kitic, M. *et al.* (2013) T-cell activation in neuromyelitis optica lesions plays a role in their formation. *Acta Neuropathologica Communications*, **1** (1), 85.

Prineas, J.W. & Graham, J.S. (1981) Multiple sclerosis: Capping of surface immunoglobulin G on macrophages engaged in myelin breakdown. *Annals of Neurology*, **10**, 149–158.

Prineas, J.W., Kwon, E.E., Cho, E.S. *et al.* (2001) Immunopathology of secondary-progressive multiple sclerosis. *Annals of Neurology*, **50**, 646–657.

Ransohoff, R.M. & Brown, M.A. (2012) Innate immunity in the central nervous system. *Journal of Clinical Investigation*, **122** (4), 1164–71.

Ransohoff, R.M. & Engelhardt, B. (2012) The anatomical and cellular basis of immune surveillance in the central nervous system. *Nature Reviews Immunology*, **12** (9), 623–35.

Ransohoff, R.M. & Liu, L. (2007) Chemokines and chemokine receptors: Multipurpose players in neuroinflammation. *International Review of Neurobiology*, **82**, 187–204.

Sawcer, S., Hellenthal, G., Pirinen, M. *et al.* (2011) Genetic risk and a primary role for cell-mediated immune mechanisms in multiple sclerosis. *Nature*, **476** (7359), 214–9.

Saxena, A., Bauer, J., Scheikl, T. *et al.* (2008) Cutting edge: Multiple sclerosis-like lesions induced by effector CD8 T cells recognizing a sequestered antigen on oligodendrocytes. *Journal of Immunology*, **181** (3), 1617–1621.

Segel, G.B., Halterman, M.W. & Lichtman, M.A. (2011) The paradox of neutrophil's role in tissue injury. *Journal of Leukocyte Biology*, **89** (3), 359–72.

Serafini, B., Rosicarelli, B., Magliozzi, R., Stigliano, E. & Aloisi, F. (2004) Detection of ectopic B-cell follicles with germinal centers in the meninges of patients with secondary progressive multiple sclerosis. *Brain Pathology*, **14**, 164–174.

Skulina, C., Schmidt, S., Dornmair, K. *et al.* (2004) Multiple sclerosis: brain-infiltrating CD8+ T cells persist as clonal expansions in the cerebrospinal fluid. *Proceedings of the National Academy of Sciences of the United States of America*, **101** (8), 2428–33.

Smith, A.M. & Dragunow, M. (2014) The human side of microglia. *Trends in Neurosciences*, **37** (3), 125–135.

Steiner, O., Coisne, C., Cecchelli, R. *et al.* (2010) Differential roles for endothelial ICAM-1, ICAM-2 and VCAM-1 in shear-resistant T-cell arrest, polarization and directed crawling on blood brain barrier endothelium. *Journal of Immunology*, **185**, 4846–55.

Stubbe, T., Ebner, F., Richter, D. *et al.* (2013) Regulatory T cells accumulate and proliferate in ischemic hemisphere for up to 30 days after MCAP. *Journal of Cerebral Blood Flow and Metabolism*, **33** (1), 37–47.

Takeshita, Y., Ransohoff, R.M. (2012) Inflammatory cell trafficking across the blood-brain-barrier: chemokine regulation and in vitro models. *Immunological Reviews*, **248**, 228–39.

Taylor, R.A. & Sansing, L.H. (2013) Microglial response after ischemic stroke and intracerebral hemorrhage. *Clinical and Developmental Immunology*, **2013**, 746068.

Trapp, B.D. & Nave, K.A. (2008) Multiple sclerosis: An immune or neurodegenerative disorder? *Annual Review of Neuroscience*, **31**, 247–2696.

Trapp, B.D., Peterson, J., Ransohoff, R.M., Rudick, R., Mork, S. & Bo, L. (1998) Axonal transection in the lesions of multiple sclerosis. *New England Journal of Medicine*, **338**, 278–285.

Trebst, C., Sorensen, T.L., Kivisakk, P. *et al.* (2001) CCR1+/CCR5+ mononuclear phagocytes accumulate in the central nervous system of patients with multiple sclerosis. *American Journal of Pathology*, **159**, 1701–1710.

Tzartos, J.S., Craner, M.J., Friese, M.A. *et al.* (2011) Il-21 and Il-21 receptor expression in lymphocytes and neurons in multiple sclerosis brain. *American Journal of Pathology*, **178**, 794–802.

Tzartos, J.S., Friese, M.A., Craner, M.J. *et al.* (2008) Interleukin 17 production in central nervous system infiltrating T cells and glial cells is associated with active disease in multiple sclerosis. *American Journal of Pathology*, **172**, 146–55.

Ulvestad, E., Williams, K., Vedeler, C. *et al.* (1994) Reactive microglia in multiple sclerosis lesions have an increased expression of receptors for the Fc part of IgG. *Journal of the Neurological Sciences*, **121**, 125–131.

Van Horssen, J., Schreibelt, G., Drexhage, J. *et al.* (2008) Severe oxidative damage in multiple sclerosis lesions coincides with enhanced antioxidant enzyme expression. *Free Radical Biology and Medicine*, **45**, 1729–1737.

Vass, K., Heininger, K., Schäfer, B., Linington, C. & Lassmann, H. (1992) Interferon-gamma potentiates antibody mediated demyelination in vivo. *Annals of Neurology*, **32**, 189–206.

Vercellino, M., Masera, S., Lorenzatti, M. *et al.* (2009) Demyelination, inflammation, and neurodegeneration in multiple sclerosis deep grey matter. *Journal of Neuropathology and Experimental Neurology*, **68**, 489–502.

Vogel, D.Y., Vereyken, E.J., Gilm, J.E. *et al.* (2013) Macrophages in inflammatory multiple sclerosis lesions have an intermediate activation status. *Journal of Neuroinflammation*, **19**, 35.

Vogelgesang, A. & Dressel, A. (2011) Immunological consequences of ischemic stroke; immunosuppression and autoimmunity. *Journal of Neuroimmunology*, **231** (1–2), 105–10.

Washington, R., Burton, J., Todd, R.R. 3rd, Newman, W., Dragovic, L. & Dore-Duffy, P. (1994) Expression of immunologically relevant endothelial cell activation antigens on isolated central nervous system microvessels from patients with multiple sclerosis. *Annals of Neurology*, **35** (1), 89–97.

Wekerle, H., Linington, C., Lassmann, H. & Meyermann, R. (1986) Cellular immune reactivity within the CNS. *Trends in Neurosciences*, **9**, 271–277.

Wiendl, H. & Hohlfeld, R. (2009) Multiple sclerosis therapeutics: unexpected outcomes clouding undisputed successes. *Neurology*, **72**, 1008–1015.

Windhagen, A., Newcombe, J., Dangond, F. *et al.* (1995) Expression of costimulatory molecules B7-1 (CD80), B7-2 (CD86), and interleukin 12 cytokine in multiple sclerosis lesions. *Journal of Experimental Medicine*, **182**, 1985–96.

Wisniewski, H.M. & Bloom, B.R. (1975) Demyelination as a nonspecific consequence of a cell-mediated immune reaction. *Journal of Experimental Medicine*, **141** (2), 346–59.

Xanthos, D.N. & Sandkühler, J. (2013) Neurogenic neuroinflammation: inflammatory CNS reactions in response to neuronal activity. *Nature Reviews Neuroscience*, **15** (1), 43–53.

Xiong, X., Gu, L., Zhang, H., Xu, B., Zhu, S. & Zhao, H. (2013) The protective effects of T cell deficiency against brain injury are ischemic model-dependent in rats. *Neurochemistry International*, **62** (3), 265–70.

Zierath, D., Schulze, J., Kunze, A. *et al.* (2013) The immunologic profile of adoptively transferred lymphocytes influences stroke outcome of recipients. *Journal of Neuroimmunology*, **263** (1–2), 28–34.

2 *In Vivo* Imaging of Glial and Immune Cell Responses in Central Nervous System Injury and Disease

Alexandre Paré[1] and Steve Lacroix[1,2]

[1] Centre de recherche du Centre hospitalier universitaire (CHU) de Québec - CHUL, Québec, QC, Canada
[2] Département de médecine moléculaire, Faculté de médecine, Université Laval, Québec, QC, Canada

Introduction

Microglia are myeloid-derived cells that migrate to the central nervous system (CNS) during development (Ginhoux *et al.*, 2010; Schulz *et al.*, 2012; Kierdorf *et al.*, 2013). Once they occupy the CNS niche, microglia extend fine processes that continuously and dynamically explore the extracellular space (Nimmerjahn *et al.*, 2005). Microglial are implicated in host defense, brain homeostasis, and synapse remodeling (Kettenmann *et al.*, 2011). Following an insult, microglia are the first cells recruited and they act rapidly to phagocyte debris, producing inflammatory mediators and recruiting and regulating blood-derived immune cells (Hanisch and Kettenmann, 2007; Ransohoff and Perry, 2009; Rivest, 2009). Inflammatory stimuli within the CNS may come from various sources, such as damage-associated molecular patterns (DAMPs) (Pineau and Lacroix, 2009), pathogen-associated molecular patterns (PAMPs) (Rivest, 2009), and protein aggregates (α-synuclein, amyloid-ß, tau) (Drouin-Ouellet and Cicchetti, 2012). Importantly, these inflammatory stimuli are common hallmarks of neurological disorders, including traumatic brain injury (TBI), spinal cord injury (SCI), cerebral ischemia, multiple sclerosis (MS), and Alzheimer's disease (AD). It is now well established that CNS inflammation can have Janus-like effects, with both beneficial and detrimental effects (Donnelly and Popovich, 2008; Doring and Yong, 2011; Gentleman, 2013), and much work has been done to find ways to regulate the immune response so as to create a regenerative environment (Popovich and Longbrake, 2008). The elaboration of therapies based on immune cell polarization is at its early stage, but a better comprehension of immune cell dynamics and mechanisms is imperative.

One powerful tool that has contributed to the advancement of knowledge in CNS inflammation is intravital imaging, which allows visualization of biological phenomena in a whole organism context in living animals and humans (Weissleder and Pittet, 2008; Pittet and Weissleder, 2011). In particular, imaging of living tissue at microscopic resolution using intravital microscopy

Neuroinflammation: New Insights into Beneficial and Detrimental Functions, First Edition. Edited by Samuel David.
© 2015 John Wiley & Sons, Inc. Published 2015 by John Wiley & Sons, Inc.

(IVM) has been extremely helpful to understand how individual cells respond to inflammatory stimuli. The recent advances in genome modification as well as the development of various transgenic animals have greatly added to the power, versatility, and popularity of this technique (Sung *et al.*, 2012; Miao, 2013). Furthermore, the development of two-photon intravital microscopy (2P-IVM), a fluorescence-based system that resembles confocal microscopy, has allowed deeper imaging of the CNS for longer periods with reduced laser-generated inflammation and photoactivation (Helmchen and Denk, 2005; Benninger *et al.*, 2008). In this chapter, we review the latest findings in the vast field of CNS inflammation that were made by means of IVM. Macroscopic imaging techniques have been the object of excellent recent reviews and will not be covered in depth in this chapter (readers are referred to Weissleder and Pittet, 2008; Ntziachristos, 2010).

Intravital Microscopy in the CNS and Its Challenges

IVM has truly lived a golden age since the early 2000s: commercial systems have been developed at relatively low costs, the availability of transgenic animal models has increased exponentially, and literature reporting IVM has exploded in countless research fields. The popularity of IVM comes from its ability to study complex cellular behaviors and mechanisms in a whole organism context, a major advantage over *in vitro* or *ex vivo* studies in which cells are either isolated in an artificial environment or fixed in time and space, respectively. As both the brain and spinal cord are accessible and relatively easy to stabilize because they are enclosed by bone structures, IVM has been particularly useful for studying disorders affecting the CNS, including trauma (i.e., TBI, SCI, and cerebral ischemia) and neurodegenerative diseases such as MS and AD.

One of the main challenges for IVM is the surgery. Exposure of the brain or spinal cord is a critical step that must be conducted with minimal bleeding and no damage to the target tissue. Although an opening in the skull or vertebral column has proven to be extremely valuable for data acquisition during a single imaging session, it is less compatible with the idea of performing chronic imaging, as bone will eventually regrow. An alternative to the removal of a piece of skull (craniotomy) or vertebral column (laminectomy) is thinned bone preparations (Drew *et al.*, 2010; Yang *et al.*, 2010). Since 2012, the IVM field has seen the emergence of a number of methods that consist of installing a window on top of the exposed brain or spinal cord to prevent tissue degradation and to allow for repeated imaging up to several weeks following implementation (Farrar *et al.*, 2012; Fenrich *et al.*, 2012; Nimmerjahn, 2012; Ritsma *et al.*, 2013). One important shortcoming of these types of windows, however, is the need to inject animals with potent anti-inflammatory drugs (e.g., dexamethasone) to reduce fibrosis and improve optical clarity. These substances have a significant impact on CNS physiology and can be a confounding factor in some areas of research involving animal models of CNS inflammation, as recently shown by Fenrich *et al.* using the most widely used model of MS, experimental autoimmune encephalomyelitis (EAE) (Fenrich *et al.*, 2013). In the latter study, the average time to onset was delayed by 4 days in EAE mice implanted with the chronic window and injected with corticosteroid. However, no change was noted with regard to disease severity. In contrast, we found that a single imaging session through an opening in the vertebral bones influences neither EAE onset nor disease severity (Aubé *et al.*, 2014). Thus, chronic window implementation is probably not yet optimal, and many technical concepts are under investigation to overcome its limitations. Another important challenge is the issue of intrinsic movement artifacts that are caused by cardiac and respiratory cycles and muscular and vascular tone, which will inevitably impair IVM imaging. This problem is currently being solved with the development of technologies that can be used to reduce movement artifacts in real time (Laffray *et al.*, 2011) or in post-acquisition (Soulet *et al.*, 2013).

Although *ex vivo* labeling of immune cells with a cell tracing compound is an easy and fairly efficient way to track cells (Coisne and Engelhardt, 2010), imaging of microglia and blood-derived immune cells is usually achieved using transgenic fluorescent reporter mouse lines, including CX$_3$CR1-EGFP-*ki* and Lys-EGFP-*ki* mice (Faust *et al.*, 2000; Jung *et al.*, 2000). Additional mouse strains have also been used to visualize other types of leukocytes (e.g., lymphocytes, dendritic cells, and platelets), blood vessels, astrocytes, oligodendrocytes, and neurons/axons (Feng *et al.*, 2000; Mempel *et al.*, 2004; Hirrlinger *et al.*, 2005). The most used mouse models for studying neuroinflammation are listed in Table 2.1. For cell structure labeling, Romanelli *et al.* (2013) listed a variety of commercially available fluorescent dyes that allow visualization of the nucleus, mitochondria, myelin, and many others.

Other IVM techniques such as positron emission tomography (PET) and magnetic resonance imaging (MRI) have also been used to study signs of neuroinflammation, such as blood–brain

Table 2.1 List of fluorescent mouse models commonly used to study the role of glia and immune cells in the CNS using intravital microscopy

Mouse strain	Mutation	Targeted cell types	Reference
Immune cells			
CX$_3$CR1-eGFP	Knock-in	Microglia, monocytes/macrophages	Jung *et al.*, 2000
LysM-eGFP	Knock-in	Neutrophils, monocytes/macrophages and perivascular macrophages	Faust *et al.*, 2000
PU.1-eGFP	Knock-in	Myeloid progenitors and B cells (intermediate expression)	Back *et al.*, 1999
C5aR-eGFP	Knock-in	Cells expressing high levels of both CD11b and Ly6C/Ly6G (Gr-1)	Dunkelberger *et al.*, 2012
Iba1-eGFP	Transgene	Microglia and macrophages	Hirasawa *et al.*, 2005
CD11c-DTR-eGFP	Transgene	CD8$^+$ and CD8$^-$ dendritic cells, subset of macrophages	Jung *et al.*, 2002
CD2-RFP	Transgene	T cells and a small subset of NK cells	Looney *et al.*, 2011
Non-immune cells			
Thy1-XFP	Transgene	Specific Thy1 strains label different axonal populations with either CFP, GFP, YFP or DsRed1	Feng *et al.*, 2000
hGFAP-eCFP	Transgene	Astrocytes	Hirrlinger *et al.*, 2005
Tie2-eGFP	Transgene	Endothelial cells	Motoike *et al.*, 2000
CNP-eGFP	Transgene	Oligodendrocytes and Schwann cells	Yuan *et al.*, 2002

Definitions: eGFP, enhanced green fluorescent protein; RFP, red fluorescent protein; CFP, cyan fluorescent protein; YFP, yellow fluorescent protein; DTR, diphteria toxin receptor; hGFAP, human glial fibrillary acidic protein; CNP, 2'-3'-cyclic nucleotide 3'-phosphodiesterase.

barrier (BBB) leakage, macrophages/microglia activation, and CNS lesions (Kannan *et al.*, 2009). For example, brain regions where microglia become activated and blood-derived macrophages are recruited can be identified by measuring the retention of $[^{11}C](R)PK11195$, a radioligand for PET imaging that specifically binds the peripheral benzodiazepine receptor. MRI is a key aspect of MS diagnosis, and its use with gadolinium enhancement allows the discrimination between demyelinated plaques, which show gadolinium leakage corresponding to BBB disruption, and other neurological conditions such as brain tumors (Traboulsee and Li, 2006). Although these imaging techniques offer the distinct advantage of being able to sample the entire CNS many times relatively quickly without having to perform invasive surgery, the spatial resolution that they achieved is relatively poor compared to 2P-IVM (Fig. 2.1).

In Vivo Imaging of the CNS Following Sterile Injury

Traumatic Brain and Spinal Cord Injury

It has been suspected for years that injured neural cells release DAMPs that rapidly trigger neuroinflammation (reviewed by Pineau and Lacroix (2009)). However, it is only with the advent of IVM imaging that a thorough analysis of cell behaviors became possible in the living rodent brain and spinal cord in both normal and injured conditions. Using time-lapse 2P-IVM, two pioneering studies demonstrated that microglia respond in a matter of seconds to minutes to a laser-induced or mechanical brain injury, firstly by extending their processes and then cell bodies toward the site of injury (Davalos *et al.*, 2005; Nimmerjahn *et al.*, 2005). Davalos *et al.* further demonstrated that the formation of a nucleotide gradient, primarily constituted of adenosine triphosphate (ATP), adenosine diphosphate (ADP), and uridine triphosphate (UTP), is crucial to the attraction of microglia. At least two other IVM studies have since confirmed the importance of the nucleotide gradient for microglial response (Haynes *et al.*, 2006; Dibaj *et al.*, 2010). Importantly, nucleotide-mediated microglial chemotaxis, but not baseline motility, is highly dependent on the purinergic receptor $P2Y_{12}$ (Haynes *et al.*, 2006). The vasodilatory molecule nitric oxide (NO) also participates in microglial migration through the formation of the nucleotide gradient (Dibaj *et al.*, 2010). An important open question is whether recognition of these signals by microglia leads to the production of molecules in the lesion environment, such as cytokines, which could regulate inflammation and astroglial and fibrotic responses.

High-resolution imaging of severed CNS axons has revealed that they undergo two successive degradation processes, namely, acute axonal degeneration (AAD; also referred to as axonal dieback) and Wallerian degeneration (WD). By using IVM, AAD was found to occur within 30 min of the axonal injury and described as the retraction of both proximal and distal axonal ends over hundreds of micrometers (~300 µm on average) (Kerschensteiner *et al.*, 2005). In this situation, the AAD can reach major axonal branch and cause unlesioned segments to degenerate as well. About 30 h after injury, WD launches and causes fragmentation of the distal part of the axon, while the proximal axonal segment starts to regenerate but grows blindly and inefficiently (Kerschensteiner *et al.*, 2005). The former observation is in line with earlier findings by Coleman *et al.* who, by using either tissue sections or nerve explants from Thy1-YFP transgenic mice, reported that axonal fragmentation in the distal peripheral (sciatic) nerve stump occurs between

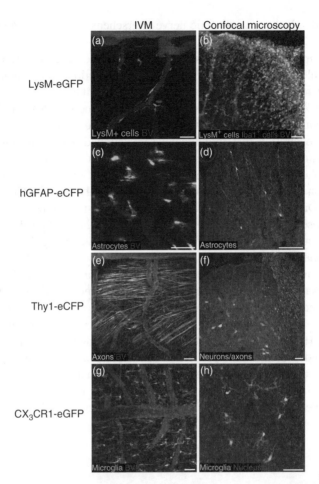

Figure 2.1 Two-photon intravital microscopy and confocal immunofluorescence in transgenic mice in which cell-specific promoters drive GFP or CFP expression. (a, c, e, and g) Two-photon intravital microscopy (2P-IVM) imaging of LysM-positive (+) cells (green in a), astrocytes (cyan in c), axons (cyan in e), and microglia (green in g) in the spinal cord of promoter-specific transgenic mice. Blood vessels (BV) were labeled through tail vein injection of either Texas red-dextran or Qdot705 (red color). Note that eGFP is not expressed in microglia in the CNS of LysM-eGFP mice (a). (b, d, f, and h) Confocal images of spinal cord sections obtained from the transgenic mice mentioned previously. (b) Infiltration of blood-derived LysM$^+$ cells (green) in the inflamed (EAE) CNS of a LysM-eGFP mouse. Macrophages/microglia and blood vessels were immunostained with antibodies directed against Iba1 (red) and CD31 (blue), respectively. The absence of colocalization between the LysM and Iba1 signals reinforces the idea that the LysM-eGFP mouse line can be used to track hematogenous myeloid cells specifically, as recently suggested by the Debakan laboratory (Mawhinney *et al.*, 2012). (d and f) Confocal imaging of astrocytes (d) and neurons/axons (f) expressing eCFP in the spinal cord of hGFAP-eCFP and Thy1-eCFP-23 transgenic mice, respectively. (h) Confocal imaging of microglia expressing eGFP in the spinal cord of CX$_3$CR1-eGFP mice. The blue signal in H shows counterstaining with the nuclear dye DAPI. Scale bars: 50 μm. (*See insert for color representation of this figure.*)

36 and 44 h after injury (Beirowski *et al.*, 2004, 2005). AAD and WD share degenerative mechanisms, as both types of degeneration are either largely delayed or abolished in mice harboring the Wallerian degeneration slow mutation (Wld^s) or treated with calpain inhibitiors. Notably, a number of IVM studies have demonstrated that blocking calcium (Ca^{2+}) release from intra-axonal Ca^{2+} stores or inhibiting calcium-dependant proteases such as calpain prevents

AAD in the injured spinal cord and optic nerve (Kerschensteiner *et al.*, 2005; Knöferle *et al.*, 2010; Stirling *et al.*, 2014).

By sealing the injured CNS, the astroglial and fibrotic scars (Sofroniew, 2009; Göritz *et al.*, 2011; Soderblom *et al.*, 2013) confer a natural protection against potentially neurotoxic molecules that are released by infiltrating blood-borne immune cells (Faulkner *et al.*, 2004; Göritz *et al.*, 2011). Accordingly, injury- and inflammatory-induced scarring is a major obstacle to axonal regeneration (Yiu and He, 2006). This long-standing view has recently been challenged by the demonstration that individual laser-sectioned axons are able to regenerate in glial-rich areas (Canty *et al.*, 2013). Similarly, crushed dorsal root axons regenerate beyond the astrocyte–peripheral nervous system (PNS) interface at the dorsal root entry zone, often in close association with astrocytic processes, before collapsing in CNS areas containing oligodendrocytes (Di Maio *et al.*, 2011). It must be emphasized, however, that the amount of scarring seen in these two models cannot be compared to what is typically observed after TBI or SCI. One of the current limits of 2P-IVM with respect to studying the effects of scarring on inflammation, secondary degeneration, and axonal regeneration in SCI has been its inability to image deep enough into spinal cord tissue to reach the interface between the astroglial scar and lesion border. The same problem holds true and is perhaps more critical for the fibrotic scar as it forms deeper in the spinal cord, that is, within the lesion core. A future challenge of 2P-IVM will therefore be to attain higher penetration depths in CNS tissue, using longer wavelength lasers for example. However, this will necessitate the development of near-infrared and infrared fluorescent dyes and proteins with properties suitable for *in vivo* imaging and eventually a complete change of the fleet of fluorescent mouse models that are currently being used by the neuroscience community. Another alternative is to develop mechanical TBI and SCI models that are more adapted to 2P-IVM, with a focal injury inflicted on the surface of the brain or spinal cord.

Cerebral Ischemia

Cerebral ischemia is a condition that features a reduction of available oxygen (hypoxia), the recruitment of immune cells in the infarcted area and edema (Iadecola and Anrather, 2011; Khatri *et al.*, 2012). *In vivo* two-photon imaging of cortical axons during middle cerebral artery occlusion (MCAO) in mice has revealed early changes in fine dendritic structures in areas of reduced blood flow (Li and Murphy, 2008; Murphy *et al.*, 2008). Murphy *et al.* (2008) reported that the number of dendrites undergoing blebbing, a precursor sign of dendritic damage and spine loss, increases dramatically shortly after occlusion and is associated with reduced synaptic activity (Li and Murphy, 2008). Of importance for the clinical outcome is the observation that, depending on the MCAO duration, recovery of fine dendritic structures is observed in the penumbra area after 20–30 min of reperfusion.

The effects of a stroke are not only limited to neurons, but also affect surrounding supporting cells, which may ultimately influence neuronal responses. Using a bioluminescent mouse reporter model, Lalancette-Hebert *et al.* (2009) showed that MCAO triggers a rapid activation of microglia that is sustained up to 3 months after stroke. Selective depletion of proliferating macrophages and microglia was found to increase infarct area and neuronal apoptosis (Lalancette-Hébert *et al.*, 2007). The same study further demonstrated that activated/proliferating microglia found in close proximity to the ischemic lesion are an important source of the neurotrophic factor insulin-like growth factor 1 (IGF-1). By using a similar IVM bioluminescent method in the neonatal ischemic brain, endothelial cells of the BBB and perivascular astrocytes were also shown to become rapidly activated, demonstrating nuclear factor κB (NF-κB) activity as early as 6 h after MCAO (Kielland *et al.*, 2011). Using real-time MRI, Breckwoldt *et al.* (2008) demonstrated increased levels of myeloperoxidase (MPO) activity and MPO-related oxidation at 3 days after stroke, a response that remained elevated for about 3 weeks. Together, these studies suggest that neurons, immune cells, glia, and other supporting cells are interacting in complex ways after cerebral ischemia, with evidence both in favor and against a role for neuroinflammation in the pathophysiology of stroke (Iadecola and Anrather, 2011). Better insight into these interactions and the early dynamic events occurring in the CNS after stroke is therefore necessary if we aim to clarify the importance of neuroinflammation and to develop therapies on the basis of its modulation. In this regard, 2P-IVM could be a very useful tool to study if, and how, immune cells participate in the secondary damage produced by ischemia and the ensuing tissue-regenerative and repair processes.

In Vivo Imaging of the CNS in Disorders with an Inflammatory Component

Multiple Sclerosis (MS) and Its Animal Model Experimental Autoimmune Encephalomyelitis (EAE)

MS is a chronic degenerative disease of the CNS in which immune cells cross the BBB and direct a self-reactive attack against myelin and axons. MS primarily affects young adults living in the northern hemisphere (Ramagopalan and Sadovnick, 2011). Despite the abundance of literature on the subject, the exact causes of the disease and what triggers it remain ill-defined. A major obstacle to obtaining an undistorted picture of the series of events leading to MS lies in the fact that, until recently, we were entirely dependent on data acquired post-mortem. In contrast to intravital imaging, post-mortem analysis offers only limited snapshots at a single time point. Since 2001, however, the diagnosis of MS has been revolutionized by the integration of leading-edge imaging technologies and, as such, is not based on only the clinical history of neurological episodes separated in time and space. Using real-time MRI, it is now possible to visualize BBB disruption and neuroinflammation through gadolinium enhancement and to assess the integrity of CNS myelin sheaths through T2-weighted MRI (Sormani *et al.*, 2009). These values can be used to determine the stage of the disease by counting the number of combined active lesions and estimating brain volume atrophy. MRI has also been used as an important tool to follow disease progression and measure the effect of a treatment on relapses in clinical trials (Sormani and Bruzzi, 2013). However, although the contribution of MRI to MS is undeniable, its contribution to understanding the precise mechanisms involved in disease pathogenesis has been mitigated by its poor spatial resolution and the absence of contrast agents that would help measure key disease biomarkers.

In vivo imaging of the blood–spinal cord barrier (BSCB) using 2P-IVM has revealed that its disruption is one of the earliest events occurring in the CNS during EAE (Davalos *et al.*, 2012). This leakage was found to allow the passage of blood proteins such as fibrinogen, which induces rapid microglial response toward the spinal cord vasculature through the myeloid cell receptor CD11b/CD18. Blocking fibrin formation or neutralizing the interaction between fibrinogen and CD11b/CD18 was further shown to inhibit perivascular microglial clustering and axonal damage. Our own 2P-IVM work has extended these findings by showing that neutrophils mediate BSCB disruption in EAE, an event that precedes EAE onset (Aubé *et al.*, 2014). Importantly, neutrophil depletion delayed EAE onset and reduced disease severity. Thus, from these studies, we can conclude that BSCB disruption precedes disease onset. Monitoring the integrity of the BSCB/BBB using IVM must therefore be regarded as an important tool to study the inflammatory events that precede the appearance of clinical symptoms.

Earlier IVM studies had also reported that leukocyte recruitment to the CNS precedes the appearance of clinical symptoms, with a maximal response observed at the peak of EAE (Kerfoot and Kubes, 2002; Dos Santos *et al.*, 2005). The transmigration of immune cells into the spinal cord and brain of animals with EAE is regulated by active processes. Leukocyte trafficking is a tightly coordinated process requiring cytokines and chemokines and binding to different subsets of cell adhesion molecules (CAMs) that are increased *de novo* in inflamed tissues (Ley *et al.*, 2007). Key among these CAMs are E- and P-selectins, P-selectin glycoprotein ligand-1 (PSGL-1), vascular cell adhesion molecule (VCAM)-1, intercellular cell adhesion molecule (ICAM)-1, lymphocyte function-associated antigen-1 (LFA-1), and the $\alpha_4\beta_1$ integrin, all of which were shown by IVM to be involved in the transmigration of autoreactive T cells and/or antigen-presenting cells (APCs) across the BBB/BSCB during EAE (Kerfoot and Kubes, 2002; Piccio *et al.*, 2002; Bauer *et al.*, 2009; Jain *et al.*, 2010). As recently suggested by Prat *et al.* using post-mortem brain tissue samples from EAE mice and patients with MS, it is likely that many other CAMs will be added to a long list that already includes activated leukocyte cell adhesion molecule (ALCAM), Ninjurin-1, and melanoma cell adhesion molecule (MCAM), to only name a few (Cayrol *et al.*, 2008; Ifergan *et al.*, 2011; Larochelle *et al.*, 2012).

After transmigration across the CNS endothelium, CD4 T cell motility and crawling in the perivascular space are mediated by CXCR4 (Siffrin *et al.*, 2009). As demonstrated in EAE rats, reactivation of T cells by APCs occurs in the perivascular space surrounding the microvessels at a time before the entry of autoreactive T cells into the CNS (Pesic *et al.*, 2013). Another area where reactivation occurs during EAE is in the leptomeningeal space, as revealed using transgenic mice in which a calcium indicator was inserted into T cells (Mues *et al.*, 2013). When T cells reach the CNS parenchyma, they patrol through a rostrocaudal axis in search for their specific antigen (Kim *et al.*, 2010). Monitoring the T cell velocity using IVM has revealed that the average speed of autoreactive T cells in the CNS is reduced as the clinical score increases or as they recognize their cognate antigen (Flügel *et al.*, 2007; Siffrin *et al.*, 2010). Siffrin *et al.* (2010) also reported that autoreactive Th17 cells make close contact with axons for longer periods than Th1 cells, which resulted in an aberrant elevation in intraneuronal calcium levels and ultimately in axonal damage. IVM of transferred MBP-reactive GFP+ T cells in nonimmunized rats revealed that T cells acquire a more pathogenic phenotype, that is, reach the CNS parenchyma and induce EAE faster, when they migrate to the lungs and bronchus-associated lymphoid tissue (BALT), a process that occurs in the first 48 h after transfer (Odoardi *et al.*, 2012). Moreover, infusion of antigen during those first 48 h greatly suppressed EAE development, as T cells were "locked" in the lungs and BALT (Flügel *et al.*, 2007). Conversely, clinical symptoms of EAE were amplified when antigen infusion was done when T cells had already reached the CNS parenchyma. After leaving the lungs, autoreactive T cells accumulate in the subarachnoidal space surrounding the spinal cord, where the majority of them crawl along pial vessels (Bartholomäus *et al.*, 2009). Interestingly, crawling of autoreactive T cells along leptomeningial vessels is not restricted to CNS-antigen-specific T cells, but only T cells specific for CNS antigen can enter the CNS parenchyma. An important future avenue of research will therefore be to identify the signals underlying trafficking of autoreactive T cells from the blood into the CNS parenchyma.

Although the main focus of research on EAE has been directed toward T lymphocytes, other bone marrow-derived cells have been linked to the pathophysiology (Bauer *et al.*, 1995; Almolda *et al.*, 2011; Codarri *et al.*, 2013; Rawji and Yong, 2013). Using IVM, microglia and macrophages have been associated with axonal damage through the production of reactive oxygen species (ROS) (Nikić *et al.*, 2011; Davalos *et al.*, 2012). Although these studies demonstrated a toxic role for microglia and macrophages in EAE, accumulating evidence suggests that these cells may also exert beneficial effects depending on the manner in which they are activated (for review, see Rawji and Yong (2013)). For example, microglia and macrophages that are polarized into an anti-inflammatory M2 phenotype can promote oligodendrocyte differentiation and remyelination through the release of trophic factors such as activin-A (Miron *et al.*, 2013). As we showed using mouse models of peripheral and central axon injury, macrophages/microglia can also support axonal regeneration through the clearance of inhibitory myelin debris, release of neurotrophins, and regulation of angiogenesis and vascular remodeling (Barrette *et al.*, 2008).

Neutrophils also play an active role in demyelinating neuroinflammatory diseases. Using IVM, we recently found that neutrophils mediate BSCB disruption during EAE in mice, a phenomenon that precedes the infiltration of macrophages and T cells in the spinal cord parenchyma (Aubé *et al.*, 2014). Moreover, we showed that neutrophils are closely apposed to the vasculature in CNS areas associated with increased BBB/BSCB leakage in the MS brain and the neuromyelitis optica (NMO) spinal cord. Langer *et al.* (2012) found that platelet depletion reduced EAE severity and the rolling and firm adhesion of leukocytes. IVM has also been used to study the involvement of specific chemokines in EAE and neuroinflammation (reviewed by Teixeira *et al.* (2010)). BBB/BSCB breakdown is therefore a key feature of EAE, MS, and other demyelinating neuroinflammatory diseases. Importantly, and as shown in Fig. 2.2, this phenomenon is associated with blood-derived immune cell recruitment and activity.

Other than for MS diagnosis, MRI has also been used to study EAE lesions in rodents (Denic *et al.*, 2011). Serres *et al.* (2009) showed that demyelinated plaques or lesions in the CNS can rapidly be reactivated after systemic lipopolysaccharide (LPS) injection (Serres *et al.*, 2009). In addition, the injection of magnetically labeled antibody has allowed to localize (on a macroscopic scale) and investigate the roles of T cells (Luchetti *et al.*, 2011; Wuerfel *et al.*, 2011), B cells (Kap *et al.*, 2011), and monocytes/macrophages (Engberink *et al.*, 2010) in EAE rodents and primates. Other aspects of the immune response in MS and EAE are covered in greater detail in Chapters 1 and 3.

Alzheimer's Disease (AD)

AD is a neurological disorder that features the accumulation of amyloid-ß (Aß) peptides and neurofibrillary tangles in the CNS, leading to the formation of senile plaques, destruction of neurons, and cognitive loss. Besides these hallmarks, inflammation is commonly observed in the brain

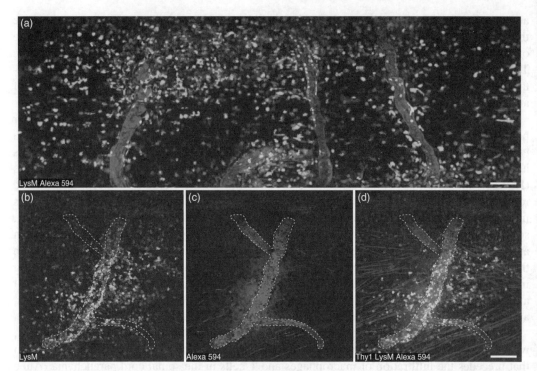

Figure 2.2 Two-photon intravital microscopy in mice shows massive recruitment of blood-derived immune cells and blood–spinal cord barrier (BSCB) leakage during EAE. (a) Peripheral LysM+ cells, which are mainly composed of neutrophils, rapidly infiltrate the spinal cord at EAE onset and are primarily localized along blood vessels. Blood vessels were labeled through tail vein injection of the fluorescent tracer Alexa-594 (Alexa Fluor® 594 hydrazide, sodium salt; in red) before imaging session. (b–d) *In vivo* permeability of the BSCB to the low molecular weight (760 Da) tracer Alexa-594 indicates that BSCB disruption and leakage coincide with the infiltration of LysM+ cells at EAE onset. Note the high colocalization between LysM+ cell infiltration (b) and Alexa-594 egress (c) outside of blood vessels (defined by the white dashed lines). (d) Merge of LysM (green) and Alexa-594 (red) channels with CFP-labeled axons (cyan/blue) imaged in the spinal cord of an LysM-eGFP; Thy1-eCFP-23 mouse. Scale bars, 50 μm. (*See insert for color representation of this figure.*)

of mouse models and individuals with AD (Wyss-Coray, 2006). Whether neuroinflammation contributes to the pathology or is a consequence of it remains, however, a subject of intense research. As will be discussed in the following section, the combination of powerful IVM techniques to recently developed methodologies allows to stain Aß deposits *in vivo*, via local or systemic delivery of Aß-specific fluorescent antibodies or dyes such as thioflavin S, Congo Red, and its derivative methoxy-XO4 (Kelényi, 1967; Bacskai *et al.*, 2001; Klunk *et al.*, 2002; Bertoncini and Celej, 2011). These approaches have led to remarkable advancements in the fundamental understanding of how neuroinflammation influences AD, and vice versa.

The biological effects of Aß peptides on neurons are still not well defined, but evidence accumulated using IVM has shown that they induce changes in axons, dendrites and synapses (for review, see Liebscher and Meyer-Luehmann (2012)), as well as stimulate the production of neurotoxic molecules such as ROS (Garcia-Alloza *et al.*, 2006). Using transcranial 2P-IVM in APP/PS1 transgenic mice, Tsai *et al.* (2004) have shown that neuronal branches passing inside or within approximately 15 μm of Aß deposits undergo abnormal changes such as atrophy and swelling, eventually resulting in spine, dendritic, and axonal loss. Aß deposits can also be found in vascular walls in the CNS, a condition seen in most cases of AD and named cerebral amyloid angiopathy (CAA). As revealed by IVM in APP transgenic mice, Robbins *et al.* (2006) have shown that accumulation of new vascular Aß deposits occurs primarily through propagation of existing deposits. Interestingly, mild chronic cerebral hypoperfusion in mice induced deposition of intravenously injected human Aß first in cerebrovascular walls and then in CNS parenchyma, linking cerebral ischemia to CAA and the development of parenchymal Aß plaques (ElAli *et al.*, 2013). Whether this holds true in AD in humans remains, however, an open question, a question that research aims to answer through the development of new imaging methods and agents for visualizing CAA *in vivo* in humans.

With respect to neuroinflammation, a number of *in vivo* imaging studies have shown that macrophages/microglia activation occurs in multiple regions of the brain in patients with AD (Kannan *et al.*, 2009; Schuitemaker *et al.*, 2013), yet macrophages/microglia activation does not always correlate perfectly with Aß accumulation (Yokokura *et al.*, 2010). Using real time 2P-IVM in APP/PS1 transgenic mice crossed with either CX_3CR1-EGFP or Iba1-EGFP mice, Aß plaques were shown to form within 24 h (Bolmont *et al.*, 2008; Meyer-Luehmann *et al.*, 2008). This response was followed by the recruitment of microglia toward newly formed Aß plaques, within 1–2 days of their appearance. The observations of the two studies diverge, however, with regard to the potential of microglia for clearance of Aß deposits. While Meyer-Luehmann *et al.* (2008) did not observe any plaques being cleared by microglia, Bolmont *et al.* (2008) found that microglia located in the vicinity of plaques internalized particles that were stained by the systemically injected fluorescent Aß probe, methoxy-X04. Nevertheless, both studies agree that microglia could help restrict the growth of Aß plaques, thus perhaps explaining why plaque size does not change much after initial formation. Several independent groups have also suggested that if properly activated using immunotherapies, microglia can help reduce the Aß load through enhanced phagocytic capacity (Bacskai *et al.*, 2001; Michaud *et al.*, 2013b). Monocytes also have the natural ability to clear Aß plaques within the lumen of the brain vasculature (Michaud *et al.*, 2013a), but similarly to microglia could exert inflammation-related negative effects as well during AD (Gentleman, 2013). The basis for these apparently contradictory roles of microglia and monocytes/macrophages during AD could depend on the nature of the stimuli present within the vasculature and CNS. Along this line, one important challenge for IVM will be the development of new fluorescent reporter mouse models that will make it possible to distinguish the various polarization phenotypes of immune cell subsets in real time *in vivo*.

Time-lapse 2P-IVM of macrophages/microglia at multiple time points within the same animals has shown that the fractalkine receptor CX_3CR1 regulates phagocytosis of oligomeric and protofibrillar Aß, but not preexisting fibrillar congophilic amyloid plaques (Liu *et al.*, 2010). Specifically, the group showed that microglia from CX_3CR1-knockout mice carrying combined APP Swedish and Indiana mutations proliferate more and have an overall greater phagocytic capacity for oligomeric and protofibrillar Aß than wild-type microglia. It should be pointed out, however, that deletion of the CX_3CR1 gene did not affect the degree of neuronal or synaptic injury around amyloid plaques.

IVM has also been used to study the effects of Aβ vaccination and passive administration of Aβ-specific antibodies on the pathogenesis of AD and CAA (Holtzman *et al.*, 2002). For example, this technology was essential for demonstrating that a single administration of anti-Aβ antibody at the site of craniotomy, directly underneath the cranial window, was sufficient to induce clearance of Aß deposits from the brain cortex and blood vessels in AD transgenic mice (Bacskai *et al.*, 2001; Prada *et al.*, 2007). It should be noted, however, that the clearance reported by Prada *et al.* (2007) was rather modest and short-lived (i.e., 1 week), yet chronic injection of the antibody for 2 weeks led to greater and more persistent clearance of CAA. Treatment of mice overexpressing mutant human APP with the anti-Aß antibody was found to promote the formation of dendritic spines away from plaques (>50 μm) within 1 h of local delivery, suggesting acute recovery of synaptic density (Spires-Jones *et al.*, 2009). Furthermore, antibody delivery increased the association between microglia and Aß plaques at 3 days after treatment, implicating a role for microglia in Aß clearance (Koenigsknecht-Talboo *et al.*, 2008). These IVM observations in AD mouse models were key for pushing forward immunotherapies on the basis of Aβ clearance in clinical trials. Unfortunately, these trials revealed that Aβ-specific antibodies are ineffective at improving cognition in patients with AD, even causing harmful effects (e.g., meningoencephalitis, autoimmunity, brain microhemorrhages, and edema) in some of them (Liu *et al.*, 2012). The possibility that Aβ-targeted immunotherapy may lead to adverse effects such as microhemorrhages and increased CAA had previously been recognized by Wilcock and Colton (2009).

Despite the disappointing results of these human trials, it should be pointed out that PET Aβ imaging using PiB showed reduced Aβ brain levels in patients with AD carrying the apolipoprotein E (APOE) ε4 allele following treatment with a humanized anti-Aβ antibody (Salloway *et al.*, 2014). These findings are intriguing, especially considering that Holmes *et al.* (2008) made similar post-mortem observations in the brain of patients with AD enrolled in a placebo-controlled trial of immunization with Aβ$_{42}$. Thus, although success has been mixed, the fact remains that only these well-organized trials will allow testing in humans the pathogenetic hypotheses developed in animal models. As highlighted previously, intravital imaging techniques could be a fast, effective, and noninvasive way of testing these hypotheses in real time in humans.

Conclusion

Studying the role of glial and immune cells and inflammatory processes in CNS disorders is a dynamic, evolving process. After all, less than a decade ago, it was not known that microglia are in constant movement in the CNS; discriminating monocyte-derived macrophages from microglia was impossible because of the absence of specific markers for either of these cell types; it was also unclear whether inflammation is a cause or consequence of neuronal loss, mainly because observations made in post-mortem material are static in time and space. However, recent years have seen the emergence of innovative, cutting-edge imaging technologies that now allow to visualize in real time *in vivo* the sequence of events taking place at a microscopic (cellular) scale. When combined to recent advances in genetic engineering, which enabled the creation of transgenic mouse models in which specific cells and elements can be made fluorescent and visible by microscopy, IVM has become a tool of choice to address the above-mentioned issues.

As presented in this chapter, many groundbreaking studies have used IVM to establish findings that could not have been addressed otherwise. For example, imaging the trafficking of peripheral immune cells across the BBB/BSCB toward the CNS parenchyma is one of the most certain ways to discriminate monocyte-derived macrophages from microglia. Another way of distinguishing both cell types in the normal CNS is to perform imaging of fluorescently labeled resident microglia through a thinned skull preparation, whereas the LysM-eGFP mouse line can be used to track hematogenous myeloid cells specifically in inflammatory conditions. IVM also allows to visualize neuronal/axonal and myelin damage in space and time on a microscopic scale and to correlate findings with other characteristic features of the disorder such as BBB/BSCB disruption, immune cell infiltration, and even the production of potentially neurotoxic molecules such as reactive oxygen and nitrogen species. As the sequence of events leading to neuronal/axonal damage and demyelination is not fully elucidated, considerable insights could be gathered from studies in which the dynamic nature of the disorder is taken into account, with minimal disturbance to the fragile environment that is the CNS. Live animal imaging offers such attributes, providing extensive temporal and spatial context in order to assess specific biological questions regarding the pathological elements at play and their relationship with the actual development of the disease. Moreover, nonterminal imaging protocols in which animals are not sacrificed at the end of imaging sessions can be used. This model provides information otherwise impossible to gather in terms of what happens before the appearance of clinical symptoms in mouse models of CNS disorders such as MS/EAE and AD, because of the inherent kinetic uncertainty relative to disease initiation and development. In conclusion, IVM has enabled us to address key gaps in neuroimmunology that had remained unexplained until recently. As knowledge and technology are evolving rapidly, it can be expected that in years to come, the molecular signals regulating immune cell phenotype and function will be identified and the effects of inflammation on CNS functions during injury and disease processes be finally elucidated.

Acknowledgments

The work leading to this book chapter was supported by grants from the Natural Sciences and Engineering Research Council of Canada (Grant number 298516-2010) and Wings for Life Spinal Cord Research Foundation (Project number 48, Contract number WFL-CA-006/11) to S.L. Salary support was provided by the Fonds de recherche du Québec en Santé (SL) and a doctoral studentship from the Multiple Sclerosis Society of Canada (AP). We thank Benoit Aubé for the 2P-IVM images of EAE spinal cords. We also thank Nicolas Vallières, Nadia Fortin, and Martine Lessard for their invaluable technical assistance.

References

Almolda, B., Gonzalez, B. & Castellano, B. (2011) Antigen presentation in EAE: Role of microglia, macrophages and dendritic cells. *Frontiers in Bioscience : a Journal and Virtual Library*, **16**, 1157–1171.

Aubé, B., Lévesque, S.A., Paré, A. *et al.* (2014) Neutrophils mediate blood−spinal cord barrier disruption in demyelinating neuroinflammatory diseases. *Journal of Immunology*, **193**, 2438–2454.

Bacskai, B.J., Kajdasz, S.T., Christie, R.H. *et al.* (2001) Imaging of amyloid-beta deposits in brains of living mice permits direct observation of clearance of plaques with immunotherapy. *Nature Medicine*, **7**, 369–372.

Back, J., Dierich, A., Bronn, C., Kastner, P. & Chan, S. (2004) PU.1 determines the self-renewal capacity of erythroid progenitor cells. *Blood*, **103**, 3615–3623.

Barrette, B., Hébert, M.-A., Filali, M. *et al.* (2008) Requirement of myeloid cells for axon regeneration. *Journal of Neuroscience*, **28**, 9363–9376.

Bartholomäus, I., Kawakami, N., Odoardi, F. *et al.* (2009) Effector T cell interactions with meningeal vascular structures in nascent autoimmune CNS lesions. *Nature*, **461**, 94–98.

Bauer, J., Huitinga, I., Zhao, W., Lassmann, H., Hickey, W.F. & Dijkstra, C.D. (1995) The role of macrophages, perivascular cells, and microglial cells in the pathogenesis of experimental autoimmune encephalomyelitis. *Glia*, **15**, 437–446.

Bauer, M., Brakebusch, C., Coisne, C. *et al.* (2009) Beta1 integrins differentially control extravasation of inflammatory cell subsets into the CNS during autoimmunity. *Proceedings of the National Academy of Sciences*, **106**, 1920–1925.

Beirowski, B., Adalbert, R., Wagner, D. *et al.* (2005) The progressive nature of Wallerian degeneration in wild-type and slow Wallerian degeneration (WldS) nerves. *BMC Neuroscience*, **6**, 6.

Beirowski, B., Berek, L., Adalbert, R. *et al.* (2004) Quantitative and qualitative analysis of Wallerian degeneration using restricted axonal labelling in YFP-H mice. *Journal of Neuroscience Methods*, **134**, 23–35.

Benninger, R.K.P., Hao, M. & Piston, D.W. (2008) Multi-photon excitation imaging of dynamic processes in living cells and tissues. *Reviews of Physiology, Biochemistry and Pharmacology*, **160**, 71–92.

Bertoncini, C.W. & Celej, M.S. (2011) Small molecule fluorescent probes for the detection of amyloid self-assembly in vitro and in vivo. *Current Protein and Peptide Science*, **12**, 205–220.

Bolmont, T., Haiss, F., Eicke, D. *et al.* (2008) Dynamics of the microglial/amyloid interaction indicate a role in plaque maintenance. *Journal of Neuroscience*, **28**, 4283–4292.

Breckwoldt, M.O., Chen, J.W., Stangenberg, L. *et al.* (2008) Tracking the inflammatory response in stroke in vivo by sensing the enzyme myeloperoxidase. *Proceedings of the National Academy of Sciences*, **105**, 18584–18589.

Canty, A.J., Huang, L., Jackson, J.S. *et al.* (2013) In-vivo single neuron axotomy triggers axon regeneration to restore synaptic density in specific cortical circuits. *Nature Communications*, **4**, 2038.

Cayrol, R., Wosik, K., Berard, J.L. *et al.* (2008) Activated leukocyte cell adhesion molecule promotes leukocyte trafficking into the central nervous system. *Nature Immunology*, **9**, 137–145.

Codarri, L., Greter, M. & Becher, B. (2013) Communication between pathogenic T cells and myeloid cells in neuroinflammatory disease. *Trends in Immunology*, **34**, 114–119.

Coisne, C. & Engelhardt, B. (2010) Preclinical testing of strategies for therapeutic targeting of human T-cell trafficking in vivo. *Methods in Molecular Biology (Clifton, NJ)*, **616**, 268–281.

Davalos, D., Grutzendler, J., Yang, G. *et al.* (2005) ATP mediates rapid microglial response to local brain injury in vivo. *Nature Neuroscience*, **8**, 752–758.

Davalos, D., Ryu, J.K., Merlini, M. *et al.* (2012) Fibrinogen-induced perivascular microglial clustering is required for the development of axonal damage in neuroinflammation. *Nature Communications*, **3**, 1227.

Denic, A., Macura, S.I., Mishra, P., Gamez, J.D., Rodriguez, M. & Pirko, I. (2011) MRI in rodent models of brain disorders. *Neurotherapeutics*, **8**, 3–18.

Di Maio, A., Skuba, A., Himes, B.T. *et al.* (2011) In vivo imaging of dorsal root regeneration: rapid immobilization and presynaptic differentiation at the CNS/PNS Border. *Journal of Neuroscience*, **31**, 4569–4582.

Dibaj, P., Nadrigny, F., Steffens, H. *et al.* (2010) NO mediates microglial response to acute spinal cord injury under ATP control in vivo. *Glia*, **58**, 1133–1144.

Donnelly, D.J. & Popovich, P.G. (2008) Inflammation and its role in neuroprotection, axonal regeneration and functional recovery after spinal cord injury. *Experimental Neurology*, **209**, 378–388.

Doring, A. & Yong, V.W. (2011) The good, the bad and the ugly. Macrophages/microglia with a focus on myelin repair. *Frontiers in Bioscience*, **3**, 846–856.

Dos Santos, A.C., Barsante, M.M., Esteves Arantes, R.M., Bernard, C.C.A., Teixeira, M.M. & Carvalho-Tavares, J. (2005) CCL2 and CCL5 mediate leukocyte adhesion in experimental autoimmune encephalomyelitis—An intravital microscopy study. *Journal of Neuroimmunology*, **162**, 122–129.

Drew, P.J., Shih, A.Y., Driscoll, J.D. *et al.* (2010) Chronic optical access through a polished and reinforced thinned skull. *Nature Methods*, **7**, 981–984.

Drouin-Ouellet, J. & Cicchetti, F. (2012) Inflammation and neurodegeneration: The story 'retolled'. *Trends in Pharmacological Sciences*, **33**, 542–551.

Dunkelberger, J., Zhou, L., Miwa, T. & Song, W.C. (2012) C5aR expression in a novel GFP reporter gene knockin mouse: implications for the mechanism of action of C5aR signaling in T cell immunity. *Journal of Immunology*, **188**, 4032–4042.

ElAli, A., Thériault, P. & Rivest, S. (2013) Mild chronic cerebral hypoperfusion induces neurovascular dysfunction, triggering peripheral beta-amyloid brain entry and aggregation. *Acta Neuropathologica Communications*, **1**, 75.

Engberink, R.D.O., van der Pol, S.M.A., Walczak, P. *et al.* (2010) Magnetic resonance imaging of monocytes labeled with ultrasmall superparamagnetic particles of iron oxide using magnetoelectroporation in an animal model of multiple sclerosis. *Molecular Imaging*, **9**, 268–277.

Farrar, M.J., Bernstein, I.M., Schlafer, D.H., Cleland, T.A., Fetcho, J.R. & Schaffer, C.B. (2012) Chronic in vivo imaging in the mouse spinal cord using an implanted chamber. *Nature Methods*, **9**, 297–302.

Faulkner, J.R., Herrmann, J.E., Woo, M.J., Tansey, K.E., Doan, N.B. & Sofroniew, M.V. (2004) Reactive astrocytes protect tissue and preserve function after spinal cord injury. *Journal of Neuroscience*, **24**, 2143–2155.

Faust, N., Varas, F., Kelly, L.M., Heck, S. & Graf, T. (2000) Insertion of enhanced green fluorescent protein into the lysozyme gene creates mice with green fluorescent granulocytes and macrophages. *Blood*, **96**, 719–726.

Feng, G., Mellor, R.H., Bernstein, M. *et al.* (2000) Imaging neuronal subsets in transgenic mice expressing multiple spectral variants of GFP. *Neuron*, **28**, 41–51.

Fenrich, K.K., Weber, P., Rougon, G. & Debarbieux, F. (2013) Implanting glass spinal cord windows in adult mice with experimental autoimmune encephalomyelitis. *Journal of Visualized Experiments*, **82**, e50826.

Fenrich, K.K., Weber, P., Hocine, M., Zalc, M., Rougon, G. & Debarbieux, F. (2012) Long-term in vivo imaging of normal and pathological mouse spinal cord with subcellular resolution using implanted glass windows. *Journal of physiology*, **590**, 3665–3675.

Flügel, A., Odoardi, F., Nosov, M. & Kawakami, N. (2007) Autoaggressive effector T cells in the course of experimental autoimmune encephalomyelitis visualized in the light of two-photon microscopy. *Journal of Neuroimmunology*, **191**, 86–97.

Garcia-Alloza, M., Dodwell, S.A., Meyer-Luehmann, M., Hyman, B.T. & Bacskai, B.J. (2006) Plaque-derived oxidative stress mediates distorted neurite trajectories in the Alzheimer mouse model. *Journal of Neuropathology and Experimental Neurology*, **65**, 1082–1089.

Gentleman, S.M. (2013) Review: Microglia in protein aggregation disorders: Friend or foe? *Neuropathology and Applied Neurobiology*, **39**, 45–50.

Ginhoux, F., Greter, M., Leboeuf, M. *et al.* (2010) Fate mapping analysis reveals that adult microglia derive from primitive macrophages. *Science*, **330**, 841–845.

Göritz, C., Dias, D.O., Tomilin, N., Barbacid, M., Shupliakov, O. & Frisén, J. (2011) A pericyte origin of spinal cord scar tissue. *Science*, **333**, 238–242.

Hanisch, U.-K. & Kettenmann, H. (2007) Microglia: Active sensor and versatile effector cells in the normal and pathologic brain. *Nature Neuroscience*, **10**, 1387–1394.

Haynes, S.E., Hollopeter, G., Yang, G. *et al.* (2006) The P2Y12 receptor regulates microglial activation by extracellular nucleotides. *Nature Neuroscience*, **9**, 1512–1519.

Helmchen, F. & Denk, W. (2005) Deep tissue two-photon microscopy. *Nature Methods*, **2**, 932–940.

Hirasawa, T., Ohsawa, K., Imai, Y., Ondo, Y., Akazawa, C., Uchino, S. & Kohsaka, S. (2005) Visualization of microglia in living tissues using Iba1-EGFP transgenic mice. *Journal of Neuroscience Research*, **81**, 357–362.

Hirrlinger, P.G., Scheller, A., Braun, C. *et al.* (2005) Expression of reef coral fluorescent proteins in the central nervous system of transgenic mice. *Molecular and Cellular Neurosciences*, **30**, 291–303.

Holmes, C., Boche, D., Wilkinson, D. *et al.* (2008) Long-term effects of Abeta42 immunisation in Alzheimer's disease: follow-up of a randomised, placebo-controlled phase I trial. *Lancet*, **372**, 216–223.

Holtzman, D.M., Bales, K.R., Paul, S.M. & DeMattos, R.B. (2002) Abeta immunization and anti-Abeta antibodies: Potential therapies for the prevention and treatment of Alzheimer's disease. *Advanced Drug Delivery Reviews*, **54**, 1603–1613.

Iadecola, C. & Anrather, J. (2011) The immunology of stroke: from mechanisms to translation. *Nature Medicine*, **17**, 796–808.

Ifergan, I., Kebir, H., Terouz, S. *et al.* (2011) Role of Ninjurin-1 in the migration of myeloid cells to central nervous system inflammatory lesions. *Annals of Neurology*, **70**, 751–763.

Jain, P., Coisne, C., Enzmann, G., Rottapel, R. & Engelhardt, B. (2010) Alpha4beta1 integrin mediates the recruitment of immature dendritic cells across the blood–brain barrier during experimental autoimmune encephalomyelitis. *Journal of Immunology*, **184**, 7196–7206.

Jung, S., Aliberti, J., Graemmel, P. *et al.* (2000) Analysis of fractalkine receptor CX3CR1 function by targeted deletion and green fluorescent protein reporter gene insertion. *Molecular and Cellular Biology*, **20**, 4106–4114.

Jung, S., Unutmaz, D., Wong, P., Sano, G., De los Santos, K., Sparwasser, T., Wu, S., Vuthoori, S., Ko, K., Zavala, F., Pamer, E.G., Littman, D.R. & Lang, R.A. (2002) In vivo depletion of CD11c+ dendritic cells abrogates priming of CD8+ T cells by exogenous cell-associated antigens. *Immunity*, **17**, 211–220.

Kannan, S., Balakrishnan, B., Muzik, O., Romero, R. & Chugani, D. (2009) Positron emission tomography imaging of neuroinflammation. *Journal of Child Neurology*, **24**, 1190–1199.

Kap, Y.S., Bauer, J., Nv, D. *et al.* (2011) B-cell depletion attenuates white and gray matter pathology in marmoset experimental autoimmune encephalomyelitis. *Journal of Neuropathology and Experimental Neurology*, **70**, 992–1005.

Kelényi, G. (1967) Thioflavin S fluorescent and Congo red anisotropic stainings in the histologic demonstration of amyloid. *Acta Neuropathologica*, **7**, 336–348.

Kerfoot, S.M. & Kubes, P. (2002) Overlapping roles of P-selectin and alpha 4 integrin to recruit leukocytes to the central nervous system in experimental autoimmune encephalomyelitis. *Journal of Immunology*, **169**, 1000–1006.

Kerschensteiner, M., Schwab, M.E., Lichtman, J.W. & Misgeld, T. (2005) In vivo imaging of axonal degeneration and regeneration in the injured spinal cord. *Nature Medicine*, **11**, 572–577.

Kettenmann, H., Hanisch, U.K., Noda, M. & Verkhratsky, A. (2011) Physiology of microglia. *Physiological Reviews*, **91**, 461–553.

Khatri, R., McKinney, A.M., Swenson, B. & Janardhan, V. (2012) Blood-brain barrier, reperfusion injury, and hemorrhagic transformation in acute ischemic stroke. *Neurology*, **79**, S52–57.

Kielland, A., Camassa, L.M.A., Døhlen, G. *et al.* (2011) NF-κB activity in perinatal brain during infectious and hypoxic-ischemic insults revealed by a reporter mouse. *Brain Pathology*, **22**, 499–510.

Kierdorf, K. *et al.* (2013) Microglia emerge from erythromyeloid precursors via Pu.1- and Irf8-dependent pathways. *Nature Neuroscience*, **16**, 273–280.

Kim, J.V., Jiang, N., Tadokoro, C.E. *et al.* (2010) Two-photon laser scanning microscopy imaging of intact spinal cord and cerebral cortex reveals requirement for CXCR6 and neuroinflammation in immune cell infiltration of cortical injury sites. *Journal of Immunological Methods*, **352**, 89–100.

Klunk, W.E., Bacskai, B.J., Mathis, C.A. *et al.* (2002) Imaging Abeta plaques in living transgenic mice with multiphoton microscopy and methoxy-X04, a systemically administered Congo red derivative. *Journal of Neuropathology and Experimental Neurology*, **61**, 797–805.

Knöferle, J., Koch, J.C., Ostendorf, T. *et al.* (2010) Mechanisms of acute axonal degeneration in the optic nerve in vivo. *Proceedings of the National Academy of Sciences of United States of America*, **107**, 6064–6069.

Koenigsknecht-Talboo, J., Meyer-Luehmann, M., Parsadanian, M. *et al.* (2008) Rapid microglial response around amyloid pathology after systemic anti-A antibody administration in PDAPP mice. *Journal of Neuroscience*, **28**, 14156–14164.

Laffray, S., Pagès, S., Dufour, H., De Koninck, P., De Koninck, Y. & Côté, D. (2011) Adaptive movement compensation for in vivo imaging of fast cellular dynamics within a moving tissue. *PloS one*, **6**, e19928.

Lalancette-Hebert, M., Phaneuf, D., Soucy, G., Weng, Y.C. & Križ, J. (2009) Live imaging of Toll-like receptor 2 response in cerebral ischaemia reveals a role of olfactory bulb microglia as modulators of inflammation. *Brain*, **132**, 940–954.

Lalancette-Hébert, M., Gowing, G., Simard, A., Weng, Y.C. & Križ, J. (2007) Selective ablation of proliferating microglial cells exacerbates ischemic injury in the brain. *Journal of Neuroscience*, **27**, 2596–2605.

Langer, H.F. Choi, E.Y., Zhou, H., Schleicher, R., Chung, K.-J., Tang, Z., Göbel, K., Bdeir, K., Chatzigeorgiou, A., Wong, C., Bhatia, S., Kruhlak, M.J., Rose, J.W., Burns, J.B., Hill, K.E., Qu, H., Zhang, Y., Lehrmann, E., Becker, K.G., Wang, Y., Simon, D.I., Nieswandt, B., Lambris, J.D., Li, X., Meuth, S.G., Kubes, P. & Chavakis, T. (2012) Platelets contribute to the pathogenesis of experimental autoimmune encephalomyelitis. *Circulation Research*, **110**, 1202–1210.

Larochelle, C., Cayrol, R., Kebir, H. *et al.* (2012) Melanoma cell adhesion molecule identifies encephalitogenic T lymphocytes and promotes their recruitment to the central nervous system. *Brain*, **135**, 2906–2924.

Ley, K., Laudanna, C., Cybulsky, M.I. & Nourshargh, S. (2007) Getting to the site of inflammation: The leukocyte adhesion cascade updated. *Nature Reviews Immunology*, **7**, 678–689.

Li, P. & Murphy, T.H. (2008) Two-photon imaging during prolonged middle cerebral artery occlusion in mice reveals recovery of dendritic structure after reperfusion. *Journal of Neuroscience*, **28**, 11970–11979.

Liebscher, S. & Meyer-Luehmann, M. (2012) A peephole into the brain: Neuropathological features of Alzheimer's disease revealed by in vivo two-photon imaging. *Frontiers in Psychiatry*, **3**, 26.

Liu, Y.-H., Giunta, B., Zhou, H.-D., Tan, J. & Wang, Y.-J. (2012) Immunotherapy for Alzheimer disease: The challenge of adverse effects. *Nature Reviews Neurology*, **8**, 465–469.

Liu, Z., Condello, C., Schain, A., Harb, R. & Grutzendler, J. (2010) CX3CR1 in microglia regulates brain amyloid deposition through selective protofibrillar amyloid-phagocytosis. *Journal of Neuroscience*, **30**, 17091–17101.

Looney, M.R., Thornton, E.E., Sen, D., Lamm, W.J., Glenny, R.W. & Krummel, M.F. (2011) Stabilized imaging of immune surveillance in the mouse lung. *Nature Methods*, **8**, 91–96.

Luchetti, A., Milani, D., Ruffini, F. *et al.* (2011) Monoclonal antibodies conjugated with superparamagnetic iron oxide particles allow magnetic resonance imaging detection of lymphocytes in the mouse brain. *Molecular Imaging*, **11**, 114–125.

Mawhinney, L.A., Thawer, S.G., Lu, W.-Y. *et al.* (2012) Differential detection and distribution of microglial and hematogenous macrophage populations in the injured spinal cord of lys-EGFP-ki transgenic mice. *Journal of Neuropathology and Experimental Neurology*, **71**, 180–197.

Mempel, T.R., Scimone, M.L., Mora, J.R. & von Andrian, U.H. (2004) In vivo imaging of leukocyte trafficking in blood vessels and tissues. *Current Opinion in Immunology*, **16**, 406–417.

Meyer-Luehmann, M., Spires-Jones, T.L., Prada, C. *et al.* (2008) Rapid appearance and local toxicity of amyloid-β plaques in a mouse model of Alzheimer's disease. *Nature*, **451**, 720–724.

Miao, X. (2013) Recent advances in the development of new transgenic animal technology. *Cellular and Molecular Life Sciences: CMLS*, **70**, 815–828.

Michaud, J.-P., Bellavance, M.-A., Préfontaine, P. & Rivest, S. (2013a) Real-time in vivo imaging reveals the ability of monocytes to clear vascular amyloid Beta. *Cell Reports*, **5**, 646–653.

Michaud, J.-P., Hallé, M., Lampron, A. *et al.* (2013b) Toll-like receptor 4 stimulation with the detoxified ligand monophosphoryl lipid A improves Alzheimer's disease-related pathology. *Proceedings of the National Academy of Sciences of United States of America*, **110**, 1941–1946.

Miron, V.E., Boyd, A., Zhao, J.-W. *et al.* (2013) M2 microglia and macrophages drive oligodendrocyte differentiation during CNS remyelination. *Nature Neuroscience*, **16**, 1211–1218.

Motoike, T., Loughna, S., Perens, E., Roman, B.L., Liao, W., Chau, T.C., Richardson, C.D., Kawate, T., Kuno, J., Weinstein, B.M., Stainier, D.Y. & Sato, T.N. (2000) Universal GFP reporter for the study of vascular development. *Genesis*, **28**, 75–81.

Mues, M., Bartholomäus, I., Thestrup, T. *et al.* (2013) Real-time in vivo analysis of T cell activation in the central nervous system using a genetically encoded calcium indicator. *Nature Medicine*, **19**, 778–783.

Murphy, T.H., Li, P., Betts, K. & Liu, R. (2008) Two-photon imaging of stroke onset in vivo reveals that NMDA-receptor independent ischemic depolarization is the major cause of rapid reversible damage to dendrites and spines. *Journal of Neuroscience*, **28**, 1756–1772.

Nikić, I., Merkler, D., Sorbara, C. *et al.* (2011) A reversible form of axon damage in experimental autoimmune encephalomyelitis and multiple sclerosis. *Nature Medicine*, **17**, 495–499.

Nimmerjahn, A. (2012) Optical Window Preparation for Two-Photon Imaging of Microglia in Mice. *Cold Spring Harbor Protocols*, **2012**, pdb.prot069286.

Nimmerjahn, A., Kirchhoff, F. & Helmchen, F. (2005) Resting microglial cells are highly dynamic surveillants of brain parenchyma in vivo. *Science*, **308**, 1314–1318.

Ntziachristos, V. (2010) Going deeper than microscopy: The optical imaging frontier in biology. *Nature Methods*, **7**, 603–614.

Odoardi, F., Sie, C., Streyl, K. *et al.* (2012) T cells become licensed in the lung to enter the central nervous system. *Nature*, **488**, 675–679.

Pesic, M., Bartholomäus, I., Kyratsous, N.I., Heissmeyer, V., Wekerle, H. & Kawakami, N. (2013) 2-photon imaging of phagocyte-mediated T cell activation in the CNS. *Journal of clinical investigation*, **123**, 1192–1201.

Piccio, L., Rossi, B., Scarpini, E. *et al.* (2002) Molecular mechanisms involved in lymphocyte recruitment in inflamed brain microvessels: Critical roles for P-selectin glycoprotein ligand-1 and heterotrimeric G(i)-linked receptors. *Journal of Immunology*, **168**, 1940–1949.

Pineau, I. & Lacroix, S. (2009) Endogenous signals initiating inflammation in the injured nervous system. *Glia*, **57**, 351–361.

Pittet, M.J. & Weissleder, R. (2011) Intravital imaging. *Cell*, **147**, 983–991.

Popovich, P.G. & Longbrake, E.E. (2008) Can the immune system be harnessed to repair the CNS? *Nature Reviews Neuroscience*, **9**, 481–493.

Prada, C.M., Garcia-Alloza, M., Betensky, R.A. *et al.* (2007) Antibody-mediated clearance of amyloid-peptide from cerebral amyloid angiopathy revealed by quantitative in vivo imaging. *Journal of Neuroscience*, **27**, 1973–1980.

Ramagopalan, S.V. & Sadovnick, A.D. (2011) Epidemiology of multiple sclerosis. *Neurologic Clinics*, **29**, 207–217.

Ransohoff, R.M. & Perry, V.H. (2009) Microglial physiology: Unique stimuli, specialized responses. *Annual Review of Immunology*, **27**, 119–145.

Rawji, K.S. & Yong, V.W. (2013) The benefits and detriments of macrophages/microglia in models of multiple sclerosis. *Clinical and Developmental Immunology*, **2013**, 1–13.

Ritsma, L., Steller, E.J.A., Ellenbroek, S.I.J., Kranenburg, O., Rinkes, I.H.M.B. & van Rheenen, J. (2013) Surgical implantation of an abdominal imaging window for intravital microscopy. *Nature Protocols*, **8**, 583–594.

Rivest, S. (2009) Regulation of innate immune responses in the brain. *Nature Reviews Immunology*, **9**, 429–439.

Robbins, E.M., Betensky, R.A., Domnitz, S.B. *et al.* (2006) Kinetics of cerebral amyloid angiopathy progression in a transgenic mouse model of Alzheimer disease. *Journal of Neuroscience*, **26**, 365–371.

Romanelli, E., Sorbara, C.D., Nikić, I., Dagkalis, A., Misgeld, T. & Kerschensteiner, M. (2013) Cellular, subcellular and functional in vivo labeling of the spinal cord using vital dyes. *Nature Protocols*, **8**, 481–490.

Salloway, S., Sperling, R., Fox, N.C., Blennow, K., Klunk, W., Raskind, M., Sabbagh, M., Honig, L.S., Porsteinsson, A.P., Ferris, S., Reichert, M., Ketter, N., Nejadnik, B., Guenzler, V., Miloslavsky, M., Wang, D., Lu, Y., Lull, J., Tudor, I.C., Liu, E., Grundman, M., Yuen, E., Black, R., Brashear, H.R. & Bapineuzumab 301 and Investigators 302 Clinical Trial (2014) Two phase 3 trials of bapineuzumab in mild-to-moderate Alzheimer's disease. *New England Journal of Medicine*, **370**, 322–333.

Schuitemaker, A., Kropholler, M.A., Boellaard, R. *et al.* (2013) Microglial activation in Alzheimer's disease: An

(R)-[11C]PK11195 positron emission tomography study. *Neurobiology of Aging*, **34**, 128–136.

Schulz, C., Perdiguero, E.G., Chorro, L. *et al.* (2012) A lineage of myeloid cells independent of Myb and hematopoietic stem cells. *Science*, **336**, 86–90.

Serres, S., Anthony, D.C., Jiang, Y. *et al.* (2009) Systemic inflammatory response reactivates immune-mediated lesions in rat brain. *Journal of Neuroscience*, **29**, 4820–4828.

Siffrin, V., Brandt, A.U., Radbruch, H. *et al.* (2009) Differential immune cell dynamics in the CNS cause CD4+ T cell compartmentalization. *Brain*, **132**, 1247–1258.

Siffrin, V., Radbruch, H., Glumm, R. *et al.* (2010) In vivo imaging of partially reversible Th17 cell-induced neuronal dysfunction in the course of encephalomyelitis. *Immunity*, **33**, 424–436.

Soderblom, C., Luo, X., Blumenthal, E. *et al.* (2013) Perivascular fibroblasts form the fibrotic scar after contusive spinal cord injury. *Journal of Neuroscience*, **33**, 13882–13887.

Sofroniew, M.V. (2009) Molecular dissection of reactive astrogliosis and glial scar formation. *Trends in Neurosciences*, **32**, 638–647.

Sormani, M.P. & Bruzzi, P. (2013) MRI lesions as a surrogate for relapses in multiple sclerosis: A meta-analysis of randomised trials. *Lancet Neurology*, **12**, 669–676.

Sormani, M.P., Bonzano, L., Roccatagliata, L., Cutter, G.R., Mancardi, G.L. & Bruzzi, P. (2009) Magnetic resonance imaging as a potential surrogate for relapses in multiple sclerosis: A meta-analytic approach. *Annals of Neurology*, **65**, 268–275.

Soulet, D., Paré, A., Coste, J. & Lacroix, S. (2013) Automated filtering of intrinsic movement artifacts during two-photon intravital microscopy. *PLoS One*, **8**, 1–9.

Spires-Jones, T.L., Mielke, M.L., Rozkalne, A. *et al.* (2009) Passive immunotherapy rapidly increases structural plasticity in a mouse model of Alzheimer disease. *Neurobiology of Disease*, **33**, 213–220.

Stirling, D.P., Cummins, K., Wayne Chen, S.R. & Stys, P. (2014) Axoplasmic reticulum Ca(2+) release causes secondary degeneration of spinal axons. *Annals of neurology*, **75**, 220–229.

Sung, Y.H., Baek, I.-J., Seong, J.K., Kim, J.-S. & Lee, H.-W. (2012) Mouse genetics: Catalogue and scissors. *BMB Reports*, **45**, 686–692.

Teixeira, M.M., Vilela, M.C., Soriani, F.M., Rodrigues, D.H. & Teixeira, A.L. (2010) Using intravital microscopy to study the role of chemokines during infection and inflammation in the central nervous system. *Journal of Neuroimmunology*, **224**, 62–65.

Traboulsee, A. & Li, D. (2006) The role of MRI in the diagnosis of multiple sclerosis. *Advances in Neurology*, **98**, 125–146.

Tsai, J., Grutzendler, J., Duff, K. & Gan, W.-B. (2004) Fibrillar amyloid deposition leads to local synaptic abnormalities and breakage of neuronal branches. *Nature Neuroscience*, **7**, 1181–1183.

Weissleder, R. & Pittet, M.J. (2008) Imaging in the era of molecular oncology. *Nature*, **452**, 580–589.

Wilcock, D.M. & Colton, C.A. (2009) Immunotherapy, vascular pathology, and microhemorrhages in transgenic mice. *CNS Neurological Disorders Drug Targets*, **8**, 50–64.

Wuerfel, E., Smyth, M., Millward, J.M. *et al.* (2011) Electrostatically stabilized magnetic nanoparticles – an optimized protocol to label murine T cells for in vivo MRI. *Frontiers in Neurology*, **2**, 72.

Wyss-Coray, T. (2006) Inflammation in Alzheimer disease: Driving force, bystander or beneficial response? *Nature Medicine*, **12**, 1005–1015.

Yang, G., Pan, F., Parkhurst, C.N., Grutzendler, J. & Gan, W.-B. (2010) Thinned-skull cranial window technique for long-term imaging of the cortex in live mice. *Nature Protocols*, **5**, 201–208.

Yiu, G. & He, Z. (2006) Glial inhibition of CNS axon regeneration. *Nature Reviews Neuroscience*, **7**, 617–627.

Yokokura, M., Mori, N., Yagi, S. *et al.* (2010) In vivo changes in microglial activation and amyloid deposits in brain regions with hypometabolism in Alzheimer's disease. *European Journal of Nuclear Medicine and Molecular Imaging*, **38**, 343–351.

Yuan, X., Chittajallu, R., Belachew, S., Anderson, S., McBain, C.J. & Gallo, V. (2002) Expression of the green fluorescent protein in the oligodendrocyte lineage: a transgenic mouse for developmental and physiological studies. *Journal of Neuroscience Research*, **70**, 529–545.

PART II
Detrimental Aspects of Inflammation

3 Roles of CD4 and CD8 T Lymphocytes in Multiple Sclerosis and Experimental Autoimmune Encephalomyelitis

Nathalie Arbour and Alexandre Prat

Department of Neurosciences, Université de Montréal, Centre de Recherche du Centre Hospitalier de l'Université de Montréal, Montreal, QC, Canada

Introduction

Multiple sclerosis (MS) is the prototypic inflammatory disorder of the human central nervous system (CNS). In 2013, it was estimated that 2.3 million people live with MS worldwide (Multiple Sclerosis International Federation, 2013). MS is characterized by multifocal areas of myelin sheath destruction, oligodendrocyte death, axonal damage, and glia cell activation. Clinically, the disease is characterized by recurrent and transient episodes of handicap, including loss of vision, balance, and mobility, and by painful sensory symptoms. The etiology of MS remains elusive; however, genetics and environmental factors are thought to contribute to the susceptibility and to the development of this disease (Koch *et al.*, 2013). Nevertheless, it is well established that the immune system participates directly in the destruction of myelin and nervous cells (Wu and Alvarez, 2011) (also see Chapter 1). Traditional genetic linkage analyses as well as more recent genome-wide association studies of MS have identified numerous disease-associated variants in genes related to immune functions (Sawcer *et al.*, 2014). Moreover, the abundance of immune cells and their products in CNS lesions or in the cerebrospinal fluid (CSF) of patients with MS supports the concept that MS is an autoimmune disorder (Wu and Alvarez, 2011). In most MS cases, demyelination is associated with a local accumulation of myeloid cells and T lymphocytes (Lucchinetti *et al.*, 2000; Lassmann *et al.*, 2012) (see Chapter 1 for more details). Finally, immune-modulatory and immune-suppressive treatments have been shown to improve clinical outcomes and disease course of MS (Cross and Naismith, 2014), establishing that the immune system plays a key role in the pathology of MS. This chapter presents an overview of the current knowledge on the roles of T lymphocytes in the pathobiology of both MS and its most common animal models, experimental autoimmune encephalomyelitis (EAE).

Neuroinflammation: New Insights into Beneficial and Detrimental Functions, First Edition. Edited by Samuel David.
© 2015 John Wiley & Sons, Inc. Published 2015 by John Wiley & Sons, Inc.

T Lymphocytes: Central Immune Cells

T lymphocytes contribute to the adaptive immune responses providing long-term protection. CD4 T lymphocytes play important roles in orchestrating multiple immune responses, whereas CD8 T lymphocytes are crucial in controlling intracellular pathogens and neoplastic cells. CD4 T lymphocytes, also called helper T cells (Th), recognize via their T cell receptor (TCR) antigens that are presented by molecules of the major histocompatibility complex (MHC) class II. Similarly, CD8 T lymphocytes, also called cytotoxic T cells (Tc), recognize antigens that are presented by MHC class I molecules. Differentiation and activation of naïve T lymphocytes require at least two signals provided by professional antigen-presenting cells (APCs): (i) TCR activation on peptide-MHC class complex engagement; (ii) co-stimulation signal through CD28. Such efficient stimulation triggers a complex cascade of intracellular signaling driving the maturation, proliferation, and production of immune mediators by T lymphocytes. Moreover, in response to specific environmental cues such as cytokines provided by APCs or cells of the local inflammatory milieu, T lymphocytes differentiate into specific subsets, each associated with distinct features (transcription factors, cytokines, etc.) (Sallusto et al., 2012). Three main subsets of Th and Tc lymphocytes bearing different effector functions have been described in the basis of their cytokine secretion profile: Th1/Tc1 [e.g., interferon-γ (IFNγ)], Th2/Tc2 [e.g., interleukin (IL)-4], and Th17/Tc17 (e.g., IL-17). Other subsets have been described, including regulatory CD4 or CD8 T lymphocytes; however, classification into distinct populations is complex in part due to the heterogeneity and plasticity of different subsets (Sallusto et al., 2012). A portion of activated T lymphocytes also acquires cytotoxic properties such as stores of lytic enzymes (perforin and granzymes) or killing receptors (e.g., FasL). Finally, a fraction of the activated T lymphocytes persists as central or effector memory cells; these memory cells provide long-term protection with augmented and more rapid responses on secondary challenge.

Autoreactive T Lymphocytes

Self-reactive T lymphocytes are part of the mature immune repertoire of healthy humans (Walker and Abbas, 2002). CD4 and CD8 T lymphocytes recognizing myelin antigens such as myelin basic protein (MBP), proteolipid protein (PLP), and myelin oligodendrocyte glycoprotein (MOG) are detected with similar or increased proportion in the blood of patients with MS as compared to healthy controls (Sospedra and Martin, 2005; Elong Ngono et al., 2012). However, an important number of studies advocate that myelin-specific T lymphocytes obtained from patients with MS bear different properties than those isolated from healthy donors: greater secretion of proinflammatory cytokines [IL-2, IFN-γ, and tumor necrosis factor (TNF)], enhanced frequency of high-avidity T lymphocytes, activated phenotype, and accumulation in the CSF (Sospedra and Martin, 2005). With the ultimate goal of inhibiting MBP-specific T lymphocytes, patients with MS were challenged with an altered MBP peptide. Unfortunately, in a subset of treated patients such injections induced the expansion of MBP-specific T lymphocytes accompanied by the development of numerous new CNS inflammatory lesions and clinical relapses (Bielekova et al., 2000). The dramatic outcome of this clinical trial provided the in vivo evidence that human myelin-reactive T lymphocytes are pathogenic in patients with MS.

A large body of evidence gathered from EAE models demonstrates that myelin-specific T lymphocytes that have been activated in the periphery can induce a CNS demyelinating disease. Active immunization of animals with myelin protein or immunodominant myelin peptides emulsified in complete Freund's adjuvant can induce EAE in several animal species (Baxter, 2007). Alternatively, the adoptive transfer of activated myelin-specific CD4 or CD8 T lymphocytes is sufficient to induce the demyelinating disorder in naïve recipients (Fletcher et al., 2010; Mars et al., 2011). Moreover, the activation and clonal expansion of T lymphocytes bearing a TCR specific for myelin epitopes that are distinct from the first targeted antigen, a phenomenon described as epitope spreading, can cause disease relapses (McRae et al., 1995; McMahon et al., 2005). The induction of immune tolerance for myelin peptides can prevent the occurrence of relapses in EAE models (Baxter, 2007) supporting the notion that T lymphocytes recognizing myelin antigens are involved not only in disease initiation, but also in disease progression. Interestingly, a phase I trial in patients with MS to induce antigen-specific tolerance to several myelin peptides has shown safety and tolerability (Lutterotti et al., 2013); whether inducing tolerance to myelin antigens using this approach will alter MS clinical course remains to be established.

As the activation of naïve T lymphocytes requires an efficient contact with professional APCs, we can speculate that activated CNS-specific autoreactive T lymphocytes in patients with MS have encountered APCs efficiently presenting CNS-derived antigens. Although the brain and spinal cord do not have defined lymphatic channels as observed in most organs, there is still lymphatic drainage for the CSF and the interstitial fluid of the brain parenchyma to the cervical lymph nodes (Laman and Weller, 2013). Dendritic cells, which are professional APCs, can travel from the CNS via the rostral migratory stream to the cervical lymph nodes where peripheral T lymphocytes could be exposed to CNS antigens (Mohammad et al., 2014). Indeed, cervical lymph nodes obtained from patients with MS and animals (marmosets and mice) affected with EAE contain mature APCs that have engulfed myelin or neuronal antigens, supporting the notion that they can activate T lymphocytes (Laman and Weller, 2013). Transgenic mice expressing a TCR specific for myelin epitopes can spontaneously develop EAE symptoms; experimental data suggest that these autoreactive T lymphocytes are first activated in the cervical lymph nodes where at least some CNS antigens are constitutively presented (Goverman, 2009). Moreover, CD8 T lymphocytes that have been activated by cervical lymph node APCs presenting CNS antigens acquire specific integrin (e.g., CD103) that will direct these cells preferentially back to the brain where the antigens were initially gathered (Masson et al., 2007). Once in the CNS, activated T lymphocytes can be reactivated locally by numerous APCs (macrophages, microglia, and dendritic cells) present in human and mouse lesions (Fig. 3.1) (Goverman, 2009). Two-photon imaging has shown that fluorescently labeled T lymphocytes can move from blood vessels to the CNS under inflamed conditions, regardless of their antigen specificity. However, only those that are specific for CNS antigens and have been in contact with local resident APCs presenting such antigen are locally reactivated and consequently licensed to enter the parenchyma (Bartholomaus et al., 2009). Activation of the second wave of CNS-specific T lymphocytes contributing to the perpetuation of disease could take place in lymph nodes and/or within the inflamed CNS. Indeed, removal of CNS draining lymph nodes attenuated the relapse severity in a chronic EAE model (van Zwam et al., 2009). In addition, a subset of dendritic cells within the inflamed brain of EAE

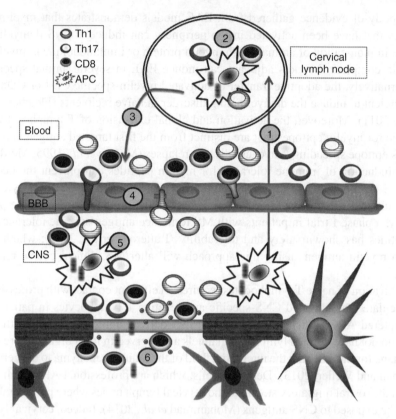

Figure 3.1   Roles of T lymphocytes in the pathogenesis of MS and EAE. (1) Although the brain and spinal cord do not have defined lymphatic channels, there is still lymphatic drainage for the CSF and the interstitial fluid of the brain parenchyma to the cervical lymph nodes (Laman and Weller, 2013). Dendritic cells, which are professional APCs, can travel from the CNS to the cervical lymph nodes. (2) Cervical lymph nodes obtained from patients with MS and animals affected with EAE contain mature APCs that have engulfed myelin or neuronal antigens such that they can activate T lymphocytes (Laman and Weller, 2013). (3) Activated T lymphocytes acquire cell surface activation markers and exit from the lymph node to the peripheral blood. CD4 and CD8 T lymphocytes recognizing myelin or neuronal antigen are detected in the blood of human donors. In patients with MS, CNS-specific autoreactive T lymphocytes (Th1, Th17, and CD8) bear enhanced activation properties compared to those obtained from healthy controls. (4) Activated T lymphocytes, regardless of their antigen specificity, acquire chemokine receptors, adhesion molecules, and integrins that favor their extravasation across the BBB (Goverman, 2009). (5) Once in the CNS, activated T lymphocytes can be reactivated locally by APC (macrophages, microglia, and dendritic cells) present in human and mouse lesions. Only those that are specific for CNS antigens and have been in contact with local APC presenting such antigen are locally reactivated and consequently licensed to enter the parenchyma (Bartholomaus *et al.*, 2009). (6) Th1 and Th17 CD4 lymphocytes and CD8 T lymphocytes as well as their secreted products (e.g., IFNγ, IL-17, and GM-CSF) are detected in CNS lesions of patients with MS (Kebir *et al.*, 2009; Fletcher *et al.*, 2010).

mice has been shown to present myelin antigens to naïve CD8 T lymphocytes leading to their efficient activation (Ji *et al.*, 2013). A better understanding of the aberrant activation of self-reactive T lymphocytes in the context of MS and EAE will provide invaluable tools to design therapies specifically geared toward these detrimental cells.

From Peripheral Activation to CNS Extravasation

The blood–brain barrier (BBB) controls the entry of cells and molecules into the CNS and thus maintains CNS homeostasis and the optimal microenvironment for neuronal functions. Under physiological conditions, only a limited number of peripheral immune cells including T lymphocytes cross the BBB in a process called immune surveillance of the CNS (Larochelle et al., 2011). Numerous studies using the EAE models have documented that myelin-specific T lymphocytes activated in the periphery acquire cell surface activation markers such as chemokine receptors, adhesion molecules, and integrins that favor their extravasation across the BBB (Fig. 3.1) (Goverman, 2009). Lymphocytes undergo firm adhesion on interaction between cell adhesion molecules (CAMs) expressed by the BBB cells and their cognate ligands expressed by leukocytes (Larochelle et al., 2011). On activation with inflammatory cytokines, endothelial cells of the BBB express intercellular adhesion molecule (ICAM)-1 and vascular cell adhesion molecule (VCAM)-1, which mediate, at least in part, the adhesion and transmigration to the CNS of T lymphocytes expressing the cognate integrin ligands: $\alpha L\beta 2$ [lymphocyte function-associated antigen 1 (LFA-1)] and $\alpha 4\beta 1$ [very late antigen-4 (VLA-4)], respectively (Larochelle et al., 2011). The efficacy of Natalizumab (a humanized antibody that blocks VLA-4) therapy in MS emphasizes that the interaction between activated T lymphocytes and the BBB is a crucial step in the formation of MS lesions (Polman et al., 2006). However, the increased risk of severe infections (e.g., JC-virus-induced progressive multifocal leukoencephalopathy) in patients treated with biological agents (e.g., Natalizumab, Efalizumab) broadly blocking immune cell extravasation (Major, 2010) has highlighted the need to develop tools to impair the migration of specific subsets of lymphocytes. We have demonstrated that other CAMs: activated leukocyte cell adhesion molecule (ALCAM) and melanoma cell adhesion molecule (MCAM) are upregulated in active MS and EAE lesions and that blockade of either of these molecules restricts the transmigration of CD4 T lymphocytes across the BBB and consequently dampens EAE severity (Cayrol et al., 2008; Larochelle et al., 2012). Moreover, MCAM identifies a subset of activated CD4 T lymphocytes producing elevated levels of inflammatory mediators (e.g., IL-17, GM-CSF) compared to cells devoid of this marker (Larochelle et al., 2012).

The contribution of specific chemokine receptors to the migration of activated T lymphocytes into the CNS has also been investigated. Human and mouse Th17 lymphocytes preferentially express CCR6, a chemokine receptor for CCL20, which is abundantly detected in the choroid plexus under normal physiological and MS inflamed conditions (Reboldi et al., 2009). However, the exact influence of CCR6 on autoimmune CNS inflammation remains the matter of debate, as conflicting reports demonstrated that CCR6-deficient mice are either resistant to EAE (Reboldi et al., 2009) or have more severe EAE (Elhofy et al., 2009; Villares et al., 2009). Explanations for these important discrepancies remain to be established. Nevertheless, it is well recognized and well demonstrated that activated T lymphocytes express elevated levels of several molecules (CAMs, integrins, chemokine receptors, etc.) that can favor their migration from the periphery to the CNS.

Role of CD4 T Lymphocytes in MS and EAE: Th1 versus Th17

Activated myelin-specific CD4 T lymphocytes secreting IFNγ are sufficient to transfer disease into naïve mice (Fletcher *et al.*, 2010), and injection of IFNγ to patients with MS led to aggravated symptoms (Panitch *et al.*, 1987a, 1987b). These seminal observations were the impetus for the concept that myelin-specific IFNγ-producing Th1 lymphocytes are responsible for disease induction in MS and its animal models. However, publications in the 1990s challenged the view that these IFNγ-producing cells are the main culprits in disease pathogenesis. Indeed, IFNγ or IFNγ receptor-deficient mice are susceptible to EAE induction with a more severe course, and injection of antibodies neutralizing IFNγ enhances disease severity (Steinman, 2007). Subsequently, a new Th cell subset called Th17 has been identified; these lymphocytes secrete several cytokines including IL-17A, IL-17F, IL-21, and IL-22. Similarly to Th1 lymphocytes, adoptive transfer of myelin-specific Th17 lymphocytes is also sufficient to induce EAE in naïve recipient mice (Fletcher *et al.*, 2010). However, mice deficient for either of the characteristic cytokines of this cell subset (IL-17, IL-21, and IL-22) are still susceptible to EAE (Codarri *et al.*, 2013). In contrast, granulocyte-macrophage colony-stimulating factor (GM-CSF), which is produced by both activated myelin-specific Th1 and Th17 lymphocytes is now considered to be a critical factor involved in autoimmune CNS inflammation (Codarri *et al.*, 2013). Indeed, mice deficient in GM-CSF are resistant to EAE; administration of GM-CSF worsens disease symptoms, whereas injection of blocking antibodies even after disease onset decreases disease severity (Codarri *et al.*, 2013).

Elevated amounts of Th1 (IFNγ) and Th17 cytokines (IL-17, IL-22) as well as GM-CSF are detected in the CSF and CNS lesions of patients with MS, especially during the active phase of the disease (Kebir *et al.*, 2009; Mellergard *et al.*, 2010). Tzartos *et al.* (2008) and Kebir *et al.* (2007) have shown that more than 70% of T lymphocytes in acute and chronic MS lesions expresses IL-17 (Fig. 3.1). We have shown that activated CD4 T lymphocytes simultaneously producing IFNγ and IL-17 are present in MS brain tissue, are preferentially expanded from blood lymphocytes obtained from relapsing MS patients, and demonstrate a greater capacity to cross the human BBB (Kebir *et al.*, 2009). Moreover, key cytokines involved in the differentiation of Th1 and/or Th17 cell subsets such as IL-12 and IL-23 are expressed at greater levels in the CSF and/or CNS of patients with MS compared to controls (Li *et al.*, 2007). Unfortunately, attempts to block both IL-12 and IL-23 using an antibody targeting the shared p40 subunit of these two cytokines did not lead to clinical improvement in patients with MS (Segal *et al.*, 2008), although this approach has been successful for treating other autoimmune diseases (Kumar *et al.*, 2013). Interestingly, a phase Ib/IIa trial in patients with rheumatoid arthritis receiving a human monoclonal antibody to GM-CSF has shown some efficacy (Behrens *et al.*, 2014), and the safety of this antibody in patients with MS is being tested in a phase 1 trial (source: www.clinicaltrials.org). Additional clinical trials will be necessary to determine whether any therapy targeting specific cytokines could be beneficial to patients with MS.

Observations in animal models suggest that the relative importance of Th1 versus Th17 immune responses dictates the localization of CNS inflammation (Pierson *et al.*, 2012). Indeed, strong Th1 responses characterized by an elevated production of IFNγ cause a massive infiltration in the spinal cord accompanied by classical EAE symptoms (e.g., flaccid tail and hindlimb paralysis) (Stromnes *et al.*, 2008). In contrast, encephalitogenic T lymphocytes producing mainly IL-17 and less IFNγ infiltrate preferentially the brain parenchyma and cause the atypical EAE symptoms (e.g., head tilt, spinning, and axial rotation) (Stromnes *et al.*, 2008). Several factors can cause an impact on the preferential CNS infiltration of encephalitogenic T lymphocytes such as genetic background, myelin epitope targeted, cytokines provided by professional APCs, and local cytokine receptor expression in CNS areas (Pierson *et al.*, 2012). Data obtained from patients with MS suggest that the predominance of either Th1 or Th17 responses can also contribute to the disease heterogeneity with variations in clinical course, response to immunomodulators, and localization of CNS lesions (Axtell *et al.*, 2010; Pierson *et al.*, 2012). It is now well established that Th1 and Th17 CD4 lymphocytes are both involved in the initiation of MS and EAE (Fig. 3.1) (Kebir *et al.*, 2007, 2009; Stromnes *et al.*, 2008). Moreover, subsets of CD4 T lymphocytes bearing cytotoxic properties can also participate in the tissue damage. We have shown that CD4 T lymphocytes expressing NKG2C as well as other markers (e.g., CD56, NKG2D, and granzyme B) are enriched in the peripheral blood of patients with MS, are detected in CNS MS lesions, and are able to kill human oligodendrocytes, which express HLA-E, the cognate ligand of NKG2C (Zaguia *et al.*, 2013). A better understanding of the various immune molecules and mechanisms expressed by T lymphocytes to attack the CNS will provide essential insight into the heterogeneity observed in patients with MS and could identify biomarkers to efficiently and specifically target the immune mediators causing the CNS damage (Pierson *et al.*, 2012).

Role of CD8 T Lymphocytes in MS and EAE

An extensive body of evidence from EAE models points to the role of CD4 T lymphocytes in disease pathogenesis (Fletcher *et al.*, 2010). However, an anti-CD4-depleting antibody did not yield any clinical benefits to patients with MS (Lindsey *et al.*, 1994; Rep *et al.*, 1997; van Oosten *et al.*, 1997), implying that CD4 T lymphocytes are not the only actors involved in MS pathogenesis. Multiple lines of evidence suggest that CD8 T lymphocytes also participate in the typical CNS damage observed in patients with MS (Mars *et al.*, 2011). CD8 T lymphocytes are detected in perivascular and parenchymal MS lesions and often reach or surpass in abundance CD4 T lymphocytes (Mars *et al.*, 2011). Even in early stages, CD8 T lymphocytes are detected in cortical demyelinating MS lesions (Lucchinetti *et al.*, 2011). The presence of CD8 T lymphocytes in MS lesions positively correlates with the extent of axonal damage (Bitsch *et al.*, 2000; Kuhlmann *et al.*, 2002). Interestingly, we and others (Kebir *et al.*, 2007; Tzartos *et al.*, 2008; Ifergan *et al.*, 2011) reported an enrichment of IL-17-producing CD8 T lymphocytes (i.e., Tc17) in MS lesions.

It is possible to determine the clonal diversity of T lymphocytes present in a specific compartment by a spectratyping analysis of the complementarity-determining region 3 of the TCR, as each clone bears a distinct sequence. The presence of a limited number of clones in a specific compartment suggests that T lymphocytes did not randomly enter this site, but rather antigen-specific T lymphocytes preferentially infiltrated this organ. Different groups analyzed the TCR of CD8 T lymphocytes from the blood, CSF, and/or the brain of patients with MS. Most CD8 T lymphocytes recovered from MS lesions belonged to a few clones (Babbe *et al.*, 2000; Junker *et al.*, 2007). Moreover, clones of CD8 T lymphocytes isolated from the CNS (CSF and/or tissue) of patients with MS persist over time in patients studied longitudinally (Jacobsen *et al.*, 2002; Skulina *et al.*,

2004). In contrast, the repertoire of the infiltrating CD4 T lymphocytes in the CNS of patients with MS is heterogeneous (Mars et al., 2011). These studies strongly suggest that infiltrating CD8 T lymphocytes in the CNS of patients with MS selectively enter this organ. Unfortunately, the antigen specificity of these infiltrating CD8 T lymphocytes remains still unknown.

Under basal physiological conditions, CNS cells including neurons, oligodendrocytes, and astrocytes express low levels of MHC class I molecules, which are recognized by CD8 T lymphocytes. However, upregulated MHC class I is observed on resident CNS cells in MS lesions (Hoftberger et al., 2004) even in the initial phases of the disease (Ransohoff and Estes, 1991; Gobin et al., 2001). These observations support the notion that infiltrating CD8 T lymphocytes can directly interact with resident CNS cells. Indeed, CD8 T lymphocytes are frequently observed in close proximity to oligodendrocytes and demyelinated axons (Mars et al., 2011). Finally, autoreactive CD8 T cells can induce EAE with pathological features (e.g., demyelination) reminiscent of human MS disease (Huseby et al., 2001; Sun et al., 2001; Friese and Fugger, 2005). Recent data support the notion that both CD4 and CD8 T lymphocytes work in concert to cause the autoimmune attack observed in EAE (Huber et al., 2013). Additional investigations on the interplay between CD4 and CD8 T lymphocytes during different phases of MS and EAE could shed light on the complex and heterogeneous immune mechanisms involved in the disease pathobiology.

Regulatory T Lymphocytes in MS and EAE

Both CD4 and CD8 T lymphocytes with regulatory properties have been described (Jadidi-Niaragh and Mirshafiey, 2011). These cells are crucial to maintain peripheral tolerance and prevent autoimmune attacks; they are capable of restricting functions of a wide spectrum of immune cells, including CD4 and CD8 T lymphocytes, natural killer (NK) cells, and APCs (e.g., monocytes, macrophages, and dendritic cells) (Lowther and Hafler, 2012). Numerous studies performed in the EAE models have demonstrated that regulatory T lymphocytes can control the development and severity of this disease and could also promote the recovery phase (Lowther and Hafler, 2012). Defects in regulatory functions and migratory properties, but not necessarily in the frequency of regulatory CD4 T lymphocytes, have been documented in patients with MS compared to healthy donors (Lowther and Hafler, 2012).

Subsets of CD8 T lymphocytes with regulatory properties have been reported. However, it is difficult to evaluate whether these cells are really regulatory, because specific markers (e.g., CD25, CD122, and CD56) or cytokines [IL-10 or transforming growth factor beta (TGFβ)] associated with regulatory CD8 T lymphocytes (Jiang and Chess, 2004; Hu et al., 2013) are also hallmarks of activated effector CD8 T lymphocytes (Willing and Friese, 2012). It has been suggested that CD8 T lymphocytes can kill myelin-specific CD4 T lymphocytes in a HLA-E restricted manner (Correale and Villa, 2008) and that treatment of patients with MS with glatiramer acetate, a synthetic copolymer of four amino acids, can augment the capacity of CD8 T lymphocytes to destroy CD4 T lymphocytes via an HLA-E-dependent mechanism among others (Tennakoon et al., 2006). Overall, impaired immune regulatory functions in both CD4 and CD8 T cell compartments have been reported in patients with MS. However, the mechanisms used by different human T cell subsets to regulate detrimental autoimmune responses and the causes underlying potential defects in such regulatory cells remain largely unresolved.

Conclusions

In the last decades, the scientific community has taken giant steps forward to elucidate the complexity of the immune mechanisms implicated in the pathogenesis of MS. Subsets of T lymphocytes (e.g., Th1, Th17, and CD8), cytokines (e.g., GM-CSF), and mechanisms have been identified and characterized. There is now an impressive body of evidence supporting the notion that both CD4 and CD8 T lymphocytes contribute to the pathogenesis of MS (Fig. 3.1). Moreover, the roles of specific T cell subsets as well as other immune factors (e.g., B lymphocytes) have been unraveled. Additional rodent models have been developed to mirror at least part of the complex human disease; these models have provided valuable insights to investigate the causes underlying disease heterogeneity in patients. Despite these phenomenal advances, the exact etiology of MS remains undefined and no cure is available. Therefore, researchers will need to pursue their investigations to dissect the numerous potential immune mechanisms participating in this inflammatory disease of the CNS.

Acknowledgments

N.A. holds a New Investigator Salary Award from the Canadian Institutes of Health Research, and A.P. is a Research Scholar from the Fonds de recherche du Québec Santé.

References

Axtell, R.C., de Jong, B.A., Boniface, K. *et al.* (2010) T helper type 1 and 17 cells determine efficacy of interferon-beta in multiple sclerosis and experimental encephalomyelitis. *Nature Medicine*, **16**, 406–412.

Babbe, H., Roers, A., Waisman, A. *et al.* (2000) Clonal expansions of CD8(+) T cells dominate the T cell infiltrate in active multiple sclerosis lesions as shown by micromanipulation and single cell polymerase chain reaction. *Journal of Experimental Medicine*, **192**, 393–404.

Bartholomaus, I., Kawakami, N., Odoardi, F. *et al.* (2009) Effector T cell interactions with meningeal vascular structures in nascent autoimmune CNS lesions. *Nature*, **462**, 94–98.

Baxter, A.G. (2007) The origin and application of experimental autoimmune encephalomyelitis. *Nature Reviews Immunology*, **7**, 904–912.

Behrens, F., Tak, P.P., Ostergaard, M. *et al.* (2014) MOR103, a human monoclonal antibody to granulocyte-macrophage colony-stimulating factor, in the treatment of patients with moderate rheumatoid arthritis: results of a phase Ib/IIa randomised, double-blind, placebo-controlled, dose-escalation trial. *Annals of the Rheumatic Diseases*. doi:10.1136/annrheumdis-2013-204816

Bielekova, B., Goodwin, B., Richert, N. *et al.* (2000) Encephalitogenic potential of the myelin basic protein peptide (amino acids 83–99) in multiple sclerosis: results of a phase II clinical trial with an altered peptide ligand. *Nature Medicine*, **6**, 1167–1175.

Bitsch, A., Schuchardt, J., Bunkowski, S., Kuhlmann, T. & Bruck, W. (2000) Acute axonal injury in multiple sclerosis. Correlation with demyelination and inflammation. *Brain*, **123**, 1174–1183.

Cayrol, R., Wosik, K., Berard, J.L. *et al.* (2008) Activated leukocyte cell adhesion molecule promotes leukocyte trafficking into the central nervous system. *Nature Immunology*, **9**, 137–145.

Codarri, L., Greter, M. & Becher, B. (2013) Communication between pathogenic T cells and myeloid cells in neuroinflammatory disease. *Trends in Immunology*, **34**, 114–119.

Correale, J. & Villa, A. (2008) Isolation and characterization of CD8+ regulatory T cells in multiple sclerosis. *Journal of Neuroimmunology*, **195**, 121–134.

Cross, A.H. & Naismith, R.T. (2014) Established and novel disease-modifying treatments in multiple sclerosis. *Journal of Internal Medicine*, **275**, 350–363.

Elhofy, A., Depaolo, R.W., Lira, S.A., Lukacs, N.W. & Karpus, W.J. (2009) Mice deficient for CCR6 fail to control chronic experimental autoimmune encephalomyelitis. *Journal of Neuroimmunology*, **213**, 91–99.

Elong Ngono, A., Pettre, S., Salou, M. *et al.* (2012) Frequency of circulating autoreactive T cells committed to myelin determinants in relapsing-remitting multiple sclerosis patients. *Clinical Immunology*, **144**, 117–126.

Fletcher, J.M., Lalor, S.J., Sweeney, C.M., Tubridy, N. & Mills, K.H. (2010) T cells in multiple sclerosis and experimental autoimmune encephalomyelitis. *Clinical and Experimental Immunology*, **162**, 1–11.

Friese, M.A. & Fugger, L. (2005) Autoreactive CD8+ T cells in multiple sclerosis: a new target for therapy? *Brain*, **128**, 1747–1763.

Gobin, S.J., Montagne, L., Van Zutphen, M., Van Der Valk, P., Van Den Elsen, P.J. & De Groot, C.J. (2001) Upregulation of transcription factors controlling MHC expression in multiple sclerosis lesions. *Glia*, **36**, 68–77.

Goverman, J. (2009) Autoimmune T cell responses in the central nervous system. *Nature Reviews Immunology*, **9**, 393–407.

Hoftberger, R., Aboul-Enein, F., Brueck, W. *et al.* (2004) Expression of major histocompatibility complex class I molecules on the different cell types in multiple sclerosis lesions. *Brain Pathology*, **14**, 43–50.

Hu, D., Weiner, H.L. & Ritz, J. (2013) Identification of cytolytic CD161-CD56+ regulatory CD8 T cells in human peripheral blood. *PLoS One*, **8**, e59545.

Huber, M., Heink, S., Pagenstecher, A. *et al.* (2013) IL-17A secretion by CD8+ T cells supports Th17-mediated autoimmune encephalomyelitis. *Journal of Clinical Investigation*, **123**, 247–260.

Huseby, E.S., Liggitt, D., Brabb, T., Schnabel, B., Ohlen, C. & Goverman, J. (2001) A pathogenic role for myelin-specific cd8(+) t cells in a model for multiple sclerosis. *Journal of Experimental Medicine*, **194**, 669–676.

Ifergan, I., Kebir, H., Alvarez, J.I. *et al.* (2011) Central nervous system recruitment of effector memory CD8+ T lymphocytes during neuroinflammation is dependent on alpha4 integrin. *Brain*, **134**, 3560–3577.

Jacobsen, M., Cepok, S., Quak, E. *et al.* (2002) Oligoclonal expansion of memory CD8+ T cells in cerebrospinal fluid from multiple sclerosis patients. *Brain*, **125**, 538–550.

Jadidi-Niaragh, F. & Mirshafiey, A. (2011) Regulatory T-cell as orchestra leader in immunosuppression process of multiple sclerosis. *Immunopharmacology and Immunotoxicology*, **33**, 545–567.

Ji, Q., Castelli, L. & Goverman, J.M. (2013) MHC class I-restricted myelin epitopes are cross-presented by Tip-DCs that promote determinant spreading to CD8(+) T cells. *Nature Immunology*, **14**, 254–261.

Jiang, H. & Chess, L. (2004) An integrated view of suppressor T cell subsets in immunoregulation. *Journal of Clinical Investigation*, **114**, 1198–1208.

Junker, A., Ivanidze, J., Malotka, J. *et al.* (2007) Multiple sclerosis: T-cell receptor expression in distinct brain regions. *Brain*, **130**, 2789–2799.

Kebir, H., Ifergan, I., Alvarez, J.I. *et al.* (2009) Preferential recruitment of interferon-gamma-expressing TH17 cells in multiple sclerosis. *Annals of Neurology*, **66**, 390–402.

Kebir, H., Kreymborg, K., Ifergan, I. *et al.* (2007) Human TH17 lymphocytes promote blood-brain barrier disruption and central nervous system inflammation. *Nature Medicine*, **13**, 1173–1175.

Koch, M.W., Metz, L.M., Agrawal, S.M. & Yong, V.W. (2013) Environmental factors and their regulation of immunity in multiple sclerosis. *Journal of Neurological Sciences*, **324**, 10–16.

Kuhlmann, T., Lingfeld, G., Bitsch, A., Schuchardt, J. & Bruck, W. (2002) Acute axonal damage in multiple sclerosis is most extensive in early disease stages and decreases over time. *Brain*, **125**, 2202–2212.

Kumar, N., Narang, K., Cressey, B.D. & Gottlieb, A.B. (2013) Long-term safety of ustekinumab for psoriasis. *Expert Opinion on Drug Safety*, **12**, 757–765.

Laman, J.D. & Weller, R.O. (2013) Drainage of cells and soluble antigen from the CNS to regional lymph nodes. *Journal of Neuroimmune Pharmacology*, **8**, 840–856.

Larochelle, C., Alvarez, J.I. & Prat, A. (2011) How do immune cells overcome the blood brain barrier in multiple sclerosis? *FEBS Letters*, **585**, 3770–3780.

Larochelle, C., Cayrol, R., Kebir, H. *et al.* (2012) Melanoma cell adhesion molecule identifies encephalitogenic T lymphocytes and promotes their recruitment to the central nervous system. *Brain*, **135**, 2906–2924.

Lassmann, H., van Horssen, J. & Mahad, D. (2012) Progressive multiple sclerosis: pathology and pathogenesis. *Nature Reviews Neurology*, **8**, 647–656.

Li, Y., Chu, N., Hu, A., Gran, B., Rostami, A. & Zhang, G.X. (2007) Increased IL-23p19 expression in multiple sclerosis lesions and its induction in microglia. *Brain*, **130**, 490–501.

Lindsey, J.W., Hodgkinson, S., Mehta, R., Mitchell, D., Enzmann, D. & Steinman, L. (1994) Repeated treatment with chimeric anti-CD4 antibody in multiple sclerosis. *Annals of Neurology*, **36**, 183–189.

Lowther, D.E. & Hafler, D.A. (2012) Regulatory T cells in the central nervous system. *Immunology Reviews*, **248**, 156–169.

Lucchinetti, C., Bruck, W., Parisi, J., Scheithauer, B., Rodriguez, M. & Lassmann, H. (2000) Heterogeneity of multiple sclerosis lesions: implications for the pathogenesis of demyelination. *Annals of Neurology*, **47**, 707–717.

Lucchinetti, C.F., Popescu, B.F., Bunyan, R.F. *et al.* (2011) Inflammatory cortical demyelination in early multiple sclerosis. *New England Journal of Medicine*, **365**, 2188–2197.

Lutterotti, A., Yousef, S., Sputtek, A. *et al.* (2013) Antigen-specific tolerance by autologous myelin peptide-coupled cells: a phase 1 trial in multiple sclerosis. *Science Translational Medicine*, **5**, 188ra175.

Major, E.O. (2010) Progressive multifocal leukoencephalopathy in patients on immunomodulatory therapies. *Annual Review of Medicine*, **61**, 35–47.

Mars, L.T., Saikali, P., Liblau, R.S. & Arbour, N. (2011) Contribution of CD8 T lymphocytes to the immuno-pathogenesis of multiple sclerosis and its animal models. *Biochimica et Biophysica Acta*, **1812**, 151–161.

Masson, F., Calzascia, T., Di Berardino-Besson, W., de Tribolet, N., Dietrich, P.Y. & Walker, P.R. (2007) Brain microenvironment promotes the final functional maturation of tumor-specific effector CD8+ T cells. *Journal of Immunology*, **179**, 845–853.

McMahon, E.J., Bailey, S.L., Castenada, C.V., Waldner, H. & Miller, S.D. (2005) Epitope spreading initiates in the CNS in two mouse models of multiple sclerosis. *Nature Medicine*, **11**, 335–339.

McRae, B.L., Vanderlugt, C.L., Dal Canto, M.C. & Miller, S.D. (1995) Functional evidence for epitope spreading in the relapsing pathology of experimental autoimmune encephalomyelitis. *Journal of Experimental Medicine*, **182**, 75–85.

Mellergard, J., Edstrom, M., Vrethem, M., Ernerudh, J. & Dahle, C. (2010) Natalizumab treatment in multiple sclerosis: marked decline of chemokines and cytokines in cerebrospinal fluid. *Multiple Sclerosis*, **16**, 208–217.

Mohammad, M.G., Tsai, V.W., Ruitenberg, M.J. *et al.* (2014) Immune cell trafficking from the brain maintains CNS immune tolerance. *Journal of Clinical Investigation*, **124**, 1228–1241.

Multiple Sclerosis International Federation. (2013). Atlas of MS 2013. http://www.msif.org/includes/documents/cm_docs/2013/m/msif-atlas-of-ms-2013-report.pdf?f=1 (accessed 6 November 2014).

Panitch, H.S., Hirsch, R.L., Haley, A.S. & Johnson, K.P. (1987a) Exacerbations of multiple sclerosis in patients treated with gamma interferon. *Lancet*, **1**, 893–895.

Panitch, H.S., Hirsch, R.L., Schindler, J. & Johnson, K.P. (1987b) Treatment of multiple sclerosis with gamma interferon: exacerbations associated with activation of the immune system. *Neurology*, **37**, 1097–1102.

Pierson, E., Simmons, S.B., Castelli, L. & Goverman, J.M. (2012) Mechanisms regulating regional localization of inflammation during CNS autoimmunity. *Immunology Reviews*, **248**, 205–215.

Polman, C.H., O'Connor, P.W., Havrdova, E. *et al.* (2006) A randomized, placebo-controlled trial of natalizumab for relapsing multiple sclerosis. *New England Journal of Medicine*, **354**, 899–910.

Ransohoff, R.M. & Estes, M.L. (1991) Astrocyte expression of major histocompatibility complex gene products in multiple sclerosis brain tissue obtained by stereotactic biopsy. *Archives of Neurology*, **48**, 1244–1246.

Reboldi, A., Coisne, C., Baumjohann, D. *et al.* (2009) C-C chemokine receptor 6-regulated entry of TH-17 cells into the CNS through the choroid plexus is required for the initiation of EAE. *Nature Immunology*, **10**, 514–523.

Rep, M.H., van Oosten, B.W., Roos, M.T., Ader, H.J., Polman, C.H. & van Lier, R.A. (1997) Treatment with depleting CD4 monoclonal antibody results in a preferential loss of circulating naive T cells but does not affect IFN-gamma secreting TH1 cells in humans. *Journal of Clinical Investigation*, **99**, 2225–2231.

Sallusto, F., Impellizzieri, D., Basso, C. *et al.* (2012) T-cell trafficking in the central nervous system. *Immunology Reviews*, **248**, 216–227.

Sawcer, S., Franklin, R.J. & Ban, M. (2014) *Multiple sclerosis genetics*. Neurol, Lancet.

Segal, B.M., Constantinescu, C.S., Raychaudhuri, A. *et al.* (2008) Repeated subcutaneous injections of IL12/23 p40 neutralising antibody, ustekinumab, in patients with relapsing-remitting multiple sclerosis: a phase II, double-blind, placebo-controlled, randomised, dose-ranging study. *Lancet Neurology*, **7**, 796–804.

Skulina, C., Schmidt, S., Dornmair, K. *et al.* (2004) Multiple sclerosis: brain-infiltrating CD8+ T cells persist as clonal expansions in the cerebrospinal fluid and blood. *Proceedings of the National Academy of Sciences of the United States of America*, **101**, 2428–2433.

Sospedra, M. & Martin, R. (2005) Immunology of multiple sclerosis. *Annual Review of Immunology*, **23**, 683–747.

Steinman, L. (2007) A brief history of T(H)17, the first major revision in the T(H)1/T(H)2 hypothesis of T cell-mediated tissue damage. *Nature Medicine*, **13**, 139–145.

Stromnes, I.M., Cerretti, L.M., Liggitt, D., Harris, R.A. & Goverman, J.M. (2008) Differential regulation of central nervous system autoimmunity by T(H)1 and T(H)17 cells. *Nature Medicine*, **14**, 337–342.

Sun, D., Whitaker, J.N., Huang, Z. *et al.* (2001) Myelin antigen-specific CD8+ T cells are encephalitogenic and produce severe disease in C57BL/6 mice. *Journal of Immunology*, **166**, 7579–7587.

Tennakoon, D.K., Mehta, R.S., Ortega, S.B., Bhoj, V., Racke, M.K. & Karandikar, N.J. (2006) Therapeutic induction of regulatory, cytotoxic CD8+ T cells in multiple sclerosis. *Journal of Immunology*, **176**, 7119–7129.

Tzartos, J.S., Friese, M.A., Craner, M.J. *et al.* (2008) Interleukin-17 production in central nervous system-infiltrating T cells and glial cells is associated with active disease in multiple sclerosis. *American Journal of Pathology*, **172**, 146–155.

van Oosten, B.W., Lai, M., Hodgkinson, S. *et al.* (1997) Treatment of multiple sclerosis with the monoclonal anti-CD4 antibody cM-T412: Results of a randomized, double-blind, placebo-controlled, MR-monitored phase II trial. *Neurology*, **49**, 351–357.

van Zwam, M., Huizinga, R., Heijmans, N. *et al.* (2009) Surgical excision of CNS-draining lymph nodes reduces relapse severity in chronic-relapsing experimental autoimmune encephalomyelitis. *Journal of Pathology*, **217**, 543–551.

Villares, R., Cadenas, V., Lozano, M. *et al.* (2009) CCR6 regulates EAE pathogenesis by controlling regulatory CD4+ T-cell recruitment to target tissues. *European Journal of Immunology*, **39**, 1671–1681.

Walker, L.S. & Abbas, A.K. (2002) The enemy within: Keeping self-reactive T cells at bay in the periphery. *Nature Reviews Immunology*, **2**, 11–19.

Willing, A. & Friese, M.A. (2012) CD8-mediated inflammatory central nervous system disorders. *Current Opinion in Neurology*, **25**, 316–321.

Wu, G.F. & Alvarez, E. (2011) The immunopathophysiology of multiple sclerosis. *Neurologic Clinics*, **29**, 257–278.

Zaguia, F., Saikali, P., Ludwin, S. *et al.* (2013) Cytotoxic NKG2C+ CD4 T cells target oligodendrocytes in multiple sclerosis. *Journal of Immunology*, **190**, 2510–2518.

4 Microglia and Macrophage Responses and Their Role after Spinal Cord Injury

Antje Kroner, Andrew D. Greenhalgh, and Samuel David

Department of Neurology and Neurosurgery, Faculty of Medicine, Centre for Research in Neuroscience, The Research Institute of the McGill University Health Centre, Montreal, Quebec, Canada

Introduction

Injuries to the spinal cord result in an inflammatory response that is initiated rapidly within minutes and is prolonged for several months. Traumatic injury to the spinal cord results in a core area of tissue damage, which expands over time due to several factors, including ischemia, hemorrhage, and inflammation. This expansion of the lesion referred to as "secondary damage" is preventable and is a prime target for therapeutic intervention. However, not all aspects of the inflammatory response are harmful, as inflammation after injury is a natural response of injured tissues to fight infections, clear damaged tissue, and initiate wound healing and repair. In many non-CNS (central nervous system) tissues including the peripheral nervous system, the inflammatory response is terminated effectively and is accompanied by tissue repair and restoration of function. However, in the CNS, this response is inadequately resolved, resulting in secondary damage. In addition, unlike other tissues, the CNS has a limited capacity for repair and regeneration. The injured adult mammalian spinal cord is unable to replace lost neurons, initiate regeneration of damaged axons, and effectively remyelinate axons, resulting in permanent loss of function. Therefore, reducing inflammation-induced secondary damage that expands the size of the lesion after spinal cord injury (SCI) is a worthy therapeutic goal. The objective of any anti-inflammatory therapy for SCI, however, should be to modulate those aspects of the response that cause tissue damage while permitting its beneficial effects for fighting infections and promoting wound repair, rather than blocking or preventing all inflammatory responses.

Inflammation in the injured spinal cord is mainly mediated by resident microglia and macrophages from the peripheral circulation that enter the damaged tissue. Before discussing this, it might be instructive to take a broad look at the other cellular and molecular changes that occur immediately after injury. Trauma to the CNS results in tearing and damage to neuronal cell bodies, axons, glia, and blood vessels leading to hemorrhage. The immediate damage to blood vessels leads to ischemia and the entry of red blood cells (RBCs) and blood components, such

Neuroinflammation: New Insights into Beneficial and Detrimental Functions, First Edition. Edited by Samuel David.
© 2015 John Wiley & Sons, Inc. Published 2015 by John Wiley & Sons, Inc.

as fibrinogen, which can influence microglia responses. Edema that ensues from this damage to the vasculature is one of the first consequences of injury. This is followed within a few hours by the entry of neutrophils [polymorphonuclear leukocytes (PMNs)]. In SCI, neutrophils reach their maximum numbers in the injured tissue at 24 h after injury and are eliminated over the period of the next week. The entry of neutrophils is followed by the entry of macrophages from the peripheral circulation (Kigerl *et al.*, 2006). These cells enter the spinal cord starting about day 2–3, reach maximum numbers by 7–10 days, and remain in the spinal cord for months in rodents (Kigerl *et al.*, 2006) and even years in humans (Pruss *et al.*, 2011) (see Chapter 17 for discussion on nonresolving inflammation in the CNS). For the most part, the sequence and timing of these cellular changes after SCI are similar in rodents and humans (Fleming *et al.*, 2006; Kigerl *et al.*, 2006). This sequence of events, that is, vascular damage, edema, PMN infiltration, and macrophage entry is a general phenomenon that is also seen after damage to other tissues (Serhan, 2010). At later times after SCI, the adaptive immune response involving B and T lymphocytes may also be triggered (Ankeny and Popovich, 2009), but this will not be discussed in this chapter. In this chapter, we will focus our attention on the innate immune response involving microglia and macrophages after SCI and the factors and cell types that orchestrate this response. Because many of these changes have been studied in other regions of the CNS, we will discuss these mechanisms within the broader context of CNS injury and focus on spinal cord where evidence is available.

Microglial Responses to Injury

Process Extension and Cell Body Motility

Resident microglia are the first cell type to respond to CNS injury within the first few minutes (Fig. 4.1). This is before the entry of circulating monocytes and macrophages that begin to enter after 2–3 days. Microglia, similarly to resident macrophages in other tissues, monitor the tissue for pathogens, injury, and other perturbations (Davalos *et al.*, 2005; Dibaj *et al.*, 2010). Microglia are process-bearing cells that vary in their branching complexity and density in different regions of the CNS. After small laser lesions or stab wounds in the cerebral cortex, two-photon imaging revealed that microglia surrounding the lesion respond by extending cytoplasmic processes toward the lesion within 10–15 min (Davalos *et al.*, 2005; Hines *et al.*, 2009). These microglial processes form a dense network tightly surrounding the lesion within 30–60 min (Davalos *et al.*, 2005; Hines *et al.*, 2009), with similar responses also seen *in vivo* in spinal cord white matter (Dibaj *et al.*, 2010). In the cortex where there is a high density of microglia with cells almost touching each other, there is no movement of microglial cell bodies. In contrast, in spinal cord white matter where microglia numbers are less dense, microglial cell bodies migrate toward the lesion within 2 h, appearing to do so in some cases along degenerating axons (Dibaj *et al.*, 2010). Interestingly, the formation of the dense network of microglial processes around the lesion appears to be a protective response, as preventing it by selective laser ablation of surrounding microglia, or blocking process extension pharmacologically leads to significant expansion of the size of the lesion. Later, astrocytes line the wound and reform the glia limitans that seals the injured CNS parenchyma from the external non-CNS environment (Li and

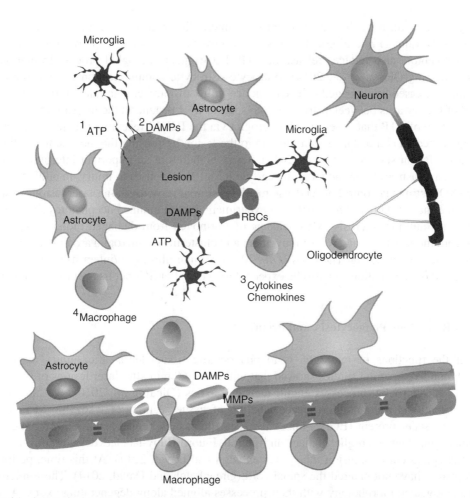

Figure 4.1 Schematic showing some of the signaling molecules that mediate microglia and monocyte-derived macrophage responses after CNS injury. (1) The earliest response of microglia to injury is mediated by ATP released by astrocytes near the lesion site. (2) Subsequently DAMPs released by damaged cells in this region signal via TLRs on microglia as well as on astrocytes and neurons to release proinflammatory mediators including cytokines, and reactive oxygen species (ROS) via NFκB signaling that can cause damage to neurons and glia. (3) Cytokines together with chemokines induce the recruitment of leukocytes from the peripheral circulation that include neutrophils and monocyte-derived macrophages into the CNS parenchyma. (4) The entry of these leukocytes into the CNS requires the action of MMPs that degrade the ECM around blood vessels, leading to the release of additional DAMPs and a further round of activation of TLRs on CNS glia at the injury site and the expression of cytokines and proinflammatory mediators. Inflammation therefore can proceed for prolonged periods after injury. (*See insert for color representation of this figure.*)

David, 1996). Whether such microglial responses also occur in large lesions such as spinal cord contusion injuries and whether the early microglial responses to such injuries are protective are currently not known.

The rapid microglial process extension in response to injury is mediated by adenosine triphosphate (ATP) binding to P2Y12 G-protein coupled purinergic receptors (Davalos *et al.*, 2005; Haynes *et al.*, 2006). The ATP required is released by astrocytes after injury, as blocking astrocytic connexin hemichannels can abrogate microglia process extension toward the lesion (Fig. 4.1) (Davalos *et al.*, 2005). Recent studies show that noncytotoxic activation of neuronal NMDA receptors also induces release of ATP that triggers microglial process formation via P2Y12 (Dissing-Olesen *et al.*, 2014). Astrocyte–astrocytic communication is also important. Glutamate released by damaged cells can induce influx of intracellular calcium (Ca^{2+}) and the spread of Ca^{2+} waves between astrocytes that spreads over distances; the increase in Ca^{2+} leads to the release of ATP that is sensed by microglia via the P2Y12 receptors (Sieger *et al.*, 2012). Microglia located at a distance then migrate to the lesion by sensing the increasing gradient of ATP at the lesion site (Sieger *et al.*, 2012). There is therefore an important interplay between microglia and astrocytes in inducing the early microglial responses to injury. In addition, nitric oxide (NO) acting via control of ATP also mediates similar responses after laser lesions in spinal cord white matter (Dibaj *et al.*, 2010). In experimental autoimmune encephalomyelitis (EAE), a model of multiple sclerosis (MS), leakage of fibrinogen from damaged blood vessel in the spinal cord induces rapid and robust movement and clustering of microglia around blood vessels that result in axonal damage (Davalos *et al.*, 2012). Similar fibrinogen/integrin-mediated axonal damage and demyelination can also be expected to occur after SCI but has yet to be studied.

Process Retraction, Phagocytosis, and Proliferation

One of the functions of microglia is to phagocytose tissue debris after injury or disease. Two-photon live imaging studies showed that within 30–60 min after laser lesions of the mouse spinal cord, microglial processes engulf damaged axons (Dibaj *et al.*, 2010). We have shown with conventional immunofluorescence labeling of tissue sections of lysozyme M enhanced green fluorescent protein (EGFP)-knockin mice, which tags hematogenous macrophages but not microglia, that microglia contact and engulf Fluoro-Ruby-labeled degenerating axons 1 day after spinal cord contusion injury (Greenhalgh and David, 2014). At this time, peripheral macrophages have not entered the spinal cord (Greenhalgh and David, 2014). These microglia have an elongated morphology with their processes aligned along degenerating axons. As they transition to the next step of phagocytosis, microglia often retract their processes and become ameboid. Recent studies have provided some insights into the mechanisms underlying this process. High levels of NO were reported to convert ramified microglia to ameboid microglia and their migration toward the lesion in laser-induced lesions in the spinal cord (Dibaj *et al.*, 2010). More recently, the transcription factor Runx1, a regulator of myeloid cell proliferation and differentiation, was reported to be expressed in amoeboid microglia during development, is downregulated in ramified microglia, and is upregulated in the ameboid microglia in the adult spinal cord after injury (Zusso *et al.*, 2012).

Microglia increase in number at the site of injury and disease. This increase in numbers is by cell proliferation, which has been shown in the spinal cord in a variety of injury and disease models such as after spinal cord contusion injury (Greenhalgh and David, 2014), peripheral nerve injury (Echeverry *et al.*, 2008), and in experimental autoimmune encephalomyelitis (Remington *et al.*, 2007). Macrophages from the peripheral circulation are not thought to contribute to the long-term microglial pool after CNS injury or disease (Ajami *et al.*, 2007, 2011; Mildner *et al.*, 2007). In addition to microglial activation, proliferation, and phagocytic activity, the early changes in the injured tissue lead to the production of chemokines, cytokines, and other factors by various CNS cells that promote the infiltration of circulating immune cells including neutrophils and monocytes/macrophages into the injured spinal cord.

Interactions between Microglia and Other Cell Types in Signaling Responses to Injury

Immediately after CNS injury, molecular interactions between CNS glia, neurons, and endothelial cells lead to the further activation of microglia and astrocytes and generate the signals required to recruit monocyte-derived macrophages from the peripheral circulation. Some of these signaling molecules and pathways are summarized in the following sections.

TLR Signaling and Cytokine Responses

After a traumatic injury to the CNS, signals reflecting the damage to tissue are propagated through pattern recognition receptors (PRRs). These are a class of receptor that respond to both pathogens and endogenous molecules. The endogenous molecules that initiate the inflammatory response are known as danger- or damage-associated molecular patterns (DAMPs). Molecules identified as DAMPs are diverse and include heat shock proteins, single-stranded RNA, DNA, high-mobility group box 1 (HMGB1) protein, amyloid-β, and fragments of extracellular matrix (ECM) molecules (Piccinini and Midwood, 2010). These have been reviewed elsewhere in the context of CNS injury (Kigerl et al., 2014). Many DAMPs bind to Toll-like receptors (TLRs) and signal the expression of cytokines and other factors that mediate inflammation (for discussion of other PRRs and their role in stroke see Chapter 5). TLR signaling mediates activation of pathways such as the nuclear factor-κB (NFκB) pathway that leads to expression of cytokines, cyclooxygenase-2 (COX-2), inducible nitric oxide synthase (iNOS), matrix metalloproteinases (MMPs), and others (Heiman et al., 2014). COX-2 gives rise to a variety of bioactive lipids such as prostaglandins and leukotrienes that promote inflammatory responses (David et al., 2012). Nitric oxide generated via iNOS can be cytotoxic. Furthermore, MMPs induce breakdown of ECM around blood vessels, facilitating increased influx of immune cells (neutrophils and macrophages) into the injured spinal cord (Noble et al., 2002). MMPs will also release more DAMPs that trigger further TLR signaling (Fig. 4.1). Heme, a breakdown product of hemoglobin from RBCs arising from hemorrhage into the tissue, acts as a DAMP and potently induces interleukin (IL)-1α, a key cytokine that mediates neuronal cell death (Chen et al., 2007; Greenhalgh et al., 2012). After the initial insult, microglia detect DAMPs within minutes (Fig. 4.1). As the lesion expands over time, more tissue is damaged, releasing more DAMPs. We have also reported recently that macrophages that enter the injured spinal cord from the peripheral circulation are more susceptible to cell death after phagocytosing tissue debris (Greenhalgh and David, 2014). These dying cells can also be a source of DAMPs. Therefore, DAMP-TLR signaling is likely to be prolonged after SCI. Quantitative real-time polymerase chain reaction (PCR) analysis showed increased expression of TLR2 and TLR4 from 3 to 14 days after SCI; it could be longer, as this was the maximum post-injury time examined (Kigerl et al., 2007). The work on SCI in TLR2 and TLR4 null mice is difficult to interpret (Kigerl et al., 2014), as differences in locomotor recovery were not seen. Further studies using conditional knockout mice or treatment with blocking antibodies will be needed to fully establish their role in SCI.

Whether through DAMP-TLR signaling or other mechanisms, the expression of cytokines IL-1β and tumor necrosis factor (TNF) is increased after SCI (Fig. 4.1). Studies on contusion injury in mice showed that the number of cells expressing TNF messenger RNA (mRNA) increased as early as 15 min after injury, reached a peak at 1 h, and remained high for the first 24 h (Pineau and Lacroix, 2007). There is also a second period of TNF mRNA expression at 14 and 28 days (the longest time point studied) (Pineau and Lacroix, 2007). During the first phase of expression, TNF mRNA is expressed in microglia, astrocytes, oligodendrocytes, and neurons, while in the second phase at 14 and 28 days, it appears to be expressed by microglia/macrophages (Pineau and Lacroix, 2007). In the injured spinal cord, TNF is expressed by macrophages and microglia as detected by fluorescence-activated cell sorting (FACS) analysis (Kroner et al., 2014). TNF immunoreactivity was also detected in microglia and neurons in injured rat spinal cord (Yang et al., 2005). Similarly, the number of IL-1β mRNA-expressing cells increases as early as 5 min after SCI and spreads over a wider area by 15 min (Pineau and Lacroix, 2007). Their numbers increase progressively between 1 and 12 h when they reach peak numbers but continue to be expressed at 24 h at reduced levels. A small second increase also occurs at 14 days (Pineau and Lacroix, 2007). In the first phase of expression, IL-1β is expressed in microglia and astrocytes, while in the second phase is expressed mainly by endothelial cells at 14 days (Pineau and Lacroix, 2007). These findings show that these cytokines are expressed by microglia and astrocytes within 5–15 min after injury, which coincides with the rapid microglial process extension toward the lesion and the early engulfment and phagocytosis of damage axons and tissue debris.

Chemokine Expression

The expressions of several chemokines are increased after SCI. These include CCL2, 3, 4, 5, 7, 8, 20, 21; CXCL1, 2, 3, 5, 8, 10, 12; and CX3CL1 (fractalkine) (Jaerve and Muller, 2012). In most cases, chemokine mRNA expression peaks rapidly within 1–12 h after injury, for example, mRNAs for CCL2, 3, 4, and CXCL2/3 increase within 15 min after SCI and peak between 3 and 6 h (Rice et al., 2007). On the basis of their receptor distribution, these chemokines are expected to have differential effects in recruiting immune cells. These chemokines combined with cytokines play a role in the influx of monocytes and macrophages from the peripheral circulation to the site of CNS injury (Fig. 4.1). A particularly important chemokine for the influx of monocytes into the CNS is CCL2 (monocyte chemoattractant protein-1), which is expressed by astrocytes, neurons, and endothelial cells (Conductier et al., 2010; Williams et al., 2014). The recruitment of immune cells is reduced after SCI in mice deficient for CCL2 receptor, CCR2, which is expressed on myelomonocytic cells (Ma et al., 2002). The functional outcome after SCI in humans is also correlated with the levels of CCL2 and CXCL8 (IL-8) in the cerebrospinal fluid (CSF) (Kwon et al., 2010). CCL2 is also involved in the migration of a population of monocyte-derived M1macrophages (Ly6C^{high}CX3CR1^{low}) into the injured spinal cord via the leptomeninges (Shechter et al., 2013b). Astrocytes in the injured spinal cord express CCL2, CXCL1, and CXCL2 between 3 and 12 h after contusion injury in mice as detected by *in situ* hybridization (Pineau *et al.*, 2010). The expression of these chemokines in astrocytes is mediated by MyD88 and IL-1 receptor 1(IL-1R1) signaling, as mice deficient in these molecules showed reduced influx of "inflammatory" monocytes (Ly6C^{high}, CX3CR1^{low}) and complete lack of neutrophils for up to 4 days after SCI, which normally peak in numbers at 1 day (Pineau *et al.*, 2010). Two types of monocytes were previously described (Geissmann *et al.*, 2008): "inflammatory" monocytes (CX3CR1^{low}, CCR2$^+$, Gr1$^{+)}$ recruited to sites of inflammation and "resident" monocytes (CX3CR1^{high}, CCR2$^-$, Gr1$^-$), which show CX3CR1-dependent recruitment into noninflamed tissues. Other work showed that treatment with a function-blocking antibody against CXCL10 after SCI reduced inflammation and was neuroprotective (Glaser *et al.*, 2004; Glaser *et al.*, 2006). Interactions of CXCL12 with its receptor CXCR4 also mediate attraction of CXCR4$^+$ macrophages after SCI (Tysseling *et al.*, 2011). As mentioned previously, expression of chemokines such as CCL2 is mediated by cytokines (such as IL-1) that are expressed early after SCI. The expression of these and other cytokines is mediated by TLR signaling.

Entry of Peripheral Macrophages and Differences with Microglia

Influx of Peripheral Macrophages into the Injured Spinal Cord

The higher levels of chemokines and cytokines at the site of injury, and the increased expression of MMPs at these sites that breakdown EMC around the blood–brain barrier, lead to the entry of immune cells from the circulation into the CNS parenchyma (Fig. 4.1). Integrins are important regulators of leukocyte migration out of the circulation. The $\alpha4\beta1$ integrin was first shown to be effective in reducing symptoms of EAE in mice (Yednock *et al.*, 1992) and has subsequently moved into the clinic for the treatment of MS (Miller *et al.*, 2003). The $\alpha4$ integrin-blocking antibody (natalizumab/Tysabri) used in the treatment of MS was tested in spinal cord compression injury in rats and found to significantly reduce the influx of neutrophils and macrophages into the injured spinal cord by about 50% and resulted in reduced tissue injury and improved locomotor recovery (Fleming *et al.*, 2008). The percentage of neutrophils and macrophages expressing $\alpha4$ and CD11d increases in humans after SCI (Bao *et al.*, 2011). Blocking another integrin $\alpha D\beta2$ (CD11d/CD18) during the early acute period after SCI also reduced transiently the influx of neutrophils (70%) and macrophages (36%) and improved functional recovery (Gris *et al.*, 2004; Saville *et al.*, 2004).

MMP-9 also influences inflammatory responses after SCI. Studies on MMP-9 null mice have shown that it plays an important role in increasing the permeability of blood–brain barrier immediately after SCI, increasing neutrophil entry, and worsening locomotor recovery (Noble *et al.*, 2002). The expression of MMP-9 increases rapidly, reaching a peak at 24 h after SCI, and is expressed mainly by glia, macrophages, neutrophils, and endothelial cells (Noble *et al.*, 2002).

Differences in the Response of Microglia and Peripheral Macrophages to Injury

Macrophages enter the injured spinal cord starting at about 2–3 days after injury and reach a peak between 7 and 10 days (Kigerl *et al.*, 2006). Before they enter into the injured CNS, microglia in the vicinity of the injury respond by extending processes along degenerating axons and begin to phagocytose degenerating material. After peripheral macrophages enter, they become the main cell type to phagocytose tissue debris, which may be, in part, dependent on C1q complement (Greenhalgh and David, 2014). Peripherally derived macrophages and resident microglia appear to process phagocytosed material differently, as tissue debris is cleared more efficiently in microglia than in macrophages *in vivo*. At day 7 after SCI, microglia proliferation is fivefold greater than peripheral macrophages, which may result in microglia dividing their phagocytic load and explain why they are less susceptible to cell death than macrophages after phagocytosis (Greenhalgh and David, 2014). There are therefore important differences in the response of microglia and peripherally derived macrophages to injury. Microglia appear to be the first responders but appear to revert back to a quiescent state after the entry of peripheral macrophages. Gene expression profiling has also revealed that microglia have a quiescent, less metabolically active profile than peripherally derived macrophages in other neurological disease states (Yamasaki *et al.*, 2014). When they become phagocytic, microglia and peripherally derived macrophages in the injured CNS are virtually indistinguishable in tissue section on the basis of their morphology and currently available antigenic markers. However, by FACS analysis, it is possible to distinguish these two cell types on the basis of the expression of $CD45^{low}Ly\text{-}6C^{low}Gr\text{-}1^{low}CX3CR1^{high}$ in microglia and $CD45^{high}Ly\text{-}6C^{high}Gr\text{-}1^{high}CX3CR1^{low}$ in peripherally derived macrophages. A recent study using gene expression profiling, quantitative mass spectrometry, and microRNA (miRNA) analysis has revealed differences in gene expression between these two cells types, as well as differences between microglia and other tissue macrophages (Butovsky *et al.*, 2014). Other earlier work has also identified several microglia-specific genes (Hickman *et al.*, 2013). The identity of six uniquely microglial genes (*P2ry12, Fcrls* – Fc receptor-like S, *C1qa, Pros1, Merk* – a tyrosine receptor kinase, and *Gas6*) was reported (Butovsky *et al.*, 2014). Antibodies to some are available; as antibodies to others become available, we may have good markers to distinguish between peripheral macrophages and microglia in histological sections and also additional markers for FACS analysis. This study also identified three miRNAs (miR-99, miR-342-3p, and 125b-5p) that are highly expressed in microglia but not in circulating blood monocytes or bone-marrow-derived macrophages and other tissue macrophages (Butovsky *et al.*, 2014). There are therefore several unique differences between microglia and peripheral macrophages. It is not known whether the expression of these genes changes after SCI.

Diverse Roles of Macrophages/Microglia in CNS Injury and Disease

There are several lines of evidence showing that macrophages/microglia have detrimental and tissue-damaging effects. In SCI, the depletion of peripheral circulating macrophages but not microglia with clodronate, which is taken up by macrophages and is toxic to these cells, results in a small but significant improvement in tissue protection and locomotor recovery (Popovich *et al.*, 1999). There is also *in vivo* evidence that the area occupied by activated macrophages coincides with areas of axonal dying back, which is the retraction of the terminal cut ends of axons. Clodronate-induced depletion of macrophages after SCI reduces axonal dying back (Horn *et al.*, 2008). In addition, *in vitro* studies also showed that interactions between macrophages and dystrophic axons cause axonal retraction. This was dependent on the state of activation of macrophages and microglia, and some axonal damage is required, as only dystrophic adult axons were susceptible (Horn *et al.*, 2008). There are also several lines of *in vitro* evidence that activated macrophages and microglia are cytotoxic and can kill neurons. This includes cell culture work showing lipopolysaccharide (LPS) activation of bone-marrow-derived macrophages and microglia being cytotoxic to cerebral cortical neurons (Kroner *et al.*, 2014); other work showing that macrophages exacerbate, but microglia protect against neuronal death in oxygen-glucose-deprived organotypic brain slices (Girard *et al.*, 2013); evidence that Kv1.3 potassium channels play a role in nicotinamide adenine dinucleotide phosphate (NADPH)-mediated respiratory burst and peroxynitrite formation and killing of cortical neurons (Fordyce *et al.*, 2005); and also Ca^{2+}-activated K^+ channel KCa3.1 contributes to microglial activation, increased production of NO and peroxynitrite, and cytotoxicity (Kaushal *et al.*, 2007). Other evidence shows that microglia may also execute neuronal death by phagocytosing stressed-but-viable neurons (Brown and Neher, 2014). Defining the role of microglia after SCI is vital as, after thoracic contusion injury, increased cytokine expression and microglial activation extend for up to 10 spinal segments into the lumbar cord and contribute to the development of pain and deficits in motor learning (Detloff *et al.*, 2008; Hansen *et al.*, 2013). However, there are also several lines of evidence showing that macrophages and microglia under certain conditions are protective and pro-regenerative. One example, cited previously, shows that microglial process extension toward laser lesions and microlesions is protective, as the lesion expands when this response is blocked (Hines *et al.*, 2009). Furthermore, there is evidence that the activation of macrophages by injection of zymosan (TLR2 ligand) into the eye promotes greater axonal regeneration of retinal neurons after optic nerve injury (Yin *et al.*, 2003) (see Chapter 12), and activated macrophage promotes remyelination (see Chapter 13). There are also several articles reporting that the transplantation of activated macrophages into different regions of the injured CNS including the spinal cord promotes axon regeneration and recovery (Lazarov-Spiegler *et al.*, 1998; Rapalino *et al.*, 1998) (see Chapter 11). These seemingly opposite effects of activated microglia/macrophages appeared puzzling, but recent evidence suggests that such differences might be due to their polarization state.

Macrophage Polarization in SCI

Evidence from other fields of immunology first showed that macrophages can be polarized along a continuum from a proinflammatory M1 phenotype at one end to a pro-repair, anti-inflammatory M2 phenotype at the other. Mantovani *et al.* called this nomenclature a " ... simplified conceptual framework to describe the plasticity of mononuclear phagocytes" (Mantovani *et al.*, 2005). Stimulation with the prototypical Th1 cytokine interferon γ (IFN-γ) or TLR signaling via LPS induces M1 macrophage polarization, in which these cells express proinflammatory cytokines (IL-12, IL-23, IL-1β, and TNF), cytotoxic mediators (iNOS and NO) and express phagocytic receptors (CD16/32), and costimulatory molecules (CD86) on the cell surface (Fig. 4.2). In contrast, stimulation with the Th2 cytokines IL-4 or IL-13 as well as other factors (IL-10, glu-cocorticoids, immunoglobulin complexes/TLR ligands) induces M2 polarization characterized

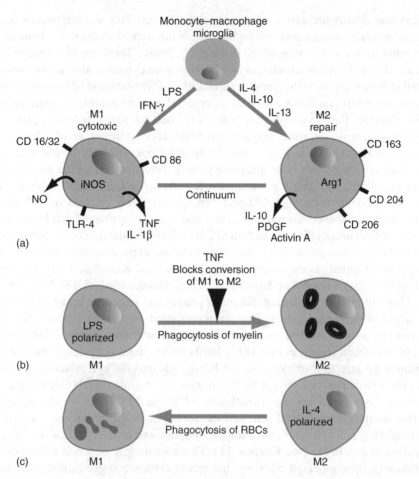

Figure 4.2 (a) Macrophages and microglia can be polarized by specific factors into a cytotoxic (proinflammatory) M1 or pro-repair (anti-inflammatory) M2 states. In the injured spinal cord, macrophages remain polarized largely in the M1 state. (b) and (c) illustrate our recent findings (Kroner *et al.*, 2014) that phagocytosis of myelin by macrophages and microglia *in vitro* induces a shift from LPS-polarized proinflammatory M1 to an anti-inflammatory M2 phenotype. This switch in phenotype can be blocked by TNF. In addition, phagocytosis of RBCs by IL-4-polarized M2 macrophages induces them to transform into proinflammatory M1 cells.

by inhibition of production of proinflammatory cytokines (TNF, IL-1β, IL-2, IL-8, IL-12, and CXCL10), expression of high levels of anti-inflammatory cytokines [IL-10 and transforming growth factor beta (TGFβ)], defective NF-κB activation, upregulation of arginase 1 (Arg1), which gives rise to polyamines, and increased expression of CD204, CD206 (Fig. 4.2) (Gordon and Taylor, 2005; David and Kroner, 2011). M2 macrophages are therefore often referred to as being anti-inflammatory cells. M1 macrophages help fight bacterial infections by phagocytosing microorganisms and killing them intracellularly. M1 cells are therefore proinflammatory in phenotype. In contrast, M2 macrophages help fight parasitic infections by generating a fibrous capsule around them and thus helping to sequester the parasites. In the context of tumors, tumor-associated macrophages are M2 polarized with immunosuppressive characteristics that allow tumor cells to evade immune attack (Mantovani et al., 2002).

In the context of SCI, the first detailed assessment of macrophage polarization reported by Popovich's group showed that although both M1 and M2 polarized macrophages are present in the injured mouse spinal cord after contusion injury, the macrophages are predominantly M1 polarized (Kigerl et al., 2009). Screening using a complementary DNA (cDNA) microarray and quantitative polymerase chain reaction (qPCR) analysis showed that M1 markers (CD16, CD32, CD86, CD64, and iNOS) are highly expressed in the first 2 weeks after SCI, whereas M2 markers (Arg1, CD163, CD206, CD14, and CD23) are expressed at a lower level (Kigerl et al., 2009). Immunofluorescence labeling of tissue sections showed a gradual reduction of Arg1 and increase of CD16/32 between 3 and 28 after SCI (Kigerl et al., 2009). Bone-marrow-derived macrophages polarized with IL-4 to a M2 phenotype in vitro and transplanted into the contused spinal cord, lost expression of M2 markers (Arg1 and CD206) after 3 days (Kigerl et al., 2009). These findings provide strong evidence that the injured spinal cord environment favors M1 polarization. A later study showed that M1 and M2 macrophages in the injured spinal cord can enter the spinal cord via two different routes and mechanisms (Shechter et al., 2013b). M1 macrophages were shown to enter the injury site from the leptomeninges via a CCL2-mediated mechanism, while M2 macrophages enter the injury site via a circuitous route, crossing from the blood into the CSF in the choroid plexus in the brain via vascular cell adhesion molecule (VCAM)/very late antigen-4 (VLA4) cell adhesion molecule interactions and the enzyme CD73. These M2 macrophages are thought to migrate along the central canal down to the site of injury (Shechter et al., 2013b). It was suggested that the CSF and the central canal provide an anti-inflammatory environment that could promote M2 polarization (see Chapter 11).

Role of Phagocytosis in Macrophage Polarization

The evidence cited previously shows that the environment of the injured spinal cord favors greater M1 polarization (Kigerl et al., 2009). TLR4 activation immediately after SCI would drive macrophages to M1 polarization. However, in vitro studies with human blood macrophages have shown that phagocytosis of myelin by LPS-stimulated macrophages reduce the expression of proinflammatory cytokines (IL-12, TNF) (Boven et al., 2006). We extended this observation using FACS analysis to show that myelin phagocytosis by LPS or LPS + IFN-γ-stimulated bone-marrow-derived M1 macrophages in vitro not only reduces TNF expression, but also reduces expression of the M1 markers CD16/32 and CD86, Ly6C and increases expression of M2 markers CD204, CD206 (Fig. 4.2) (Kroner et al., 2014). Similar effects of myelin phagocytosis on the expression of M1 and M2 markers were also seen in LPS or LPS + IFN-γ-stimulated microglia (Kroner et al., 2014). Interestingly, the myelin phagocytosis-induced switch from M1 to M2 also had a profound protective effect on neuronal cell death and neurite outgrowth in vitro, which could have important implications in vivo after SCI. Furthermore, in the context of multiple sclerosis, histological analysis has shown that macrophages containing phagocytosed myelin show reduced expression of NADPH oxidase, suggesting that myelin containing M2 macrophages also downregulate the expression of pro-oxidant molecules (Fischer et al., 2012).

In addition to phagocytosis of damaged myelin, there is also abundant phagocytosis of RBCs resulting from hemorrhage, and phagocytosis of neutrophils, which peak in numbers at 1 day after SCI and reduces markedly over the next 3–5 days. The reduction in neutrophils is due to phagocytosis by macrophages. A comparison of the changes in M1 markers following phagocytosis of myelin, RBCs, or neutrophils revealed that although phagocytosis of all three reduced the expression of CD16 and CD86, the increases in TNF induced by LPS stimulation were reduced by phagocytosis of myelin and neutrophils but not by RBCs. Furthermore, the LPS-induced increase in IL-12 is only reduced by myelin, unaffected by neutrophil but markedly increased by RBCs. These findings indicate that unlike phagocytosis of myelin and neutrophils, macrophages phagocytosing RBCs still maintain a proinflammatory profile. Thus, phagocytosis alone is not sufficient to cause a switch to an anti-inflammatory state, but what is phagocytosed also plays an important role in the transformation of M1 cells to a less inflammatory M2 phenotype.

Role of TNF in Macrophage Polarization

One of the key findings from earlier work done by Kigerl *et al.* (2009) is that the injured spinal cord environment favors M1 polarization. Why is it so, when abundant phagocytosis of myelin occurs in the injured spinal cord and should drive macrophages toward M2 polarization? Our cell culture studies show that TNF is not only a M1 cytokine, but its presence also prevents myelin phagocytosis-induced transformation of M1 macrophages to a M2 phenotype (Fig. 4.2) (Kroner *et al.*, 2014). This was confirmed *in vivo* after SCI in TNF null mice. As expected, there is greater number of M2 macrophages in the injured spinal cord of TNF null mice as compared to wild-type controls. This is significant because TNF expression is increased in two waves very early after injury and starting again from 2 to 4 weeks and possibly beyond (Pineau and Lacroix, 2007), suggesting that the TNF effect can be prolonged after SCI.

Role of Iron in Macrophage Polarization

As mentioned previously, phagocytosis of RBCs by M1 macrophages induces reduction of some M1 markers (CD16 and CD86) but still retains expression of high levels of proinflammatory cytokines (TNF and IL-12). In the injured spinal cord, a greater number of macrophages that are immunoreactive for ferritin (an iron-binding protein and a good surrogate marker for intracellular iron) also express TNF as compared to ferritin-negative macrophages (Kroner *et al.*, 2014). This finding indicates that high levels of intracellular iron favors increased TNF expression. This was further confirmed *in vivo* in SCI when mice treated with intraperitoneal injections of iron dextran showed increased TNF expression in the injured spinal cord. Thus, increased iron loading of macrophages in the injured spinal cord favors increased TNF expression.

Earlier work has shown that although there is a preponderance of M1 macrophages after SCI, M2 macrophages are also present (Kigerl *et al.*, 2009; Shechter *et al.*, 2013a). M2 macrophages are also highly phagocytic cells (David and Kroner, 2011). We therefore assessed the effects of RBC phagocytosis on M2 macrophages. RBC phagocytosis caused a rapid shift of IL-4-induced

M2 macrophages to a M1 phenotype within 16 h, that is, rapid increase in expression of M1 markers (CD16, CD86, iNOS, and TNF), and reduction of M2 markers (CD206 and Ym1) (Kroner et al., 2014). An important aspect of the effects of iron was revealed when M2 macrophages were either loaded with iron dextran or allowed to phagocytose RBCs and then transplanted into the injured spinal cord. Three days after transplantation, most cells expressed TNF and CD16, while the expression of the CD206 was markedly reduced (Kroner et al., 2014). These data clearly indicate that phagocytosis or RBC or uptake of iron from dying cells can transform M2 cells to a proinflammatory M1 phenotype (Fig. 4.2).

Taken together, these findings show that TNF can prevent the myelin phagocytosis-induced shift in polarization from M1 to M2, that increased iron levels in M1 macrophages induce increased TNF expression, and that increased iron levels in M2 macrophages induce a shift to a proinflammatory M1 state.

Role of Other Cytokines and Factors in Macrophage Phenotype

Other cytokines have also been reported to influence macrophage polarization after SCI. Blockade of IL-6 with a monoclonal antibody against the IL-6 receptor led to a significant increase of M2 markers (Arg1 and CD206) and reduction of M1 markers (iNOS and CD16/32) after SCI (Guerrero et al., 2012). Such treatment also improved locomotor recovery, tissue sparing, and reduced proinflammatory cytokine expression after (Guerrero et al., 2012). Another study investigated the influence of granulocyte-colony-stimulating factor (G-CSF) on macrophages/microglia polarization and showed increased M2 but decreased M1 markers in a microglial cell line when treated with factors from the G-CSF-treated injured spinal cord (Guo et al., 2013). Among treatments that influence macrophage polarization after SCI is the neuropeptide, Substance P. In a rat contusion injury model, intravenous treatment with Substance P led to decrease of M1 and increase of M2 polarization and improved recovery (Jiang et al., 2012). Transplantation of mesenchymal stem cells into the injured rat spinal cord also showed increase in M2 polarized macrophages, with reduction of the proinflammatory cytokines IL-6 and TNF (Nakajima et al., 2012). In another work, a subpopulation of IL-10-expressing anti-inflammatory monocyte-derived macrophages was identified that can contribute to recovery after SCI (Shechter et al., 2009). The limited recruitment of these cells is thought to underlie the limited recovery after SCI. Indirect evidence for co-inhibitory molecule PD-1 (programmed cell death 1) contributing to macrophage polarization was provided by a study that investigated SCI in PD-1 null mice, which exhibited increased M1 polarization and impaired recovery (Yao et al., 2014). In addition to these factors, enzymatic digestion of chondroitin sulfate proteoglycan (CSPG) using a chondroitinase gene therapy approach induced a strong switch toward M2 polarization after spinal cord contusion injury in rats and showed remarkable tissue protection and functional recovery (Bartus et al., 2014). Finally, recent evidence shows that mechanisms involved in the efficient remyelination of CNS axons, an event critical to functional recovery after injury, require the polarization of microglia/macrophages to an M2 phenotype (Miron et al., 2013) (see Chapter 13). These findings suggest that a variety of cytokines and other factors can influence the polarization of macrophages/microglia after SCI, raising the hope that some of these approaches can be translated to the clinic to modulate inflammation and promote recovery of function.

Concluding Remarks

Macrophages can remain in the injured spinal cord for months and even years in humans (Norenberg *et al.*, 2004; Fleming *et al.*, 2006; Pruss *et al.*, 2011). This lack of timely resolution of inflammation after SCI is unlike that seen after injuries to many other tissues. Several factors are likely to underlie this process, including the lack of a shift in macrophage polarization from M1 to M2 and the lack of an efficient active resolution program involving bioactive lipids (see Chapter 17). As inflammation can have both detrimental and beneficial effects, the aim of any therapy should be to modulate this response to steer it toward its beneficial aspects and minimize the harmful detrimental effects that cause secondary tissue damage. Work in the past 5 years has lead to a better understanding of macrophage polarization after SCI. Several strong candidates have been identified that prevent or promote a shift to M2 polarization in the injured spinal cord, and targeting these appropriately may lead to better tissue protection and recovery of function.

Acknowledgments

Work in Sam David's laboratory was supported by grants from the Canadian Institutes of Health Research (CIHR) (MOP-14828). AK was supported by Postdoctoral fellowships (PDF) from the CIHR, the CIHR Neuroinflammation Training Program (CIHR-NTP), and the Deutsche Forschungsgemeinschaft; ADG is funded by a CIHR PDF and also received support from the CIHR-NTP. We thank Margaret Attiwell for help with the illustrations.

References

Ajami, B., Bennett, J.L., Krieger, C., Tetzlaff, W. & Rossi, F.M. (2007) Local self-renewal can sustain CNS microglia maintenance and function throughout adult life. *Nature Neuroscience*, **10**, 1538–1543.

Ajami, B., Bennett, J.L., Krieger, C., McNagny, K.M. & Rossi, F.M. (2011) Infiltrating monocytes trigger EAE progression, but do not contribute to the resident microglia pool. *Nature Neuroscience*, **14**, 1142–1149.

Ankeny, D.P. & Popovich, P.G. (2009) Mechanisms and implications of adaptive immune responses after traumatic spinal cord injury. *Neuroscience*, **158**, 1112–1121.

Bao, F., Bailey, C.S., Gurr, K.R. *et al.* (2011) Human spinal cord injury causes specific increases in surface expression of beta integrins on leukocytes. *Journal of Neurotrauma*, **28**, 269–280.

Bartus, K., James, N.D., Didangelos, A. *et al.* (2014) Large-scale chondroitin sulfate proteoglycan digestion with chondroitinase gene therapy leads to reduced pathology and modulates macrophage phenotype following spinal cord contusion injury. *Journal of Neuroscience*, **34**, 4822–4836.

Boven, L.A., Van Meurs, M., Van Zwam, M. *et al.* (2006) Myelin-laden macrophages are anti-inflammatory, consistent with foam cells in multiple sclerosis. *Brain*, **129**, 517–526.

Brown, G.C. & Neher, J.J. (2014) Microglial phagocytosis of live neurons. *Nature Reviews Neuroscience*, **15**, 209–216.

Butovsky, O., Jedrychowski, M.P., Moore, C.S. *et al.* (2014) Identification of a unique TGF-beta-dependent molecular and functional signature in microglia. *Nature Neuroscience*, **17**, 131–143.

Chen, C.J., Kono, H., Golenbock, D., Reed, G., Akira, S. & Rock, K.L. (2007) Identification of a key pathway required for the sterile inflammatory response triggered by dying cells. *Nature Medicine*, **13**, 851–856.

Conductier, G., Blondeau, N., Guyon, A., Nahon, J.L. & Rovere, C. (2010) The role of monocyte chemoattractant protein MCP1/CCL2 in neuroinflammatory diseases. *Journal of Neuroimmunology*, **224**, 93–100.

Davalos, D., Grutzendler, J., Yang, G. *et al.* (2005) ATP mediates rapid microglial response to local brain injury in vivo. *Nature Neuroscience*, **8**, 752–758.

Davalos, D., Ryu, J.K., Merlini, M. *et al.* (2012) Fibrinogen-induced perivascular microglial clustering is required for the development of axonal damage in neuroinflammation. *Nature Communications*, **3**, 1227.

David, S. & Kroner, A. (2011) Repertoire of microglial and macrophage responses after spinal cord injury. *Nature Reviews Neuroscience*, **12**, 388–399.

David, S., Greenhalgh, A.D. & Lopez-Vales, R. (2012) Role of phospholipase A2s and lipid mediators in secondary damage after spinal cord injury. *Cell and Tissue Research*, **349**, 249–267.

Detloff, M.R., Fisher, L.C., McGaughy, V., Longbrake, E.E., Popovich, P.G. & Basso, D.M. (2008) Remote activation of microglia and pro-inflammatory cytokines predict the onset and severity of below-level neuropathic pain after spinal cord injury in rats. *Experimental Neurology*, **212**, 337–347.

Dibaj, P., Nadrigny, F., Steffens, H. *et al.* (2010) NO mediates microglial response to acute spinal cord injury under ATP control in vivo. *Glia*, **58**, 1133–1144.

Dissing-Olesen, L., LeDue, J.M., Rungta, R.L., Hefendehl, J.K., Choi, H.B. & MacVicar, B.A. (2014) Activation of neuronal NMDA receptors triggers transient ATP-mediated microglial process outgrowth. *Journal of Neuroscience*, **34**, 10511–10527.

Echeverry, S., Shi, X.Q. & Zhang, J. (2008) Characterization of cell proliferation in rat spinal cord following peripheral nerve injury and the relationship with neuropathic pain. *Pain*, **135**, 37–47.

Fischer, M.T., Sharma, R., Lim, J.L. *et al.* (2012) NADPH oxidase expression in active multiple sclerosis lesions in relation to oxidative tissue damage and mitochondrial injury. *Brain*, **135**, 886–899.

Fleming, J.C., Bao, F., Chen, Y., Hamilton, E.F., Relton, J.K. & Weaver, L.C. (2008) Alpha4beta1 integrin blockade after spinal cord injury decreases damage and improves neurological function. *Experimental Neurology*, **214**, 147–159.

Fleming, J.C., Norenberg, M.D., Ramsay, D.A. *et al.* (2006) The cellular inflammatory response in human spinal cords after injury. *Brain*, **129**, 3249–3269.

Fordyce, C.B., Jagasia, R., Zhu, X. & Schlichter, L.C. (2005) Microglia Kv1.3 channels contribute to their ability to kill neurons. *Journal of Neuroscience*, **25**, 7139–7149.

Geissmann, F., Auffray, C., Palframan, R. *et al.* (2008) Blood monocytes: Distinct subsets, how they relate to dendritic cells, and their possible roles in the regulation of T-cell responses. *Immunology and Cell Biology*, **86**, 398–408.

Girard, S., Brough, D., Lopez-Castejon, G., Giles, J., Rothwell, N.J. & Allan, S.M. (2013) Microglia and macrophages differentially modulate cell death after brain injury caused by oxygen-glucose deprivation in organotypic brain slices. *Glia*, **61**, 813–824.

Glaser, J., Gonzalez, R., Sadr, E. & Keirstead, H.S. (2006) Neutralization of the chemokine CXCL10 reduces apoptosis and increases axon sprouting after spinal cord injury. *Journal of Neuroscience Research*, **84**, 724–734.

Glaser, J., Gonzalez, R., Perreau, V.M., Cotman, C.W. & Keirstead, H.S. (2004) Neutralization of the chemokine CXCL10 enhances tissue sparing and angiogenesis following spinal cord injury. *Journal of Neuroscience Research*, **77**, 701–708.

Gordon, S. & Taylor, P.R. (2005) Monocyte and macrophage heterogeneity. *Nature Reviews*, **5**, 953–964.

Greenhalgh, A.D. & David, S. (2014) Differences in the phagocytic response of microglia and peripheral macrophages after spinal cord injury and its effects on cell death. *Journal of Neuroscience*, **34**, 6316–6322.

Greenhalgh, A.D., Brough, D., Robinson, E.M., Girard, S., Rothwell, N.J. & Allan, S.M. (2012) Interleukin-1 receptor antagonist is beneficial after subarachnoid haemorrhage in rat by blocking haem-driven inflammatory pathology. *Disease Models & Mechanisms*, **5**, 823–833.

Gris, D., Marsh, D.R., Oatway, M.A. *et al.* (2004) Transient blockade of the CD11d/CD18 integrin reduces secondary damage after spinal cord injury, improving sensory, autonomic, and motor function. *Journal of Neuroscience*, **24**, 4043–4051.

Guerrero, A.R., Uchida, K., Nakajima, H. *et al.* (2012) Blockade of interleukin-6 signaling inhibits the classic pathway and promotes an alternative pathway of macrophage activation after spinal cord injury in mice. *Journal of Neuroinflammation*, **9**, 40.

Guo, Y., Zhang, H., Yang, J. *et al.* (2013) Granulocyte colony-stimulating factor improves alternative activation of microglia under microenvironment of spinal cord injury. *Neuroscience*, **238**, 1–10.

Hansen, C.N., Fisher, L.C., Deibert, R.J. *et al.* (2013) Elevated MMP-9 in the lumbar cord early after thoracic spinal cord injury impedes motor relearning in mice. *Journal of Neuroscience*, **33**, 13101–13111.

Haynes, S.E., Hollopeter, G., Yang, G. *et al.* (2006) The P2Y12 receptor regulates microglial activation by extracellular nucleotides. *Nature Neuroscience*, **9**, 1512–1519.

Heiman, A., Pallottie, A., Heary, R.F. & Elkabes, S. (2014) Toll-like receptors in central nervous system injury and disease: A focus on the spinal cord. *Brain, Behavior, and Immunity*, **42C**, 232–245.

Hickman, S.E., Kingery, N.D., Ohsumi, T.K. *et al.* (2013) The microglial sensome revealed by direct RNA sequencing. *Nature Neuroscience*, **16**, 1896–1905.

Hines, D.J., Hines, R.M., Mulligan, S.J. & Macvicar, B.A. (2009) Microglia processes block the spread of damage in the brain and require functional chloride channels. *Glia*, **57**, 1610–1618.

Horn, K.P., Busch, S.A., Hawthorne, A.L., van Rooijen, N. & Silver, J. (2008) Another barrier to regeneration in the CNS: Activated macrophages induce extensive retraction of dystrophic axons through direct physical interactions. *Journal of Neuroscience*, **28**, 9330–9341.

Jaerve, A. & Muller, H.W. (2012) Chemokines in CNS injury and repair. *Cell and Tissue Research*, **349**, 229–248.

Jiang, M.H., Chung, E., Chi, G.F. *et al.* (2012) Substance P induces M2-type macrophages after spinal cord injury. *Neuroreport*, **23**, 786–792.

Kaushal, V., Koeberle, P.D., Wang, Y. & Schlichter, L.C. (2007) The Ca2+−activated K+ channel KCNN4/KCa3.1 contributes to microglia activation and nitric oxide-dependent neurodegeneration. *Journal of Neuroscience*, **27**, 234–244.

Kigerl, K.A., McGaughy, V.M. & Popovich, P.G. (2006) Comparative analysis of lesion development and intraspinal inflammation in four strains of mice following spinal contusion injury. *Journal of Comparative Neurology*, **494**, 578–594.

Kigerl, K.A., de Rivero Vaccari, J.P., Dietrich, W.D., Popovich, P.G. & Keane, R.W. (2014) Pattern recognition receptors and central nervous system repair. *Experimental Neurology*, **258C**, 5–16.

Kigerl, K.A., Lai, W., Rivest, S., Hart, R.P., Satoskar, A.R. & Popovich, P.G. (2007) Toll-like receptor (TLR)-2 and TLR-4 regulate inflammation, gliosis, and myelin sparing after spinal cord injury. *Journal of Neurochemistry*, **102**, 37–50.

Kigerl, K.A., Gensel, J.C., Ankeny, D.P., Alexander, J.K., Donnelly, D.J. & Popovich, P.G. (2009) Identification of two distinct macrophage subsets with divergent effects causing either neurotoxicity or regeneration in the injured mouse spinal cord. *Journal of Neuroscience*, **29**, 13435–13444.

Kroner, A., Greenhalgh, A.D., Zarruk, J.G., Passos Dos Santos, R., Gaestel, M. & David, S. (2014) TNF and increased intracellular iron alter macrophage polarization to a detrimental M1 phenotype in the injured spinal cord. *Neuron*, **83**, 1098–1116.

Kwon, B.K., Stammers, A.M., Belanger, L.M. *et al.* (2010) Cerebrospinal fluid inflammatory cytokines and biomarkers of injury severity in acute human spinal cord injury. *Journal of Neurotrauma*, **27**, 669–682.

Lazarov-Spiegler, O., Solomon, A.S. & Schwartz, M. (1998) Peripheral nerve-stimulated macrophages simulate a peripheral nerve-like regenerative response in rat transected optic nerve. *Glia*, **24**, 329–337.

Li, M.S. & David, S. (1996) Topical glucocorticoids modulate the lesion interface after cerebral cortical stab wounds in adult rats. *Glia*, **18**, 306–318.

Ma, M., Wei, T., Boring, L., Charo, I.F., Ransohoff, R.M. & Jakeman, L.B. (2002) Monocyte recruitment and myelin removal are delayed following spinal cord injury in mice with CCR2 chemokine receptor deletion. *Journal of Neuroscience Research*, **68**, 691–702.

Mantovani, A., Sica, A. & Locati, M. (2005) Macrophage polarization comes of age. *Immunity*, **23**, 344–346.

Mantovani, A., Sozzani, S., Locati, M., Allavena, P. & Sica, A. (2002) Macrophage polarization: Tumor-associated macrophages as a paradigm for polarized M2 mononuclear phagocytes. *Trends in Immunology*, **23**, 549–555.

Mildner, A., Schmidt, H., Nitsche, M. *et al.* (2007) Microglia in the adult brain arise from Ly-6ChiCCR2+ monocytes only under defined host conditions. *Nature Neuroscience*, **10**, 1544–1553.

Miller, D.H., Khan, O.A., Sheremata, W.A. *et al.* (2003) A controlled trial of natalizumab for relapsing multiple sclerosis. *New England Journal of Medicine*, **348**, 15–23.

Miron, V.E., Boyd, A., Zhao, J.W. *et al.* (2013) M2 microglia and macrophages drive oligodendrocyte differentiation during CNS remyelination. *Nature Neuroscience*, **16**, 1211–1218.

Nakajima, H., Uchida, K., Guerrero, A.R. *et al.* (2012) Transplantation of mesenchymal stem cells promotes an alternative pathway of macrophage activation and functional recovery after spinal cord injury. *Journal of Neurotrauma*, **29**, 1614–1625.

Noble, L.J., Donovan, F., Igarashi, T., Goussev, S. & Werb, Z. (2002) Matrix metalloproteinases limit functional recovery after spinal cord injury by modulation of early vascular events. *Journal of Neuroscience*, **22**, 7526–7535.

Norenberg, M.D., Smith, J. & Marcillo, A. (2004) The pathology of human spinal cord injury: Defining the problems. *Journal of Neurotrauma*, **21**, 429–440.

Piccinini, A.M. & Midwood, K.S. (2010) DAMPening inflammation by modulating TLR signalling. *Mediators of Inflammation*, **2010**, doi:10.1155/2010/672395.

Pineau, I. & Lacroix, S. (2007) Proinflammatory cytokine synthesis in the injured mouse spinal cord: Multiphasic expression pattern and identification of the cell types involved. *Journal of Comparative Neurology*, **500**, 267–285.

Pineau, I., Sun, L., Bastien, D. & Lacroix, S. (2010) Astrocytes initiate inflammation in the injured mouse spinal cord by promoting the entry of neutrophils and inflammatory monocytes in an IL-1 receptor/MyD88-dependent fashion. *Brain, Behavior, and Immunity*, **24**, 540–553.

Popovich, P.G., Guan, Z., Wei, P., Huitinga, I., van Rooijen, N. & Stokes, B.T. (1999) Depletion of hematogenous macrophages promotes partial hindlimb recovery and neuroanatomical repair after experimental spinal cord injury. *Experimental Neurology*, **158**, 351–365.

Pruss, H., Kopp, M.A., Brommer, B. *et al.* (2011) Non-resolving aspects of acute inflammation after spinal cord injury (SCI): Indices and resolution plateau. *Brain Pathology*, **21**, 652–660.

Rapalino, O., Lazarov-Spiegler, O., Agranov, E. *et al.* (1998) Implantation of stimulated homologous macrophages results in partial recovery of paraplegic rats. *Nature Medicine*, **4**, 814–821.

Remington, L.T., Babcock, A.A., Zehntner, S.P. & Owens, T. (2007) Microglial recruitment, activation, and proliferation in response to primary demyelination. *American Journal of Pathology*, **170**, 1713–1724.

Rice, T., Larsen, J., Rivest, S. & Yong, V.W. (2007) Characterization of the early neuroinflammation after spinal cord injury in mice. *Journal of Neuropathology and Experimental Neurology*, **66**, 184–195.

Saville, L.R., Pospisil, C.H., Mawhinney, L.A. *et al.* (2004) A monoclonal antibody to CD11d reduces the inflammatory infiltrate into the injured spinal cord: A potential neuroprotective treatment. *Journal of Neuroimmunology*, **156**, 42–57.

Serhan, C.N. (2010) Novel lipid mediators and resolution mechanisms in acute inflammation: To resolve or not? *American Journal of Pathology*, **177**, 1576–1591.

Shechter, R., London, A. & Schwartz, M. (2013a) Orchestrated leukocyte recruitment to immune-privileged sites: Absolute barriers versus educational gates. *Nature Reviews Immunology*, **13**, 206–218.

Shechter, R., London, A., Varol, C. *et al.* (2009) Infiltrating blood-derived macrophages are vital cells playing an anti-inflammatory role in recovery from spinal cord injury in mice. *PLoS Medicine*, **6**, e1000113.

Shechter, R., Miller, O., Yovel, G. *et al.* (2013b) Recruitment of beneficial M2 macrophages to injured spinal cord is orchestrated by remote brain choroid plexus. *Immunity*, **38**, 555–569.

Sieger, D., Moritz, C., Ziegenhals, T., Prykhozhij, S. & Peri, F. (2012) Long-range Ca^{2+} waves transmit brain-damage signals to microglia. *Developmental Cell*, **22**, 1138–1148.

Tysseling, V.M., Mithal, D., Sahni, V. *et al.* (2011) SDF1 in the dorsal corticospinal tract promotes CXCR4+ cell migration after spinal cord injury. *Journal of Neuroinflammation*, **8**, 16.

Williams, J.L., Holman, D.W. & Klein, R.S. (2014) Chemokines in the balance: Maintenance of homeostasis and protection at CNS barriers. *Frontiers in Cellular Neuroscience*, **8**, 154.

Yamasaki, R., Lu H., Butovsky O., Ohno N., Rietsch A.M., Cialic R., Wu P.M., Doykan C.E., Lin J., Cotleur A.C., Kidd G., Zorlu M.M., Sun N., Hu W., Liu L., Lee J.C., Taylor S.E., Uehlein L., Dixon D., Gu J., Floruta C.M., Zhu M., Charo I.F., Weiner H.L. & Ransohoff R.M. (2014) Differential roles of microglia and monocytes in the inflamed central nervous system. *Journal of Experimental Medicine*, **211**, 1533–1549.

Yang, L., Jones, N.R., Blumbergs, P.C. *et al.* (2005) Severity-dependent expression of pro-inflammatory cytokines in traumatic spinal cord injury in the rat. *Journal of Clinical Neuroscience*, **12**, 276–284.

Yao, A., Liu, F., Chen, K. *et al.* (2014) Programmed death 1 deficiency induces the polarization of macrophages/microglia to the m1 phenotype after spinal cord injury in mice. *Neurotherapeutics*, **11**, 636–650.

Yednock, T.A., Cannon, C., Fritz, L.C., Sanchez-Madrid, F., Steinman, L. & Karin, N. (1992) Prevention of experimental autoimmune encephalomyelitis by antibodies against alpha 4 beta 1 integrin. *Nature*, **356**, 63–66.

Yin, Y., Cui, Q., Li, Y. *et al.* (2003) Macrophage-derived factors stimulate optic nerve regeneration. *Journal of Neuroscience*, **23**, 2284–2293.

Zusso, M., Methot, L., Lo, R., Greenhalgh, A.D., David, S. & Stifani, S. (2012) Regulation of postnatal forebrain amoeboid microglial cell proliferation and development by the transcription factor Runx1. *Journal of Neuroscience*, **32**, 11285–11298.

5 The Complexity of the Innate Immune System Activation in Stroke Pathogenesis

María Isabel Cuartero, Ignacio Lizasoain, María Ángeles Moro, and Ivan Ballesteros

Department of Pharmacology (Medical School), Universidad Complutense de Madrid, Instituto de Investigación Hospital 12 de Octubre (i+12), Madrid, Spain

Activation of the Brain Innate Immunity After Stroke

Inflammation is recognized as an important contributor to the pathophysiology of stroke. It induces the release of reactive oxygen species (ROS) and promotes immune-derived mechanisms associated with cytotoxicity and brain damage (Chamorro *et al.*, 2012; Iadecola and Anrather, 2011). In this context, a vast number of experimental studies have explored the beneficial role of anti-inflammatory approaches to block/antagonize key proinflammatory pathways driven by cerebral ischemia (Iadecola and Anrather, 2011). Furthermore, the deleterious effect of stroke-induced inflammation has been evidenced at the clinical level, where high concentrations of proinflammatory cytokines, such as interleukin (IL)-1β, tumor necrosis factor (TNF)-α, IL-6, or adhesion molecules, such as intercellular adhesion molecule (ICAM)-1, in blood and cerebrospinal fluid of patients with stroke have been positively correlated with infarct size, neurological deterioration, and poor prognosis (Castellanos *et al.*, 2002; Tarkowski *et al.*, 1995; Vila *et al.*, 2000) (see Chapter 1 for more on stroke in humans).

Three main mechanisms are associated with the activation of the innate immune system in the brain parenchyma early after stroke. Initially, because of stress or necrosis, the brain tissue releases "danger signals." These signals activate pattern recognition receptors (PRRs), which induce an inflammatory response in resident brain cells and infiltrating leukocytes (Chamorro *et al.*, 2012). In addition, and because of ischemia-induced cell death, the loss of cell–cell interactions between neurons and microglia also promotes inflammatory signaling (Chapman *et al.*, 2000). Finally, glutamate released from damaged cells plays a key role in excitotoxicity but also activates microglia (Pocock and Kettenmann, 2007). This initial inflammatory response, illustrated in Fig. 5.1, triggers a complex interplay between the CNS and the immune system, which leads to the recruitment of blood-borne cells to the ischemic tissue contributing to further activation of immune cells, production of ROS, and increased tissue damage. Because of its contribution

Neuroinflammation: New Insights into Beneficial and Detrimental Functions, First Edition. Edited by Samuel David.
© 2015 John Wiley & Sons, Inc. Published 2015 by John Wiley & Sons, Inc.

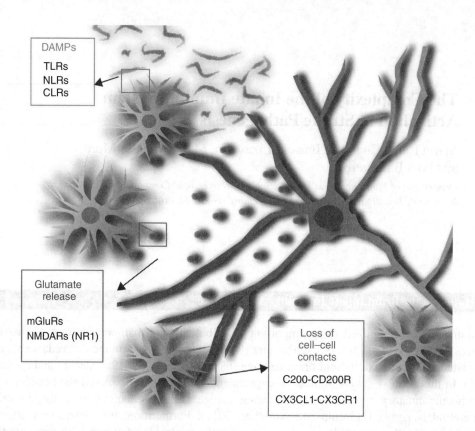

Figure 5.1   Activation of the brain innate immunity after stroke. Three main mechanisms are associated with the activation of the innate immune system in the brain parenchyma after stroke: release of "danger signals" because of stress or necrosis; loss of cell–cell interactions between neurons and microglia; and glutamate released from damaged neurons. These processes will lead to the recruitment of blood-borne cells to the ischemic tissue, contributing to further activation of immune cells, production of ROS, and increased tissue damage.

to damage, this initial phase of the inflammatory response has been termed the "killing phase." In contrast, the exact role of resident and infiltrated immune cells in resolving inflammation and mediating tissue repair after brain ischemia is still poorly understood, and the role of microglial cells and other immune cell subsets in neuroprotection should be revisited.

The Role of the Pattern Recognition Receptors on Stroke Pathogenesis

PRRs are considered to play a crucial role in the activation of the innate immune system of the brain. In the central nervous system (CNS), these receptors are primarily expressed by microglia, macrophages, and astrocytes and are activated by several pathogen-associated molecular patterns (PAMPs) or damage-associated molecular patterns (DAMPs) (Chen and Nunez, 2010). In stroke, the release of DAMPs by the ischemic tissue mediates the activation of PRRs in the CNS. Some of these pathways have been demonstrated to mediate injury following cerebral ischemia

Table 5.1 DAMPs implicated in acute inflammation after stroke and their PRR

DAMP	PRR	References
HMGB1	TLR2 and TLR4	Faraco *et al.*, 2007; Qiu *et al.*, 2010
Peroxiredoxins	TLR2 and TLR4	Shichita *et al.*, 2012
Heat shock proteins	TLR2 and TLR4	Brea *et al.*, 2011
Fibrin/fibrinogen	TLR2 and TLR4	Zhang *et al.*, 2012
Extracellular ATP	NLRs (P2X7 pathway)	Deroide *et al.*, 2013
Histone deacetylase subunit SAP130	CLRs	Suzuki *et al.*, 2013

Abbreviations: DAMP, damage-associated molecular pattern; PRR, pattern recognition receptor; HMGB1, high-mobility group box-1; TLR, Toll-like receptor; NLRs, NOD-like receptors; P2X7, purinergic receptor P2X, ligand-gated ion channel 7; CLRs, C-type lectin receptors.

(see Table 5.1). Current research will increase the number of identified PAMPs associated with stroke-elicited acute sterile inflammatory response of the brain.

Five classes of PRRs have been identified to date: Toll-like receptors (TLRs), NOD-like receptors (NLRs), RIG-I-like receptors (RLRs), C-type lectin receptors (CLRs), and absence in melanoma 2 (AIM2)-like receptors. Following ligand recognition or cellular disruption, these receptors activate downstream signaling pathways, such as nuclear factor-κB (NF-κB), mitogen-activated protein kinase (MAPK), and type I interferon pathways, which result in the upregulation of proinflammatory cytokines and chemokines associated with tissue injury after stroke (Allan *et al.*, 2005; Chamorro *et al.*, 2012; Iadecola and Anrather, 2011).

Accumulating evidence shows that post-ischemic inflammation originated by TLRs and NLRs plays critical roles in ischemic stroke. However, the functions of other PRRs are poorly understood. Recent research points to a role for *Macrophage-inducible C-type lectin* (Mincle), a receptor of the CLRs family, on the inflammatory response induced by ischemia/reperfusion (Suzuki *et al.*, 2013); however, the role of others PRRs in stroke, such as AIM2 receptors and RLRs, is still unclear. In this chapter, we will focus on the implication of TLRs and NLRs on the pathogenesis of cerebral ischemia. These receptors sense extracellular or endosomally located signals, which is the case for TLRs, or they are located within the cytoplasm and sense intracellular signals, such as the NLRs. Only NLR cytosolic receptors are involved in the formation of inflammasomes (Schroder and Tschopp, 2010).

The Role of Toll-Like Receptors (TLRs) in Stroke-Induced Inflammation

TLRs comprise a family of type I transmembrane receptors, which are characterized by an extracellular leucine-rich repeat (LRR) domain and an intracellular Toll/IL-1 receptor (TIR) domain. To date, at least 10 TLRs have been identified, and each appears to have a distinct function in innate immune recognition (Medzhitov, 2001). Most TLR ligands are conserved microbial products (i.e., PAMPs) that signal the presence of infection. In addition, DAMPs can engage TLRs to induce and amplify the inflammatory response. For example, TLR2 and TLR4 can mediate NF-κB activation initiated by the high-mobility group box-1 (HMGB1) protein (Park *et al.*, 2006), a nonhistone nuclear protein passively released by necrotic cells that mediates innate immune activation and tissue injury after stroke (Yang *et al.*, 2010).

Human TLR4 was the first characterized mammalian TLR. It is expressed in a variety of cell types, most predominantly in the cells of the immune system, including macrophages and dendritic cells (DCs). TLR4 functions as the signal-transducing receptor for lipopolysaccharides, but as indicated, DAMPs and different unrelated ligands can also activate this receptor (Doan, 2008). Evidence for the role of TLR4 in cerebral damage after stroke was obtained by studies from our research group that showed that TLR4-deficient mice had lower infarct volumes and better outcomes in neurological and behavioral tests, as well as reduced expression of stroke-induced proinflammatory mediators, such as interferon regulatory factor-1, inducible nitric oxide synthase (iNOS), and cyclooxygenase-2 (Caso et al., 2007). These findings support the idea that TLR4 signaling and activation of innate immunity are involved in brain damage and in inflammation triggered by ischemic injury.

Different groups have also shown the implication of TLR2 in tissue injury after ischemia (Lehnardt et al., 2007; Ziegler et al., 2007, 2011). These studies have shown that TLR2-deficient mice have smaller infarct volumes; furthermore, TLR2 blockade using an anti-TLR2 antibody improves neuronal survival after stroke and decreases the number of CD11b+ cells found in the infarct lesion (Ziegler et al., 2011). However, the absence of TLR2 does not affect granulocyte recruitment to the infarct region, pointing to the macrophages/microglia of the ischemic brain as potential mediators of the deleterious actions of TLR2 after stroke (Lehnardt et al., 2007).

In addition to the role of TLR4 and TLR2, the implication of TLR3 and TLR9 in ischemic damage has also been evaluated. Initial studies showed that gene knock-out mice for these receptors do not have differences in infarct volume when compared to control mice (Hyakkoku et al., 2010), suggesting that these receptors may not play a relevant role in ischemia-induced brain inflammatory response.

Role of Nucleotide-Binding Oligomerization Domain Receptors or NOD-Like Receptors (NLRs) in Stroke-Induced Inflammation

The NLR family comprises a group of intracellular receptors implicated in the recognition of PAMPs, as well as host-derived danger signals (Chen et al., 2009). On ligand activation, members of the NLR family recruit the components of multimolecular scaffolds called inflammasome (Schroder and Tschopp, 2010; Walsh et al., 2014). This molecular complex mediates the conversion of the precursor of pro-IL-1β into biologically active mature proinflammatory IL-1β, which is released into the extracellular environment contributing to acute brain injury after stroke (Allan et al., 2005). The deleterious role of the inflammasome in stroke was first suggested by the neuroprotective effect found in caspase-1 deficient mice, a crucial component of this molecular complex (Schielke et al., 1998). Evidence indicates that NLRs upregulate their expression following cerebral ischemia (Frederick Lo et al., 2008), leading to the formation of the inflammasome in the ischemic brain (Abulafia et al., 2009).

Several host signals are thought to integrate the formation of the inflammasome (Schroder and Tschopp, 2010); of them, lactic acidosis and adenosine triphosphate (ATP) release are interesting candidates to mediate its formation after stroke. Lactic acidosis occurs in the brain following a stroke, where parenchymal pH can drop as low as 6.2 (Nemoto and Frinak, 1981) and, therefore, might mediate inflammasome activation (Rajamaki et al., 2013). Acidosis may also trigger IL-1β processing in an inflammasome-independent pathway (Edye et al., 2013). In addition to acidosis, stroke induces tissue necrosis leading to the accumulation of extracellular ATP, a potent activator of the inflammasome through the P2X7 receptor pathway (Schroder and Tschopp, 2010). P2X7 antagonist treatment conferred neuroprotection in an experimental model of ischemic stroke

(Chu *et al.*, 2012). In agreement with this, recent findings indicate that the milk fat globule-EGF 8 (MFGE8), a secretory glycoprotein that binds to anionic phospholipids, extracellular matrices, and integrins, mediates a neuroprotective effect in brain ischemia by inhibition of the activity of the inflammasome. These effects are attributed to the ability of MFGE8 to limit P2X7 receptor-dependent IL-1β production (Deroide *et al.*, 2013). In this context, direct inhibition of inflammasome activation using antibodies against NRLP1, a member of the NLR family, also induces neuroprotection after stroke (Abulafia *et al.*, 2009).

Given this experimental evidence, targeting activation of the inflammasome may become an immediate possibility for stroke treatment. This is further justified because of the substantial literature on the deleterious role of IL-1β and on the protective effects associated with its blockade by interleukin 1 receptor antagonist (IL-1Ra) in stroke (Brough *et al.*, 2011).

Neuronal Loss and the Activation of Microglia

Microglia in the brain are under constant restraint and express receptors for a variety of inhibitory factors that are constitutively expressed in the brain, mostly by neurons. The most prominent ligand–receptor pairs in this respect are CD200-CD200R and CX3CL1-CX3CR1.

CD200 is a surface protein expressed in neurons that interacts with its receptor CD200R on microglia, enforcing a resting phenotype (Hoek *et al.*, 2000). Disruption of these interactions because of stroke and the expression of CD200 in macrophage-like cell subpopulations of the ischemic brain have been suggested to alter myeloid cell functions (Matsumoto *et al.*, 2007); however, there is no direct evidence of the effect of CD200-CD200R disruption on stroke outcome. In this context, recent studies point to an increased blood–brain barrier permeability in CD200-deficient mice (Denieffe *et al.*, 2013), a fact that could be associated with increased infiltration of blood-borne cells following stroke.

Regarding the CX3CL1–CX3CR1 axis, CX3CL1 or fractalkine is constitutively expressed by neurons and binds to its microglial receptor CX3CR1, leading to an inhibition of microglial activation. After neuronal injury, loss of CX3CL1 results in enhanced microglial activation in several inflammatory disease models (Cardona *et al.*, 2006). Interestingly, the lack of fractalkine or its receptor does not result in microglial neurotoxicity after stroke, but rather significantly reduces ischemic damage and inflammation (Denes *et al.*, 2008; Soriano *et al.*, 2002). These data point to possible beneficial actions of microglial activation after stroke (Hellwig *et al.*, 2013). Further evidence from fractalkine studies in cerebral ischemia has shown that its exogenous administration to ischemic rats or mice is neuroprotective but, in contrast, increases brain damage in *cx3cl1*$^{-/-}$ mice. These findings strongly indicate that the absence of constitutive CX3CL1–CX3CR1 signaling changes the outcome of microglia-mediated effects during CX3CL1 administration to the ischemic brain (Cipriani *et al.*, 2011). Taking into account these findings, microglia activation state in the healthy brain may be modulated by the CXCL1–CXCR1 axis which, in turn, will determine its activation state and functionality in the context of cerebral ischemia.

Glutamate Release and Microglia Activation

Glutamate toxicity occurs as part of the ischemic cascade in multiple pathologies of the CNS, such as trauma, stroke, or multiple sclerosis. Extracellular elevated amounts of glutamate cause neuronal death through a massive calcium influx via ionotropic glutamate receptor channels, with subsequent damage to mitochondria and activation of proapoptotic genes. The deleterious effect of glutamate has been well documented in human stroke and in animal models of cerebral ischemia. In agreement with this, experimental studies from our research group have shown the beneficial effect on stroke outcome of glutamate uptake, mediated by glutamate transporters (Hurtado *et al.*, 2008; Mallolas *et al.*, 2006), or by its clearance using peritoneal dialysis (Godino *et al.*, 2013).

In addition to its neuronal excitotoxic effects, glutamate receptors also play a role in microglia activation and neuroinflammation in various pathological conditions, including stroke (Domercq *et al.*, 2013; Pocock and Kettenmann, 2007). The implication of excitotoxicity on microglia activation was first evidenced because excitotoxic stimuli mediate a rapid cleavage of fractalkine in cultured neurons (Chapman *et al.*, 2000). Moreover, microglia express several types of glutamate receptors, including mGluRs (metabotropic glutamate receptor), NMDA(*N*-methyl-D-aspartate), and AMPA (α-amino-3-hydroxy-5-methylisoxazole-4-propanoic acid) (Pocock and Kettenmann, 2007). Activation of these receptors can mediate heterogeneous microglial functions. For example, stimulation by different subtypes of mGluRs can transform microglia into a neuroprotective (via group III mGluRs) or a neurotoxic (via group II mGluRs) phenotype (Pocock and Kettenmann, 2007). Microglial toxicity mediated by mGluRs involves the release of TNFα and FasL (Fas ligand), which trigger neuronal caspase-3 activation via TNFR1 (also known as p55) and Fas receptor, leading to neuronal death (Taylor *et al.*, 2005). In addition, agonists of metabotropic mGlu3 receptor mediate nicotinamide adenine dinucleotide phosphate (NADPH) oxidase activation promoting neurotoxicity. In contrast, antagonists of mGluR5 receptors inhibit this effect (Mead *et al.*, 2012), showing the dual role of microglial mGluRs on neuroprotection and neurotoxicity.

Myeloid Heterogeneity in Brain Ischemia

After stroke, a cascade of signals leads to the activation of resident glial cells, mainly microglia, and of perivascular macrophages, as well as to an influx of blood-derived cells recruited by cytokines, adhesion molecules, and chemokines (Chamorro *et al.*, 2012; Iadecola and Anrather, 2011). All of these cell populations are currently being associated with distinct roles in cerebral brain damage and neurodegeneration. Recent data suggest that resident microglia may be functionally distinct from blood-derived phagocytes (Prinz *et al.*, 2011). To date, various brain myeloid cells have been identified solely on the basis of their localization, morphology, and surface epitope expression. However, because of their heterogeneity, it is becoming crucial to distinguish the sources of the neuroinflammatory response after stroke to determine not only its nature and its role on brain injury, but also the effectiveness of its modulation.

Differential Role of Microglia and Blood-Borne-Derived Macrophages in Stroke Pathogenesis

The specific role of microglia and hematogenous macrophages on neurotoxicity remains unclear and is currently under debate (Hellwig *et al.*, 2013). However, accumulating evidence indicates that their origin is important.

Microglia are derived from an erythromyeloid precursor cell of embryonic hematopoiesis that persists in adult mice independently of hematopoiesis (Kierdorf *et al.*, 2013; Schulz *et al.*, 2012), making it very likely that these cells have an elaborate repertoire of brain-specific functions that may not be appropriately taken over by peripheral monocytes/macrophages. In the steady state, microglial renewal rate is low, but its number increases markedly after stroke. This is accompanied by morphological, phenotypic, and gene expression alterations and by extravasation and activation of hematogenous macrophages. Although these events play a pivotal role in the pathophysiological cascade following cerebral ischemia, the lack of reliable microglia-specific markers makes it very difficult both to discriminate between microglia and peripheral monocytes/macrophages and to allocate functions to either cell type.

Two approaches have been established to attempt to discriminate between resident and blood-borne macrophages after stroke. The first involves the tracking of infiltrating cells using bone marrow chimeric mice with labeled bone marrow cell replacement after irradiation or by *in situ* carboxyfluorescein succinimidyl ester (CFSE) labeling of blood cells (Denes *et al.*, 2007; Kokovay *et al.*, 2006; Schilling *et al.*, 2005). The second approach relies on the observation that, in contrast to macrophages, microglia express low or intermediate levels of the leukocytes marker CD45. This allows the characterization of microglia by flow cytometry using the levels of expression of CD45 in CD11b$^+$ cells, a myeloid marker similarly expressed in both resident and nonresident populations (Campanella *et al.*, 2002). Results obtained using these experimental approaches suggest that microglial proliferation is the main factor behind the increase in the number of mononuclear phagocytes seen in the ischemic brain (Denes *et al.*, 2007; Schilling *et al.*, 2005). In contrast to the classical view of the neurotoxic role of activated microglia, further studies point to a positive role of microgliosis in brain injury after stroke (Denes *et al.*, 2007; Faustino *et al.*, 2011; Lalancette-Hebert *et al.*, 2007). More importantly, this neuroprotective potential of proliferating microglia after stroke has been associated with its implication in the production of neurotrophic molecules such as insulin-like growth factor-1 (IGF-1) (Lalancette-Hebert *et al.*, 2007), which may open new therapeutic avenues in the treatment of stroke and other neurological disorders.

Furthermore, microglia are associated with the clearance of cellular debris. Its phagocytic activity in the ischemic brain predominates over that of hematogenous macrophages (Schilling *et al.*, 2005). Results from our research group have demonstrated that microglial expression of CD36, a scavenger receptor linked to the phagocytosis of apoptotic cells, is associated with the phagocytosis of apoptotic neutrophils in the ischemic tissue, contributing to resolution of inflammation and partly mediating the neuroprotective effects of rosiglitazone after stroke (Ballesteros *et al.*, 2013) (see Chapter 17 for more on resolution mediators). However, a deleterious effect of CD36 after stroke has also been shown (Cho *et al.*, 2005; Kim *et al.*, 2012). Interestingly, studies using CD36$^{-/-}$ApoE$^{-/-}$ chimeric mice indicate that CD36$^+$ monocytes contribute to ischemic injury (Kim *et al.*, 2012), suggesting that resident and peripheral myeloid cells of the brain can play opposite effects in stroke outcome despite sharing a similar phenotypical signature.

This and other data are starting to unveil the complexity of the different repertoire of functions displayed by myeloid cell subpopulations in the context of inflammation, which contrasts with the traditional and simplified view of the deleterious contribution of myeloid cell activation in brain damage after stroke, as shown in Fig. 5.2.

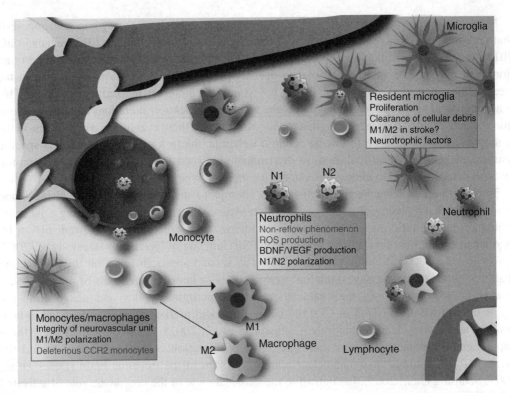

Figure 5.2 Dual role of innate immune system in stroke. The heterogeneity of immune cells population is currently being associated with distinct roles in cerebral brain damage and neurodegeneration. The study of the precise role of different subsets of monocytes, neutrophils, and brain resident macrophages in stroke will help to identify specific therapeutic targets for stroke treatment that can potentiate the benefits of innate immune responses while diminishing their deleterious effects. (*See insert for color representation of this figure.*)

The Role of Infiltrated Myeloid Cell Subsets in Stroke Pathogenesis

After disruption of cerebral blood flow, successive waves of leukocyte subsets, including neutrophils, monocytes, and lymphocytes, infiltrate into the injured brain and produce ROS, inflammatory cytokines, and matrix metalloproteinases, inducing brain damage and blood–brain barrier disruption, leading to edema, cerebral hemorrhage, and a vicious circle of continuous influx of myeloid cells (Iadecola and Anrather, 2011). However, and as previously highlighted for microglia, the effect of these cells on stroke outcome has not been completely elucidated.

Most experimental studies on the temporal dynamics of immune cells infiltration following stroke show that neutrophils are the first wave of leukocytes to infiltrate the ischemic brain. However, Gelderblom and collaborators have described that the infiltration of macrophages, lymphocytes, and DCs preceded neutrophil influx, raising an interesting possibility regarding post-stroke immunomodulation (Gelderblom *et al.*, 2009).

In this context, an important issue that needs to be clarified is which is the point of entry of the leukocytes to the brain parenchyma after stroke. Leukocyte adhesion during focal ischemia is mediated by the post-capillary venule endothelium, which expresses receptors necessary for leukocyte transmigration (Muldoon *et al.*, 2013). Recent studies suggest that meninges covering the ischemic areas appear to be the exclusive point of leukocytic entry to the brain in the early stages of ischemia (Moller *et al.*, 2014), pointing to mast cells residing in the meninges as an important factor for the early influx of neutrophils to the brain. However, platelets-neutrophils interactions within activated venules of the ischemic brain has emerge as a new mechanism to drive neutrophil migration and tissue damage after stroke (Sreeramkumar *et al.*, 2014), suggesting that different mechanisms and ports of entry are used by leukocytes to access to the ischemic brain. The translationality of these observations needs to be considered, because the use of different experimental models of stroke may differentially influence the dynamics of leukocytes recruitment to the brain. It has been discussed that a transient ischemia/reperfusion injury by means of the filament model typically produces an infarct core within the basal ganglia, whereas cortical and meningeal damage is secondary. Studies using this model have shown a delayed infiltration of neutrophils to the brain parenchyma (Gelderblom *et al.*, 2009), or no infiltration, with a preferential location of the neutrophils at the luminal surfaces or perivascular spaces of cerebral vessels (Enzmann *et al.*, 2013). In contrast, the integrity of the meninges is *per se* compromised in stroke models using craniotomy, where different studies have shown an early recruitment of these cells to the brain parenchyma (Cuartero *et al.*, 2013; Moller *et al.*, 2014). It is possible that the choice of the model of cerebral ischemia may account for the differences found in these studies.

Regarding the role of neutrophils on stroke outcome, these cells have been shown to alter microcirculatory homeostasis, causing what has been termed as the "no-reflow" phenomenon (Ames *et al.*, 1968) and, therefore, contributing to tissue damage. In addition, neutrophils have also been associated with ROS generation through the NADPH oxidase respiratory burst, which produces direct injury to the vascular endothelium and brain parenchyma. This is supported by the fact that multiple anti-inflammatory and neuroprotective strategies in stroke are accompanied with a reduced number of infiltrated neutrophils into the ischemic tissue (Segel *et al.*, 2011). Moreover, depletion of neutrophils after cerebral ischemia has been shown to induce neuroprotection (Cuartero *et al.*, 2013; Murikinati *et al.*, 2010). In agreement with this view of the detrimental role of neutrophils after stroke, several studies have found a clear correlation between the degree of neutrophil infiltration and the severity of the neurological injury. However, other studies point to neutrophilia as a marker rather than a participant in the pathological response. This view is supported by evidence that associates these cells with the production of several growth factors, including brain-derived neurotrophic factor (BDNF) and vascular-endothelial growth factor (VEGF), (Hao *et al.*, 2007; Segel *et al.*, 2011) and by evidence that shows an impaired correlation between neutrophils and damage after granulocyte-colony stimulating factor (G-CSF) treatment, a cytokine associated with the induction of neutrophilia but with a neuroprotective effect in stroke (Strecker *et al.*, 2010).

In addition to an early infiltration of neutrophils, massive infiltration of exogenous macrophages has been reported to reach a peak 24–48 h after ischemia (Denes *et al.*, 2007; Schilling *et al.*, 2005). These early infiltrated blood-borne macrophages likely emanate from CCR2+ peripheral blood monocytes. This monocytic subpopulation rapidly enters injured tissue, differentiates into macrophages or DCs, and plays a deleterious role in many CNS diseases such as autoimmune multiple sclerosis (Ajami *et al.*, 2011; Mildner *et al.*, 2007). In agreement with the deleterious role of CCR2+ monocytes on CNS pathologies, mice lacking the chemokine receptor CCR2 were protected against cerebral ischemia/reperfusion injury and had a reduced number of monocytes and neutrophils in the ischemic tissue (Dimitrijevic *et al.*, 2007). However, recent studies have associated CCR2+ monocytes with the maintenance of the integrity of the neurovascular unit following brain ischemia (Gliem *et al.*, 2012), pointing to a dual role of these cells in brain injury after stroke.

Thus, taking all these observations into consideration, it is plausible that monocytes and neutrophils, and by extension, microglia, have protective and harmful effects in the ischemic brain depending on additional cues that influence the highly regulated process of myeloid activation after stroke. These cues can be linked to the ability of myeloid cells to change their phenotype in response to their microenvironment, displaying different functions from cytotoxicity to tissue repair and immunomodulation.

Activation States on Myeloid Cells: Contribution to Stroke Outcome

Monocyte/macrophage lineages display a remarkable plasticity and can change their physiology in response to their microenvironment, giving rise to different populations of cells with distinct functions (Gordon and Martinez, 2010). To easily classify them, two main groups designated as M1 (classically activated) and M2 (alternatively activated) have been proposed (see Chapter 4 for more on macrophage polarization). M1 activation is mainly associated with cytotoxicity, and it is thought to play an important role in the killing phase of the inflammatory response, whereas polarization of macrophages toward an M2 phenotype mainly promotes tissue repair and trophic functions (Gordon and Martinez, 2010). Thus, polarization toward either of these states may be crucial for the participation of mononuclear phagocytes, including resident microglia, in inflammatory brain damage.

Reorienting and reshaping a deranged macrophage polarization from a cytotoxic profile to a profile that supports immune modulation and tissue repair may constitute the basis of macrophage therapeutic targeting in stroke.

As discussed, initial cell death after ischemia is mainly associated with necrosis, leading to the release of *danger signals* that induce the expression of proinflammatory molecules, such as TNF, IL-1β, adhesion molecules, and inducible enzymes, such as iNOS (Iadecola and Anrather, 2011). These molecules fall within the context of M1 macrophage activation, as its production by macrophages indicates that they may have experienced a polarization toward a proinflammatory and cytotoxic phenotype. Although ischemia-induced upregulation of proinflammatory mediators has been extensively reported, it is becoming accepted that the expression of markers of M2 polarization is also upregulated after brain ischemia (Cuartero *et al.*, 2013; Frieler *et al.*, 2011; Hu *et al.*, 2012; Perego *et al.*, 2011; Zarruk *et al.*, 2012). This has been attributed not only to an increased infiltration of alternative activated (M2) blood-borne monocytes into the brain parenchyma (Perego *et al.*, 2011), but also to the ability of microglia/macrophages to assume an M2 phenotype at early stages of ischemic stroke (Hu *et al.*, 2012). However, the specific mechanisms that mediate their recruitment or their re-education *in situ* are not completely understood. Of note, the coexistence of cells in different activation states and mixed phenotypes has been observed in different pathological conditions *in vivo*, a reflection of dynamic changes and complex tissue-derived signals (Sica and Mantovani, 2012).

Different studies have focussed on the characterization of M2 microglia/macrophages after stroke. Frieler and collaborators (2011) showed that specific-myeloid mineralocorticoid receptor (MR) gene knock-out mice presented an upregulated expression of M1 markers while partially preserving the ischemia-induced expression of M2 markers. This effect correlated with a better stroke outcome in $MR^{-/-}$ mice, which was linked to a lower ratio of M1/M2-polarized myeloid cells within the brain of these mice (Frieler *et al.*, 2011). Other studies have shown that a decreased M1/M2 ratio is linked to neuroprotection (Xu *et al.*, 2012). Furthermore, the neuroprotective effect of JWH-133, a selective cannabinoid receptor 2 (CB2R) agonist, is associated with its inhibitory effect on both M1/M2 activation states of macrophages, suggesting that JWH-133-mediated neuroprotection is due to the inhibition of microglia activation and not to an M2 polarization (Zarruk *et al.*, 2012). Therefore, a clear delineation between the specific effects of M1/M2 modulation in cerebral ischemia has not already been well established, and the causality between M2 polarization and neuroprotection needs to be further characterized in order to dissect the beneficial and detrimental roles of M1/M2 myeloid cell subpopulations after stroke.

Other studies have shown that microglia/macrophages assume an M2 phenotype at early stages of ischemic stroke but gradually transform into the M1 phenotype in peri-infarct regions. This transition from an initial "healthy" M2 phenotype to a "sick" M1 phenotype was associated with bad outcome, as suggested by *in vitro* experiments of neurotoxicity using conditioned media from M1 or M2 macrophages (Hu *et al.*, 2012).

In addition to macrophages, neutrophils also display functional heterogeneity *in vivo* and a capacity to change their phenotype after *in vitro* cytokine exposure (Mantovani *et al.*, 2011), a function that makes them plastic cells, capable of responding to extracellular stimuli in a context-dependent manner. This was recently highlighted in cancer, where tumor-associated neutrophils were shown to acquire a pro-tumor phenotype (N2) characterized by the expression of arginase I, CCL2, and CCL5 (Fridlender *et al.*, 2009). In stroke, studies from our group indicate that neutrophils in the ischemic brain form a heterogeneous population that express well-established markers of M2 macrophage polarization. In addition, N2 neutrophils of the ischemic tissue mediate their own clearance by macrophages/microglia, a fact that may promote resolution of inflammation after stroke (Cuartero *et al.*, 2013) (also see Chapter 17).

Concluding Remarks

Taking together the multiple implications of brain innate immune activation following a stroke, it is evident that, during the inflammatory cascade, there exists causality between the presence of specific innate immune cells subsets and the final neuronal fate. This will have an impact not only on stroke outcome, but also on the whole process of resolution of inflammation, and by extension, on subsequent effects on tissue repair and neurogenesis. Future research in stroke immunology needs to focus on a detailed analysis of these specific relationships between innate immunity and neurons, paying attention to the characterization of the cell subsets that mediate these effects. New techniques and animal models are now emerging for this analysis. Studies to dissect cell-to-cell interactions, the characterization of novel cell phenotypes, and the study of the precise role of these cell subsets on stroke will help in the identification of specific therapeutic targets for stroke treatment that can potentiate the benefits of innate immune responses while diminishing their deleterious effects.

References

Abulafia, D.P., de Rivero Vaccari, J.P., Lozano, J.D., Lotocki, G., Keane, R.W. & Dietrich, W.D. (2009) Inhibition of the inflammasome complex reduces the inflammatory response after thromboembolic stroke in mice. *Journal of Cerebral Blood Flow and Metabolism*, **29**, 534–544.

Ajami, B., Bennett, J.L., Krieger, C., McNagny, K.M. & Rossi, F.M. (2011) Infiltrating monocytes trigger EAE progression, but do not contribute to the resident microglia pool. *Nature Neuroscience*, **14**, 1142–1149.

Allan, S.M., Tyrrell, P.J. & Rothwell, N.J. (2005) Interleukin-1 and neuronal injury. *Nature Reviews. Immunology*, **5**, 629–640.

Ames, A. 3rd, Wright, R.L., Kowada, M., Thurston, J.M. & Majno, G. (1968) Cerebral ischemia. II. The no-reflow phenomenon. *American Journal of Pathology*, **52**, 437–453.

Ballesteros, I., Cuartero, M.I., Pradillo, J.M. *et al.* (2013) *Rosiglitazone-induced CD36 up-regulation resolves inflammation by PPARgamma and 5-LO-dependent pathways*. Vol. **95**. Journal of Leukocyte Biology, pp. 587–598.

Brea, D., Blanco, M., Ramos-Cabrer, P. *et al.* (2011) Toll-like receptors 2 and 4 in ischemic stroke: Outcome and therapeutic values. *Journal of Cerebral Blood Flow and Metabolism*, **31**, 1424–1431.

Brough, D., Tyrrell, P.J. & Allan, S.M. (2011) Regulation of interleukin-1 in acute brain injury. *Trends in Pharmacological Sciences*, **32**, 617–622.

Campanella, M., Sciorati, C., Tarozzo, G. & Beltramo, M. (2002) Flow cytometric analysis of inflammatory cells in ischemic rat brain. *Stroke*, **33**, 586–592.

Cardona, A.E., Pioro, E.P., Sasse, M.E. *et al.* (2006) Control of microglial neurotoxicity by the fractalkine receptor. *Nature Neuroscience*, **9**, 917–924.

Caso, J.R., Pradillo, J.M., Hurtado, O., Lorenzo, P., Moro, M.A. & Lizasoain, I. (2007) Toll-like receptor 4 is involved in brain damage and inflammation after experimental stroke. *Circulation*, **115**, 1599–1608.

Castellanos, M., Castillo, J., Garcia, M.M. *et al.* (2002) Inflammation-mediated damage in progressing lacunar infarctions: A potential therapeutic target. *Stroke*, **33**, 982–987.

Cipriani, R., Villa, P., Chece, G. *et al.* (2011) CX3CL1 is neuroprotective in permanent focal cerebral ischemia in rodents. *Journal of Neuroscience*, **31**, 16327–16335.

Cuartero, M.I., Ballesteros, I., Moraga, A. *et al.* (2013) N2 neutrophils, novel players in brain inflammation after stroke: Modulation by the PPARgamma agonist rosiglitazone. *Stroke*, **44**, 3498–3508.

Chamorro, A., Meisel, A., Planas, A.M., Urra, X., van de Beek, D. & Veltkamp, R. (2012) The immunology of acute stroke. *Nature Reviews Neurology*, **8**, 401–410.

Chapman, G.A., Moores, K., Harrison, D., Campbell, C.A., Stewart, B.R. & Strijbos, P.J. (2000) Fractalkine cleavage from neuronal membranes represents an acute event in the inflammatory response to excitotoxic brain damage. *Journal of Neuroscience*, **20**, RC87.

Chen, G., Shaw, M.H., Kim, Y.G. & Nunez, G. (2009) NOD-like receptors: role in innate immunity and inflammatory disease. *Annual Review of Pathology*, **4**, 365–398.

Chen, G.Y. & Nunez, G. (2010) Sterile inflammation: sensing and reacting to damage. *Nature Reviews Immunology*, **10**, 826–837.

Cho, S., Park, E.M., Febbraio, M. *et al.* (2005) The class B scavenger receptor CD36 mediates free radical production and tissue injury in cerebral ischemia. *Journal of Neuroscience*, **25**, 2504–2512.

Chu, K., Yin, B., Wang, J. *et al.* (2012) Inhibition of P2X7 receptor ameliorates transient global cerebral ischemia/reperfusion injury via modulating inflammatory responses in the rat hippocampus. *Journal of Neuroinflammation*, **9**, 69.

Denes, A., Vidyasagar, R., Feng, J. *et al.* (2007) Proliferating resident microglia after focal cerebral ischaemia in mice. *Journal of Cerebral Blood Flow and Metabolism*, **27**, 1941–1953.

Denes, A., Ferenczi, S., Halasz, J., Kornyei, Z. & Kovacs, K.J. (2008) Role of CX3CR1 (fractalkine receptor) in brain damage and inflammation induced by focal cerebral ischemia in mouse. *Journal of Cerebral Blood Flow and Metabolism*, **28**, 1707–1721.

Denieffe, S., Kelly, R.J., McDonald, C., Lyons, A. & Lynch, M.A. (2013) Classical activation of microglia in CD200-deficient mice is a consequence of blood brain barrier permeability and infiltration of peripheral cells. *Brain, Behavior, and Immunity*, **34**, 86–97.

Deroide, N., Li, X., Lerouet, D. *et al.* (2013) MFGE8 inhibits inflammasome-induced IL-1beta production and limits postischemic cerebral injury. *Journal of Clinical Investigation*, **123**, 1176–1181.

Dimitrijevic, O.B., Stamatovic, S.M., Keep, R.F. & Andjelkovic, A.V. (2007) Absence of the chemokine receptor CCR2 protects against cerebral ischemia/reperfusion injury in mice. *Stroke*, **38**, 1345–1353.

Doan, T. (2008) *Immunology. Lippincott's Illustrated Reviews*. Wolters Kluwer Health/Lippincott Williams & Wilkins, Philadelphia.

Domercq, M., Vazquez-Villoldo, N. & Matute, C. (2013) Neurotransmitter signaling in the pathophysiology of microglia. *Frontiers in Cellular Neuroscience*, **7**, 49.

Edye, M.E., Lopez-Castejon, G., Allan, S.M. & Brough, D. (2013) Acidosis drives damage-associated molecular pattern (DAMP)-induced interleukin-1 secretion via a caspase-1-independent pathway. *Journal of Biological Chemistry*, **288**, 30485–30494.

Enzmann, G., Mysiorek, C., Gorina, R. *et al.* (2013) The neurovascular unit as a selective barrier to polymorphonuclear granulocyte (PMN) infiltration into the brain after ischemic injury. *Acta Neuropathologica*, **125**, 395–412.

Faraco, G., Fossati, S., Bianchi, M.E. *et al.* (2007) High mobility group box 1 protein is released by neural cells upon different stresses and worsens ischemic neurodegeneration in vitro and in vivo. *Journal of Neurochemistry*, **103**, 590–603.

Faustino, J.V., Wang, X., Johnson, C.E. *et al.* (2011) Microglial cells contribute to endogenous brain defenses after acute neonatal focal stroke. *Journal of Neuroscience*, **31**, 12992–13001.

Frederick Lo, C., Ning, X., Gonzales, C. & Ozenberger, B.A. (2008) Induced expression of death domain genes NALP1 and NALP5 following neuronal injury. *Biochemical and Biophysical Research Communications*, **366**, 664–669.

Fridlender, Z.G., Sun, J., Kim, S. *et al.* (2009) Polarization of tumor-associated neutrophil phenotype by TGF-beta: "N1" versus "N2" TAN. *Cancer Cell*, **16**, 183–194.

Frieler, R.A., Meng, H., Duan, S.Z. *et al.* (2011) Myeloid-specific deletion of the mineralocorticoid receptor reduces infarct volume and alters inflammation during cerebral ischemia. *Stroke*, **42**, 179–185.

Gelderblom, M., Leypoldt, F., Steinbach, K. *et al.* (2009) Temporal and spatial dynamics of cerebral immune cell accumulation in stroke. *Stroke*, **40**, 1849–1857.

Gliem, M., Mausberg, A.K., Lee, J.I. *et al.* (2012) Macrophages prevent hemorrhagic infarct transformation in murine stroke models. *Annals of Neurology*, **71**, 743–752.

Godino, M.d.C., Romera, V.G., Sanchez-Tomero, J.A. *et al.* (2013) Amelioration of ischemic brain damage by peritoneal dialysis. *Journal of Clinical Investigation*, **123**, 4359–4363.

Gordon, S. & Martinez, F.O. (2010) Alternative activation of macrophages: Mechanism and functions. *Immunity*, **32**, 593–604.

Hao, Q., Chen, Y., Zhu, Y. *et al.* (2007) Neutrophil depletion decreases VEGF-induced focal angiogenesis in the mature mouse brain. *Journal of Cerebral Blood Flow and Metabolism*, **27**, 1853–1860.

Hellwig, S., Heinrich, A. & Biber, K. (2013) The brain's best friend: microglial neurotoxicity revisited. *Frontiers in Cellular Neuroscience*, **7**, 71.

Hoek, R.M., Ruuls, S.R., Murphy, C.A. *et al.* (2000) Down-regulation of the macrophage lineage through interaction with OX2 (CD200). *Science*, **290**, 1768–1771.

Hu, X., Li, P., Guo, Y. *et al.* (2012) Microglia/macrophage polarization dynamics reveal novel mechanism of injury expansion after focal cerebral ischemia. *Stroke*, **43**, 3063–3070.

Hurtado, O., Pradillo, J.M., Fernandez-Lopez, D. *et al.* (2008) Delayed post-ischemic administration of CDP-choline increases EAAT2 association to lipid rafts and affords neuroprotection in experimental stroke. *Neurobiology of Disease*, **29**, 123–131.

Hyakkoku, K., Hamanaka, J., Tsuruma, K. *et al.* (2010) Toll-like receptor 4 (TLR4), but not TLR3 or TLR9, knock-out mice have neuroprotective effects against focal cerebral ischemia. *Neuroscience*, **171**, 258–267.

Iadecola, C. & Anrather, J. (2011) The immunology of stroke: From mechanisms to translation. *Nature Medicine*, **17**, 796–808.

Kierdorf, K., Erny, D., Goldmann, T. *et al.* (2013) Microglia emerge from erythromyeloid precursors via Pu.1- and Irf8-dependent pathways. *Nature Neuroscience*, **16**, 273–280.

Kim, E., Febbraio, M., Bao, Y., Tolhurst, A.T., Epstein, J.M. & Cho, S. (2012) CD36 in the periphery and brain synergizes in stroke injury in hyperlipidemia. *Annals of Neurology*, **71**, 753–764.

Kokovay, E., Li, L. & Cunningham, L.A. (2006) Angiogenic recruitment of pericytes from bone marrow after stroke. *Journal of Cerebral Blood Flow and Metabolism*, **26**, 545–555.

Lalancette-Hebert, M., Gowing, G., Simard, A., Weng, Y.C. & Kriz, J. (2007) Selective ablation of proliferating microglial cells exacerbates ischemic injury in the brain. *Journal of Neuroscience*, **27**, 2596–2605.

Lehnardt, S., Lehmann, S., Kaul, D. *et al.* (2007) Toll-like receptor 2 mediates CNS injury in focal cerebral ischemia. *Journal of Neuroimmunology*, **190**, 28–33.

Mallolas, J., Hurtado, O., Castellanos, M. *et al.* (2006) A polymorphism in the EAAT2 promoter is associated with higher glutamate concentrations and higher frequency of progressing stroke. *Journal of Experimental Medicine*, **203**, 711–717.

Mantovani, A., Cassatella, M.A., Costantini, C. & Jaillon, S. (2011) Neutrophils in the activation and regulation of innate and adaptive immunity. *Nature Reviews Immunology*, **11**, 519–531.

Matsumoto, H., Kumon, Y., Watanabe, H. *et al.* (2007) Expression of CD200 by macrophage-like cells in ischemic core of rat brain after transient middle cerebral artery occlusion. *Neuroscience Letters*, **418**, 44–48.

Mead, E.L., Mosley, A., Eaton, S., Dobson, L., Heales, S.J. & Pocock, J.M. (2012) Microglial neurotransmitter receptors trigger superoxide production in microglia; consequences for microglial-neuronal interactions. *Journal of Neurochemistry*, **121**, 287–301.

Medzhitov, R. (2001) Toll-like receptors and innate immunity. *Nature Reviews. Immunology*, **1**, 135–145.

Mildner, A., Schmidt, H., Nitsche, M. *et al.* (2007) Microglia in the adult brain arise from Ly-6ChiCCR2+ monocytes only under defined host conditions. *Nature Neuroscience*, **10**, 1544–1553.

Moller, K., Boltze, J., Posel, C., Seeger, J., Stahl, T. & Wagner, D.C. (2014) Sterile inflammation after permanent distal MCA occlusion in hypertensive rats. *Journal of Cerebral Blood Flow and Metabolism*, **34**, 307–315.

Muldoon, L.L., Alvarez, J.I., Begley, D.J. *et al.* (2013) Immunologic privilege in the central nervous system and the blood-brain barrier. *Journal of Cerebral Blood Flow and Metabolism*, **33**, 13–21.

Murikinati, S., Juttler, E., Keinert, T. *et al.* (2010) Activation of cannabinoid 2 receptors protects against cerebral ischemia by inhibiting neutrophil recruitment. *FASEB Journal*, **24**, 788–798.

Nemoto, E.M. & Frinak, S. (1981) Brain tissue pH after global brain ischemia and barbiturate loading in rats. *Stroke*, **12**, 77–82.

Park, J.S., Gamboni-Robertson, F., He, Q. *et al.* (2006) High mobility group box 1 protein interacts with multiple Toll-like receptors. *American Journal of Physiology. Cell Physiology*, **290**, C917–C924.

Perego, C., Fumagalli, S. & De Simoni, M.G. (2011) Temporal pattern of expression and colocalization of microglia/macrophage phenotype markers following brain ischemic injury in mice. *Journal of Neuroinflammation*, **8**, 174.

Pocock, J.M. & Kettenmann, H. (2007) Neurotransmitter receptors on microglia. *Trends in Neurosciences*, **30**, 527–535.

Prinz, M., Priller, J., Sisodia, S.S. & Ransohoff, R.M. (2011) Heterogeneity of CNS myeloid cells and their roles in neurodegeneration. *Nature Neuroscience*, **14**, 1227–1235.

Qiu, J., Xu, J., Zheng, Y. *et al.* (2010) High-mobility group box 1 promotes metalloproteinase-9 upregulation through Toll-like receptor 4 after cerebral ischemia. *Stroke*, **41**, 2077–2082.

Rajamaki, K., Nordstrom, T., Nurmi, K. *et al.* (2013) Extracellular acidosis is a novel danger signal alerting innate immunity via the NLRP3 inflammasome. *Journal of Biological Chemistry*, **288**, 13410–13419.

Schielke, G.P., Yang, G.Y., Shivers, B.D. & Betz, A.L. (1998) Reduced ischemic brain injury in interleukin-1 beta converting enzyme-deficient mice. *Journal of Cerebral Blood Flow and Metabolism*, **18**, 180–185.

Schilling, M., Besselmann, M., Muller, M., Strecker, J.K., Ringelstein, E.B. & Kiefer, R. (2005) Predominant phagocytic activity of resident microglia over hematogenous macrophages following transient focal cerebral ischemia: An investigation using green fluorescent protein transgenic bone marrow chimeric mice. *Experimental Neurology*, **196**, 290–297.

Schroder, K. & Tschopp, J. (2010) The inflammasomes. *Cell*, **140**, 821–832.

Schulz, C., Gomez Perdiguero, E., Chorro, L. *et al.* (2012) A lineage of myeloid cells independent of Myb and hematopoietic stem cells. *Science*, **336**, 86–90.

Segel, G.B., Halterman, M.W. & Lichtman, M.A. (2011) The paradox of the neutrophil's role in tissue injury. *Journal of Leukocyte Biology*, **89**, 359–372.

Shichita, T., Hasegawa, E., Kimura, A. *et al.* (2012) Peroxiredoxin family proteins are key initiators of post-ischemic inflammation in the brain. *Nature Medicine*, **18**, 911–917.

Sica, A. & Mantovani, A. (2012) Macrophage plasticity and polarization: In vivo veritas. *Journal of Clinical Investigation*, **122**, 787–795.

Sreeramkumar V., Adrover J.M., Ballesteros I. *et al.* (2014) Neutrophils scan for activated platelets to initiate inflammation. *Science*, **346**, 1234–1238.

Soriano, S.G., Amaravadi, L.S., Wang, Y.F. *et al.* (2002) Mice deficient in fractalkine are less susceptible to cerebral ischemia-reperfusion injury. *Journal of Neuroimmunology*, **125**, 59–65.

Strecker, J.K., Sevimli, S., Schilling, M. *et al.* (2010) Effects of G-CSF treatment on neutrophil mobilization and neurological outcome after transient focal ischemia. *Experimental Neurology*, **222**, 108–113.

Suzuki, Y., Nakano, Y., Mishiro, K. *et al.* (2013) Involvement of Mincle and Syk in the changes to innate immunity after ischemic stroke. *Scientific Reports*, **3**, 3177.

Tarkowski, E., Rosengren, L., Blomstrand, C. *et al.* (1995) Early intrathecal production of interleukin-6 predicts the size of brain lesion in stroke. *Stroke*, **26**, 1393–1398.

Taylor, D.L., Jones, F., Kubota, E.S. & Pocock, J.M. (2005) Stimulation of microglial metabotropic glutamate receptor mGlu2 triggers tumor necrosis factor alpha-induced neurotoxicity in concert with microglial-derived Fas ligand. *Journal of Neuroscience*, **25**, 2952–2964.

Vila, N., Castillo, J., Davalos, A. & Chamorro, A. (2000) Proinflammatory cytokines and early neurological worsening in ischemic stroke. *Stroke*, **31**, 2325–2329.

Walsh, J.G., Muruve, D.A. & Power, C. (2014) Inflammasomes in the CNS. *Nature Reviews Neuroscience*, **15**, 84–97.

Xu, Y., Qian, L., Zong, G. *et al.* (2012) Class A scavenger receptor promotes cerebral ischemic injury by pivoting microglia/macrophage polarization. *Neuroscience*, **218**, 35–48.

Yang, Q.W., Wang, J.Z., Li, J.C. *et al.* (2010) High-mobility group protein box-1 and its relevance to cerebral ischemia. *Journal of Cerebral Blood Flow and Metabolism*, **30**, 243–254.

Zarruk, J.G., Fernandez-Lopez, D., Garcia-Yebenes, I. *et al.* (2012) Cannabinoid type 2 receptor activation downregulates stroke-induced classic and alternative brain macrophage/microglial activation concomitant to neuroprotection. *Stroke*, **43**, 211–219.

Zhang, L., Chopp, M., Liu, X. *et al.* (2012) Combination therapy with VELCADE and tissue plasminogen activator is neuroprotective in aged rats after stroke and targets microRNA-146a and the toll-like receptor signaling pathway. *Arteriosclerosis, Thrombosis, and Vascular Biology.*, **32**, 1856–1864.

Ziegler, G., Harhausen, D., Schepers, C. *et al.* (2007) TLR2 has a detrimental role in mouse transient focal cerebral ischemia. *Biochemical and Biophysical Research Communications*, **359**, 574–579.

Ziegler, G., Freyer, D., Harhausen, D., Khojasteh, U., Nietfeld, W. & Trendelenburg, G. (2011) Blocking TLR2 in vivo protects against accumulation of inflammatory cells and neuronal injury in experimental stroke. *Journal of Cerebral Blood Flow and Metabolism*, **31**, 757–766.

6   Neuroinflammation in Aging

Ashley M. Fenn,[1]* Diana M. Norden,[1]* and Jonathan P. Godbout,[1,2]

[1] Department of Neuroscience, The Ohio State University, Columbus, OH, USA
[2] Institute for Behavioral Medicine Research, The Ohio State University, Columbus, OH, USA

Increased CNS Inflammation in Response to Immune Challenge is Adaptive and Beneficial

Inflammation typically has a negative connotation, particularly within the central nervous system (CNS). After a traumatic brain injury, for example, inflammation is responsible for life-threatening edema and hypotension. But not all brain inflammation is detrimental.

During a peripheral infection, innate immune cells become activated and release inflammatory signaling molecules called cytokines and chemokines. Inflammatory cytokines typically include interleukin (IL)-1β, IL-6, and tumor necrosis factor (TNF)α, whereas chemokines can vary depending on the stimulus. Once released, these cytokines and chemokines use both neuronal and humoral pathways to activate CNS-resident microglia. Microglia are the innate immune cell of the brain, and they interpret and propagate these peripheral inflammatory signals throughout the CNS, causing a low level of brain inflammation. This low level of inflammation results in changes in neuronal activation, leading to the physiological and behavioral components of the sickness response (Dantzer et al., 2008). For example, IL-1β, IL-6, and TNFα bind to cytokine receptors on neurons within the anterior hypothalamus to alter the activation of temperature-sensitive neurons, resulting in an increase in the temperature-set point and induction of a fever response (Shibata, 1990; Stefferl et al., 1996). Other components of sickness behavior include reduced appetite and sexual drive, increased slow wave sleep, and social avoidance. These physiological and behavioral changes are evolutionarily adaptive and necessary to reallocate the host's resources and fight infection. Indeed, when lizards (Dipsosaurus dorsalis) were challenged with an active bacterial infection and given low doses of the antipyresis sodium salicylate, mortality rate increased from 0% to 100% (Bernheim and Kluger, 1976). Thus, elevations in brain inflammation are beneficial during an active immune challenge. Brain inflammation that is exaggerated or prolonged, however, can be detrimental.

*These authors contributed equally.

The CNS Microenvironment Shifts to a Proinflammatory State with Aging

There is significant clinical and experimental evidence that inflammation within the CNS increases with age. A hallmark of brain aging is increased oxidative stress and lipid peroxidation. Therefore, one hypothesis is that the accumulation of free radical damage over time leads to increased inflammation within the brain. Consistent with this premise, microarray studies indicate that there is an overall increase in inflammatory and prooxidant genes with a reduction in growth and antioxidant genes in the brain of older rodents compared to adults (Lee *et al.*, 2010; Godbout *et al.*, 2005). An increase in free radicals is detrimental, as they cause damage to many components within the cell, including lipids, proteins, and, most importantly, DNA. In mice with deficient DNA repair capacity, genotoxic stress evokes cell cycle checkpoint responses, which lead to cell cycle arrest and senescence (Matheu *et al.*, 2007). Importantly, DNA damage occurs as part of normal brain activity (Suberbielle *et al.*, 2013). Therefore, accumulation of nuclear DNA damage has been proposed as a critical factor for aging (Hoeijmakers, 2009).

DNA damage also induces upregulation of inflammatory cytokines (Rodier *et al.*, 2009). Two of the most important and potent inflammatory cytokines are IL-1β and IL-6. Both of these cytokines are expressed at a higher level in the brain of aged rodents and humans (Godbout and Johnson, 2004). In addition, there are reductions in several regulatory molecules and anti-inflammatory cytokines including IL-10 and IL-4 (Ye and Johnson, 2001; Maher *et al.*, 2005). There are several behavioral consequences to increased inflammation within the aged brain (discussed in detail later). Therefore, there is significant interest in understanding why there is an age-associated shift in the inflammatory profile of the brain. Recent evidence indicates that the resident microglia are key contributors to the increased inflammatory state of the CNS.

Microglial Priming

Microglia are long-lived cells that show little to no turnover over the course of a lifetime (Ajami *et al.*, 2007; Ginhoux *et al.*, 2010). Microglia develop early in embryogenesis in the embryonic yolk sac and migrate to the area of the CNS around embryonic day 8.5 (Ginhoux *et al.*, 2010). There, they remain and are rarely replaced except in the circumstance of pervasive blood–brain barrier breakdown, CNS trauma, or CNS diseases including Alzheimer's disease and multiple sclerosis. The longevity of microglia makes them particularly sensitive to oxidative stress and a life time of inflammatory insults. Over time, these cells may become hyperreactive or primed. This primed phenotype is characterized by a lower threshold to "switch" to a proinflammatory state (Lull and Block, 2010). Microglial priming toward an inflammatory state may be caused by decades of activation through immune surveillance and stress responses. In support of this notion, a longitudinal study conducted in Sweden suggests that inflammatory exposure during adolescence is associated with reduced long-term survival and higher mortality rates in old age (Finch and Crimmins, 2004).

On a cellular level, microglial priming has been described using various inflammatory markers. For example, the expression of the antigen-presenting molecule major histocompatibility complex (MHC) II and complement receptor 3 (CD11b) were increased in the aged brain of humans, rodents, canines, and nonhuman primates (Frank *et al.*, 2006; VanGuilder *et al.*, 2011).

Many of these markers are present specifically on microglia of the aged brain, including MHC II (Henry *et al.*, 2009). MHC II is commonly used as a marker of microglial priming in models of both aging and injury because primed MHC-II-positive microglia produce exaggerated IL-1β following activation (Henry *et al.*, 2009). Consistent with heightened MHC II expression, other inflammatory markers are also increased in models of aging. These include scavenger receptor CD68, the integrin CD11c, toll-like receptors (TLR), and co-stimulatory molecule CD86 (B7) [for a review see Norden and Godbout (2013)]. Baseline expression of inflammatory cytokines TNFα, IL-1β, and IL-6 is also increased in brain tissue and microglia with age (Sierra *et al.*, 2007; Hickman *et al.*, 2013; Youm *et al.*, 2013). This global increase in CNS inflammation suggests that there may be a common factor responsible. Recent evidence indicates that immune sensors, such as inflammasomes, may be involved in global increases in CNS inflammation. The Nlrp3 inflammasome is an immune sensor that is activated in response to a diverse array of signals. When the Nlrp3 inflammasome was deleted, CNS inflammation was reduced in aged mice (Youm *et al.*, 2013). For example, in aged wild-type mice, the nuclear factor κB (NF-κB), IL-1β, interferon, and complement pathways were all markedly upregulated compared to adults. Although these pathways were also increased in aged Nlrp3 knockout mice compared to adults, they were significantly attenuated compared to wild-type aged mice (Youm *et al.*, 2013). These novel findings indicate that the Nlrp3 inflammasome is an upstream target that controls several age-associated increases in inflammation.

The increased markers of inflammation observed on microglia in the aged brain sets the stage for an increased or exaggerated immune response following stimulation. In support of this idea, exaggerated neuroinflammation following immune challenge has been reported in rodent models of aging. For example, peripheral injection of a gram-negative bacteria, *Escherichia coli*, or a cell wall component of gram-negative bacteria, lipopolysaccharide (LPS), caused exaggerated neuroinflammation associated with increased IL-1β and IL-6 in aged rodents compared to young adults (Godbout *et al.*, 2005; Barrientos *et al.*, 2006). In addition, elevated messenger RNA (mRNA) expression of IL-1β, TNFα, and the inflammatory-associated enzyme indoleamine 2,3-dioxygenase (IDO) was detected 24 and 72 h after LPS injection, indicating that neuroinflammation is both exaggerated and prolonged in the aged brain (Godbout *et al.*, 2008; Richwine *et al.*, 2008).

Several studies indicate that this exaggerated cytokine production is dependent on microglial activation. For example, in a study comparing adult and aged mice, primed MHC II⁺ microglia from aged mice were responsible for exaggerated levels of IL-1β protein following a peripheral challenge with LPS (Henry *et al.*, 2009). These data support the hypothesis that primed, MHC II⁺ microglia are highly responsive to immune challenge and provide a direct connection between heightened neuroinflammation and microglia. Moreover, microglia isolated from aged mice 4 h after LPS injection had increased mRNA levels of IL-1β, inducible nitric oxide synthase (iNOS), TLR2, and IDO compared to adults (Henry *et al.*, 2009). Microglial activation also persisted in aged mice compared to adult mice, leading to protracted production of inflammatory cytokines (Wynne *et al.*, 2010). These studies indicate that primed microglia are hyperactive following stimulation, resulting in exaggerated and prolonged inflammatory cytokine production.

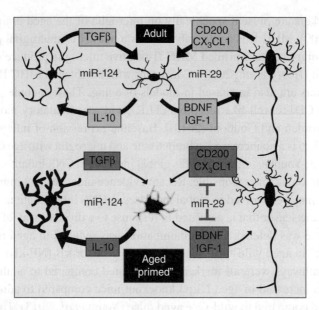

Figure 6.1 Microglia dysregulation with age. There are several regulatory factors that maintain microglia in a surveying and anti-inflammatory state including neuronal, immunological, and astrocytic regulation. As a function of age, these systems become dysregulated. Here, we highlight the significant reduction in neuronal (CD200, CX3CL1), astrocytic (TGFβ), and microRNA (reduced miR-124, increased miR-29) regulation and how this leads to reduced neuronal support by microglia (i.e., reduced neurotrophic factors) and an altered immune response (e.g., heightened release of IL-10).

Microglial Regulation

Recent evidence shows that microglia hyperactivity with age is associated with reduced regulatory pathways. There are several mechanisms within the CNS to maintain a surveying and anti-inflammatory microglia phenotype, including neuronal regulation, astrocytic regulation, and immune regulation. Within the aged brain, however, these regulatory networks begin to break down, leaving microglia primed and more responsive to activating stimuli. The breakdown of these relationships is showcased in Fig. 6.1.

Neuronal Regulation

Exaggerated or prolonged brain inflammation can have detrimental effects on neurons that are, for the most part, nonregenerative. Therefore, proper regulation of microglia is important. To maintain control of microglial activation, neurons produce several immunomodulatory factors that interact with microglia. These include but are not limited to CD200, fractalkine ligand (CX3CL1), neurotransmitters, and neurotrophins (Biber *et al.*, 2007).

CD200–CD200R
CD200 is membrane glycoprotein that is constitutively expressed on neurons. Within the CNS, the CD200 receptor (CD200R) is expressed exclusively on microglia, and the binding of CD200

ligand to CD200R plays a pivotal role of modulating microglial activation (Hoek *et al.*, 2000; Lyons *et al.*, 2007). This way, CD200 regulation keeps microglia in a resting and surveying state. The importance of CD200 regulation of microglia is evident in CD200-deficient mice that spontaneously exhibit a more activated microglia phenotype (Hoek *et al.*, 2000) with increased MHC II expression (Costello *et al.*, 2011). In CD200-deficient mice, microglial activation is exaggerated in several models of inflammation (Hoek *et al.*, 2000; Broderick *et al.*, 2002; Deckert *et al.*, 2006; Denieffe *et al.*, 2013). To escape regulation by CD200 during an inflammatory challenge such as an LPS injection, microglia downregulate CD200R (Masocha, 2009). These findings indicate that lack of CD200 regulation promotes or even exacerbates neuroinflammation.

Aging is associated with a decrease in CD200–CD200R signaling. In rodent models of aging, there were decreased levels of both CD200 and CD200R mRNA and protein (Frank *et al.*, 2006; Lyons *et al.*, 2007). In aged rats, decreased CD200 expression was accompanied by increased MHC II expression, indicating that a loss of CD200 regulation promotes a state of microglial priming (Lyons *et al.*, 2007). Thus, enhancing CD200 signaling has been tested as an intervention to reduce microglial reactivity in several models of aging. Injection of a mimetic of CD200 [neural cell adhesion molecule fibroblast growth loop (FGL)] or CD200 fusion protein into the aged brain rescued a portion of the age-related inflammatory properties of microglia (Downer *et al.*, 2009, 2010; Cox *et al.*, 2011). Overall, CD200 is important for modulating microglial activity, and impairments in CD200 signaling with age can have detrimental effects on microglia–neuron interactions.

CX_3CL1–CX_3CR1

Similar to regulation by CD200, neuronal expression of the chemokine fractalkine is an important factor for maintaining microglia in a surveying and anti-inflammatory state. Fractalkine ligand (CX_3CL1) binds to the corresponding fractalkine receptor (CX_3CR1) whose expression within the CNS is restricted to microglia (Harrison *et al.*, 1998). CX_3CL1 is constitutively expressed at high levels by neurons throughout the brain (Tarozzo *et al.*, 2003), and all microglia express the fractalkine receptor at relatively high levels (Wynne *et al.*, 2010). This widespread expression of both CX_3CL1 by neurons and CX_3CR1 on microglia indicates that fractalkine is an important immunomodulatory mechanism. In support of this idea, CX_3CR1 knockout mice have amplified and prolonged microglial activation following immune challenge (Cardona *et al.*, 2006; Corona *et al.*, 2010).

Several studies indicate reduced expression of CX_3CL1 mRNA and protein in the brain of aged rodents and humans (Wynne *et al.*, 2010; Bachstetter *et al.*, 2011; Fenn *et al.*, 2013). Central administration of CX_3CL1 attenuated the age-related increase in microglial activation and reversed the age-related decline in neurogenesis (Bachstetter *et al.*, 2011). Therefore, the alteration in fractalkine signaling during normal aging appears to be due to reduced levels of CX_3CL1. During an inflammatory challenge, however, the deficit in fractalkine regulation in the aged becomes twofold. Similar to CD200, microglia escape regulation by CX_3CL1 during an inflammatory challenge by downregulating CX_3CR1 (Wynne *et al.*, 2010). In aged mice, however, downregulation of CX_3CR1 was prolonged on microglia of aged mice compared to adult mice (Wynne *et al.*, 2010). This prolonged downregulation of CX_3CR1 corresponded with amplified and protracted expression of IL-1β and an extended sickness response. Taken together, reduced levels of CX_3CL1 and prolonged downregulation of CX_3CR1 can combine to severely impair fractalkine signaling in the aged brain, ultimately leading to a dysregulated microglial population.

TREM2 Regulation

Triggering receptor expressed on myeloid cells 2 (TREM2) is a recently identified transmembrane glycoprotein that can participate in the regulation of microglia. TREM2 has only recently been associated with general aging, but initially received attention for its role in genetic predisposition to Alzheimer's disease.

TREM2 expression is considered anti-inflammatory and may play a role in reducing microglial activation. For example, knockdown of TREM2 in cultured primary microglia significantly increased expression of inflammatory mediators including IL-12 and TNFα when microglia were co-cultured with apoptotic neurons (Takahashi et al., 2005). Related to our discussion of aging and Alzheimer's disease, exaggerated inflammatory cytokine production was coupled with a lower phagocytic capacity. Lentiviral-induced overexpression of TREM2 on primary microglia, however, significantly improved phagocytosis (Takahashi et al., 2005; Melchior et al., 2010). Thus, impairments in TREM2 may increase the risk for Alzheimer's disease because of improper clearance of amyloid-β and increased microglial activation (Jiang et al., 2013; Jonsson et al., 2013). TREM2 was recently identified as a gene that is significantly downregulated in microglia from aged mice (Hickman et al., 2013). This result indicates that loss of TREM2 expression is involved in both normal aging and neurodegenerative aging and may be a potential target of therapeutics for treatment of age-associated CNS complications.

Immune Regulation

In addition to neuronal and TREM2 regulation of microglia, anti-inflammatory immune regulation is also an important component to maintain an acute and directed inflammatory response. For example, in a normal inflammatory response, the same factors that induce transcription of inflammatory cytokines (e.g., IL-1β) will induce transcription of anti-inflammatory and regulatory mediators including interleukin-1 receptor antagonist (IL-1RA) and IL-10. In aging, it is proposed that both the expression and responsiveness to anti-inflammatory mediators are reduced.

In regards to immune regulation, it is important to discuss the different phenotypes that are induced by various immunomodulatory factors [for reviews see Mantovani et al. (2004), Mosser and Edwards (2008), and David and Kroner (2011)]. The two primary profiles are M1, or classically activated, and M2, or alternatively activated (Fig. 6.2). The M1 phenotype is induced by prototypic inflammatory stimuli and cytokines including LPS, IL-1β, interferon γ (IFN-γ), and TNFα. M1 cells are characterized by upregulation of TLR2 and TLR4 and expression of inflammatory cytokines including IL-1β, IL-6, and TNFα. The M2 phenotype is more complex and has been broken down into the M2a, M2b, and M2c profiles. An M2a, or alternative activation state, is induced by IL-4 or IL-13 and results in the upregulation of the arginase enzyme, chitinase-like receptor (Ym-1), antigen-presenting proteins (e.g., MHC II), and scavenger receptors including mannose receptor and scavenger receptor-A. M2a cells are associated with increased wound repair and the clearance of parasites. An M2b, or homeostatic phenotype, is induced by immune

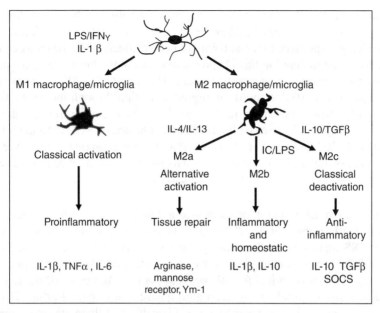

Figure 6.2 M1 and M2 microglial profiles. Microglial activation can be directed toward an M1, inflammatory state or an M2, reparative/anti-inflammatory state. The M2 phenotype can be further broken down into M2a, M2b, and M2c profiles. The stimuli that induce the M1, M2a, M2b, and M2c responses, the general roles these profiles perform, and the factors they produce are shown here.

complexes coupled with stimulation by a TLR ligand and produces high levels of both inflammatory (IL-1β) and anti-inflammatory (IL-10) cytokines. The M2c, or classical deactivation state, is induced by IL-10 and transforming growth factor beta (TGFβ) and is characterized by the lack of IL-1β expression and high IL-10 expression. These cells are important in the resolution of inflammation. A clear concept in the field of aging is that as an individual ages, these microglia phenotypes are skewed away from the M2a and M2c phenotypes toward an M1 or inflammatory phenotype (Ye and Johnson, 2001; Kumar *et al.*, 2012; Lee *et al.*, 1999). The cytokines affiliated with the M2a and M2c phenotypes and how they change with age are discussed in the following section.

IL-10–M2c

In the absence of an immune challenge, the aged brain has decreased anti-inflammatory IL-10 expression (Ye and Johnson, 2001). This is important because IL-10 has significant immunoregulatory effects in the brain (Murray, 2006). For example, direct administration of IL-10 into the brain suppressed cytokine-mediated sickness behavior (Bluthe *et al.*, 1999) and blocked IL-1β expression in the hippocampus after peripheral challenge with LPS (Lynch *et al.*, 1998). In IL-10-deficient mice, peripheral LPS challenge caused exaggerated neuroinflammation and prolonged sickness behavior compared to wild-type mice (Richwine *et al.*, 2009). Although there is pervasive support for a skew toward an M1 phenotype in microglia with age, it is also apparent that this may not always be the case. After an immune challenge, for example, microglia from aged mice release exaggerated levels of both IL-1β and IL-10 (Sierra *et al.*, 2007; Henry *et al.*,

2009). This increased IL-10 response, however, was not sufficient to restore homeostasis and inflammation persisted (Henry *et al.*, 2009; Fenn *et al.*, 2012). Recent evidence indicates that astrocytes are highly responsive to the anti-inflammatory effects of IL-10 (Norden *et al.*, 2014). Although not discussed in detail in this chapter, astrocytes in the brain are active participants in both propagating and regulating neuroinflammation (Farina *et al.*, 2007). For instance, primary astrocytes treated with IL-10 decreased microglial activation through increased TGFβ production (Norden *et al.*, 2014). Astrocytes in the aged brain have a more inflammatory phenotype (Zamanian *et al.*, 2012) with increased glial fibrillary acidic protein (GFAP) and vimentin expression (Godbout *et al.*, 2005). Therefore, current research is investigating astrocyte responsiveness to these inflammatory and anti-inflammatory signals and how this may be altered with age.

TGFβ–M2c

TGFβ is an anti-inflammatory cytokine expressed at low levels by both neurons and glial cells (Flanders *et al.*, 1991; Hamby *et al.*, 2010), and its expression is upregulated in response to a wide range of CNS insults and inflammatory challenges (Henrich-Noack *et al.*, 1996; Wynne *et al.*, 2010). TGFβ is an important regulator of microglia both during and after development. In recent studies, TGFβ was critical for microglia to populate the brain (Butovsky *et al.*, 2014) and identified as a strong regulator of microglial quiescence (Abutbul *et al.*, 2012; Butovsky *et al.*, 2014; Norden *et al.*, 2014). Therefore, it is plausible that there are impairments in TGFβ regulation of primed microglia in the aged brain. In support of this notion, comparison of the cytokine expression profile of brain tissue from immune-challenged aged and adult mice showed that TGFβ expression was increased after immune challenge only in adults (Wynne *et al.*, 2010; Tichauer *et al.*, 2013). This reduction in TGFβ could explain some of the hyperresponsiveness of aged microglia. For example, treatment with TGFβ in culture decreased IL-1β and increased CX$_3$CR1 expression in microglia (Wynne *et al.*, 2010). This finding provides a possible link between impaired TGFβ upregulation and prolonged downregulation of CX$_3$CR1.

In addition to impaired upregulation of TGFβ following immune challenge, microglia from aged mice are also less sensitive to TGFβ. A recent study found that microglia isolated from aged mice had deceased expression of TGFβ receptor compared to adults (Hickman *et al.*, 2013). Furthermore, microglial cultures established from aged mice were less sensitive to the anti-inflammatory effects of TGFβ compared to microglia from adult mice (Rozovsky *et al.*, 1998). Finally, when microglia were isolated from LPS-injected adult and aged mice, only microglia from adult mice were responsive to TGFβ treatment *ex vivo* (Tichauer *et al.*, 2013). These studies provide strong support that TGFβ-mediated regulation of microglia becomes impaired with age.

Impaired regulation of microglia by TGFβ is significant in both normal aging and age-associated neurodegenerative diseases such as Alzheimer's disease. During Alzheimer's disease, there is impaired clearance of neurotoxic amyloid-β plaques. Specifically, microglial clearance of amyloid-β plaques is impaired in aging and Alzheimer's disease (Floden and Combs, 2011). Under normal conditions, TGFβ signaling in microglia promotes an anti-inflammatory microglial phenotype that is highly phagocytic (Wyss-Coray *et al.*, 2001; Tichauer *et al.*, 2013). In aged mice, however, microglia are less sensitive to TGFβ and do not increase phagocytosis following TGFβ treatment (Tichauer *et al.*, 2013). Overall, impaired regulation of microglia by TGFβ may promote microglial priming and decrease the phagocytic efficiency of aged microglia.

IL-4–M2a

In addition to classical IL-10- and TGFβ-mediated regulation, there is increasing support for regulation of microglia by the alternative-activation (M2a) cytokine IL-4. A primary problem associated with aging is the reduction in memory and learning and general cognition. These age-associated deficits have been connected with impaired long-term potentiation (LTP) in the hippocampus (Pang and Lu, 2004; Maher *et al.*, 2005). Importantly, age-associated reductions in LTP coincide with hippocampal elevations of IL-1β and reductions in IL-4 (Cunningham *et al.*, 2009; Vereker *et al.*, 2000; Maher *et al.*, 2004, 2005; Nolan *et al.*, 2005; Loane *et al.*, 2009). Pharmacological induction of IL-4 in the hippocampus by Rosiglitazone reduced IL-1β and enhanced LTP in aged rats (Loane *et al.*, 2009; Cowley *et al.*, 2012), indicating that IL-4 may have a role in maintaining LTP and regulating the inflammatory status of the brain. In support of this notion, IL-4-deficient mice had elevated CNS inflammation and reduced learning and memory in a Morris Water maze paradigm (Derecki *et al.*, 2010).

Deficits in IL-4 signaling with age may go beyond impairments in IL-4 protein. A recent study showed that the ligand-binding receptor for IL-4, interleukin-4 receptor alpha (IL-4Rα), was reduced in the aged brain after an inflammatory challenge. In this study, a peripheral injection of LPS increased IL-4Rα expression on the surface of microglia in adult mice, but not in aged mice (Fenn *et al.*, 2012). Moreover, when LPS-activated microglia were isolated from adult and aged mice and treated *ex vivo* with IL-4, aged microglia were less sensitive to IL-4 and failed to reduce inflammatory-associated iNOS or induce the M2a factor arginase (Fenn *et al.*, 2012). Another study showed that following intrahippocampal injections of IL-4/IL-13, age mice had reduced expression of IL-4/IL-13-driven gene transcripts including FIZZ1 and IGF-1 compared to adult mice given the same injection. Expression of inflammatory-driven genes, however, was maintained in aged mice given an intrahippocampal injection of TNFα, IL-12, and IL-1β (Lee *et al.*, 1999). This study indicates that responsiveness to IL-4 may be selectively inhibited in the brain of aged mice.

Impaired responsiveness to IL-4 may be critical in the context of CNS injury. IL-4 is increased acutely after CNS trauma (Lee *et al.*, 2013; Guerrero *et al.*, 2012) and contributes to the high level of M2a responsiveness observed following injury. This M2a response is primarily characterized by the induction of arginase, which is thought to participate in endogenous repair (Wu and Morris, 1998; Barbul, 2008) and increase axonal growth and survival (Cai *et al.*, 2002). Therefore, reduced IL-4 sensitivity may lead to dampened repair and growth-supportive processes in the aged. In support of this idea, aged mice given a traumatic brain injury had reduced arginase expression, which corresponded with enhanced inflammatory gene expression, increased lesion size, and more functional deficits compared to adult mice (Kumar *et al.*, 2012). Therefore, enhancing the M2a responsiveness of microglia from aged mice may be one way to boost repair after CNS trauma and limit age-associated morbidity and mortality.

MicroRNA Regulation of the Aged CNS

A new player in the modulation of inflammation has recently arisen, microRNAs (miRs). miRs are short (19–22 nt) noncoding strands of RNA that can bind to and inhibit the translation of mRNAs (Lagos-Quintana *et al.*, 2001). Although most miRs associated with the inflammatory and immune response have been investigated in the context of peripheral inflammation, new studies have elucidated the important role of miRs in regulating CNS inflammation (Fig. 6.1).

miR-124

miR-124 is expressed at higher levels in the brain than in the periphery and is expressed in monocytes (microglia/macrophage precursors) (Cheng *et al.*, 2009; Ponomarev *et al.*, 2011). A recent study showed that if peripheral macrophages were transfected with exogenous miR-124, they became more "microglia-like" with reduced MHC II and CD45 expression (Ponomarev *et al.*, 2011). Moreover, peripheral induction of miR-124 was able to arrest macrophage and microglial activation in a model of experimental autoimmune encephalomyelitis and reduce disease pathology (Ponomarev *et al.*, 2011). This study was paramount in demonstrating that a CNS-specific phenotype can be induced by the upregulation of a single miR.

Some studies have suggested that miR-124 is reduced in the brain with age (Inukai *et al.*, 2012). Interestingly, IL-4/IL-13 pathways can induce miR-124 (Veremeyko *et al.*, 2013), suggesting that immune and miR regulatory system deficits may be closely connected in the aged brain. Altered miR-124 expression in microglia may partially explain why microglia in the aged brain become more MHC II$^+$ and take on phenotypic characteristics that are normally associated with peripheral macrophages, including a higher capacity to produce inflammatory cytokines (Ponomarev *et al.*, 2011). It is important to note that not all studies have found this age-associated decrease in miR-124 expression (Fenn *et al.*, 2013). This may be attributed to site-specific microglia priming with aging. Aging is associated with a 10–25% increase in the percentage of MHC II$^+$ cells that are considered primed or hyperreactive (Henry *et al.*, 2009). Thus, a change in miR-124 expression may only occur in this small microglia subpopulation, and gross analysis in whole brain may miss this small change (Lagos-Quintana *et al.*, 2002). Future studies examining miR-124-specific decreases in a brain-region-dependent manner are important.

miR-29

Another miR that has received attention in the field of aging is miR-29. Previous studies have demonstrated that the miR-29a/b-1 cluster is upregulated in immune cells after activation and acts as a negative regulator to suppress IFN-γ production by Th1 cells (Steiner *et al.*, 2011). Importantly, the actions of miR-29 may be dysregulated in chronic inflammatory diseases and in the aged (Smith *et al.*, 2012; Fenn *et al.*, 2013).

miR-29 is normally expressed within the CNS (Hebert *et al.*, 2008) and has been found in high levels within CNS-resident glia (Lau *et al.*, 2008; Fenn *et al.*, 2013; Ouyang *et al.*, 2013). One of the most noted changes within the brain of patients with Alzheimer's disease is the upregulation of BACE1 beta-secretase expression (Hebert *et al.*, 2008), which is associated with increased cleavage of amyloid precursor protein and the aggregation of amyloid-beta fibrils. miR-29 was found to strongly inhibit BACE1 expression *in vitro* and is markedly downregulated in patients with sporadic Alzheimer's disease (Hebert *et al.*, 2008; Shioya *et al.*, 2010). Surprisingly, the opposite was found for normal nonpathologic aging. The expression of miR-29a/b-1 was increased in the brain of aged mice and humans in the absence of neurodegenerative disease (Fenn *et al.*, 2013). This increase in miR-29a/b-1 in the aged could contribute to impaired microglial regulation and increased inflammation within the aged brain due to its targeting of CX$_3$CL1 and insulin-like growth factor (IGF)-1 (Fenn *et al.*, 2013), two microglial regulators. The discrepancy between miR-29 expression in Alzheimer's disease and normal aging is intriguing and may suggest a differential brain response during normal aging compared to active neurodegeneration.

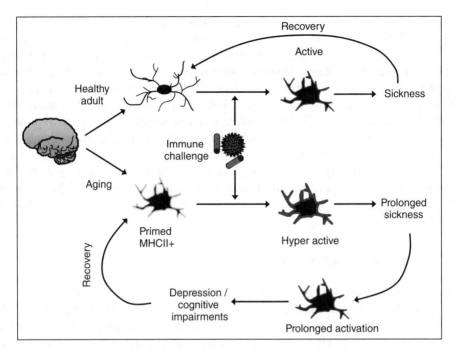

Figure 6.3   Age-associated cognitive impairments and depression result from a hyperinflammatory response by primed microglia. In normal, healthy adults, activation of the immune system by an infection or stressor results in activation of brain-resident microglia, the release of inflammatory cytokines into the CNS, and a short period of sickness (e.g., fever, lethargy, social withdrawal, and reduced appetite). Within a short period of time, however, active microglia return to a ramified and anti-inflammatory state. In the aged, however, microglia are primed at baseline. Following the same immune challenge as was experienced by adults, the primed microglia become hyperreactive and release exaggerated levels of inflammatory cytokines into the CNS. This results in a period of prolonged sickness behavior, sustained inflammation within the CNS, and the induction of neuropsychiatric complications including cognitive impairments and depression.

Immune Reactivity of Glia Contributes to Cognitive and Behavioral Deficits

Microglia priming as characterized by exaggerated inflammatory cytokine production may lead to more severe long-lasting behavioral complications in the aged. For instance, prolonged exposure to cytokines such as IL-1β and IL-6 is accompanied by behavioral complications including prolonged sickness response, depression, and cognitive impairments as shown in Fig. 6.3.

Neurodegenerative Diseases

Increased microglial priming and inflammation in the aged brain are also involved in the pathophysiology of several neurodegenerative diseases. For example, both prion disease (transmissible spongiform encephalopathies) and Alzheimer's disease show marked microglial priming associated with an increased inflammatory status of the CNS. In concert with increasing microglial activation within the hippocampus, Alzheimer's disease is characterized by a precipitous loss in cognitive function and memory (Cagnin *et al.*, 2001). Moreover, patients with Alzheimer's disease are more likely to develop psychiatric complications including depression. In a clinical study, over 75% of patients with suspected Alzheimer's disease had symptoms of depression, including apathy (Craig *et al.*, 2005), and researchers proposed that a heightened CNS inflammatory milieu was to blame. In support of this idea, challenges that activate the immune response worsen cognitive impairments and depressive symptoms in murine models of prion disease and Alzheimer's disease. For example, both central and peripheral immune challenge exacerbated brain inflammation (IL-1β and iNOS) and neuronal death in a model of prion disease (Cunningham *et al.*, 1996), and systemic challenge with LPS caused a significant increase in CNS IL-1β in transgenic Alzheimer's disease mice compared to nontransgenic controls (Sly *et al.*, 2001). The priming of microglia and their hyperactivation under inflammatory conditions may contribute to or even amplify the neurodegenerative processes of prion and Alzheimer's disease, making microglial priming an important research focus in the field of neurodegeneration (Lucin and Wyss-Coray, 2009).

Reduced Cognition as a Function of Age

Excessive or prolonged exposure to inflammatory cytokines in the brain also abrogates neuronal plasticity, resulting in cognitive impairments in aged individuals in the absence of neurodegenerative disease. For instance, increased neuroinflammation has negative effects on neurogenesis, dendritic restructuring, and LTP. With normal, nonpathologic aging, elevated neuroinflammation is associated with a steady decrease in the ability for pyramidal neurons in the granule layer of the CA1 and dentate gyrus of the hippocampus to support LTP (Lynch, 2004; Maher *et al.*, 2005). Lowering hippocampal IL-1β signaling by minocycline treatment, IL-1 receptor antagonists, or IL-4 partially rescued this impairment in LTP, indicating that lowering inflammation by inhibiting microglial activity has beneficial effects on LTP.

Age-associated declines in cognition may also result from a reduction in synaptic connections (Dickson *et al.*, 1995; Peters *et al.*, 2008; VanGuilder *et al.*, 2010). Increased synaptic connectivity is reliant on the appropriate expression and signaling of several neurotrophic factors, so called because they improve the function, growth, and survival of neurons. Of the known neurotrophins, brain-derived neurotrophic factor (BDNF) and IGF-1 have been extensively studied in the context of age and inflammation. Studies have shown that IGF-1 is significantly reduced in the aged brain, both in humans and in rodents (Sonntag *et al.*, 2005; Deak and Sonntag, 2012), but that expression of BDNF and the receptor for BDNF, TrkB, remained unchanged or are increased with advanced age (Hellweg *et al.*, 1990; Lapchak *et al.*, 1993).

Reduced IGF-1 in the aged brain is associated with reduced cognition in a host of studies. For example, intracerebroventricular injection of IGF-1 into aged rats significantly improved working memory compared to vehicle controls (Markowska *et al.*, 1998) and also improved neurogenesis (Lichtenwalner *et al.*, 2001). As mentioned earlier, a possible explanation for reduced brain IGF-1 may be increased inflammatory-associated miR-29a/b-1 in microglia. As IGF-1 can also moderate the inflammatory response of microglia (Dodge *et al.*, 2008; O'Connor *et al.*, 2008), inflammatory-induced reductions in IGF-1 would only potentiate more inflammation, creating a caustic cycle of enhanced microglia activation.

Although BDNF levels were not altered in the normal aged brain, following an inflammatory challenge, aged rats had significantly reduced BDNF expression compared to adults (Cortese *et al.*, 2011). Thus, the most significant reductions in age-associated cognition could occur after an immune challenge when multiple neurotrophic factors are suppressed.

Reduced Cognition and Increased Depression in the Aged After an Immune Challenge

Cognition

Work in basic science models of aging and inflammation indicates that impaired cognition in the aged may result from a hyperactive inflammatory response following an immune challenge. Thus, aged persons may show the most overt signs of cognitive impairment during, or in the aftermath of, sickness or stress (Fig. 6.3). In support of this notion, studies have shown that aged mice have no impairments in learning and memory at baseline, but following an acute immune challenge, memory impairments were significant compared to adults (Chen *et al.*, 2008; Barrientos *et al.*, 2009a, 2009b). If aged mice were supplemented with a diet high in resveratrol, a potent anti-inflammatory agent, then LPS-induced IL-1β levels were significantly reduced and learning and memory was restored (Abraham and Johnson, 2009).

Within the clinical literature, systemic infection is also closely associated with cognitive impairment in the elderly. For example, a study performed on nondemented patients older than the age of 70 years showed that increased circulating concentrations of C-reactive protein and TNFα negatively correlated with cognitive performance in semantic memory and visuospatial tests (Arfanakis *et al.*, 2013). Moreover, a study evaluating the rate of acute cognitive impairment in nursing hospital patients submitted to the emergency room identified that acute cognitive impairment was diagnosed in over 40% of individuals diagnosed with an acute infection, whereas only 10% of individuals had cognitive impairment if treated for cardiovascular disease (Wofford *et al.*, 1996). In further support, a recent study found that compared to older individuals without hospitalization, those who had been hospitalized for a noncritical illness had a significantly greater risk for developing long-term cognitive decline (Ehlenbach *et al.*, 2010). Thus, active infection resulting in an exaggerated neuroinflammatory response may underlie the majority of cognitive decline observed in the elderly (Fig. 6.3).

Depression

In addition to cognitive impairments, mood and depressive symptoms are also common in elderly patients. From clinical and laboratory studies of depression, a causative relationship between inflammatory cytokines and depression has been proposed. For example, it is estimated that 15–30% of the elderly develop a depressive disorder associated with disease or illness (Mulsant and Ganguli, 1999). Elderly patients who experienced a prolonged inflammatory response to influenza vaccinations also had a higher incidence of mild depressive symptoms (Glaser *et al.*, 2003). Further support for a role of inflammation in depression is evident from clinical studies where depressed patients had higher levels of IL-6 and IL-1β in their cerebrospinal fluid (Dentino *et al.*, 1999; Penninx *et al.*, 2003). Furthermore, there was a correlation between increased inflammatory cytokine expression and the severity of the depressive symptoms (Dentino *et al.*, 1999). Overall, these findings suggest that a prolonged neuroinflammatory response in the elderly may have a profound effect on depression.

Evidence from rodent models supports this hypothesis. In aged mice, an immune challenge lead to a prolonged and exaggerated sickness response characterized by protracted anorexia, lethargy, social withdrawal, and febrile response (Godbout *et al.*, 2005; Abraham *et al.*, 2008; Barrientos *et al.*, 2009a, 2009b). Central administration of an IL-1 receptor antagonist, however, rescued these age-associated behaviors (Abraham and Johnson, 2008). This finding suggests that the exaggerated sickness response in aged rodents was likely caused by the exaggerated and prolonged production of IL-1β by primed microglia. In addition to a prolonged sickness response, aged mice also developed depressive-like behavior following immune challenge. To evaluate the depressive state of rodents, resignation behavior is determined in the tail suspension test (TST) and forced swim test (FST). Protracted depressive-like behavior in the TST and FST was evident in aged but not adult mice after acute (Godbout *et al.*, 2008) and chronic (Kelley *et al.*, 2013) immune challenge. These results from rodent models support clinical findings in which elderly patients exposed to infection or illness have an increased frequency of behavioral complications including depression compared to younger adults with similar peripheral insults.

Conclusions

Aging results in the loss of integrated regulatory systems designed to maintain microglia in a surveying and anti-inflammatory state. Loss of these regulatory pathways does not come from a single source, but instead represents a global loss in regulation from neurons, astrocytes, miRs, and autocrine immune mediators. As a result, microglia in the aged brain develop a primed phenotype and become hyperinflammatory following challenge to the immune system. An exaggerated and prolonged microglial response promotes the development of neuropsychiatric complications including depression and cognitive decline. Moreover, this hyperinflammatory response can precipitate or contribute to the development of neurodegenerative diseases. Thus, efforts to restore proper microglia regulation and function may be the key to successful CNS aging.

References

Abraham, J., Jang, S., Godbout, J.P. *et al.* (2008) Aging sensitizes mice to behavioral deficits induced by central HIV-1 gp120. *Neurobiology of Aging*, **29**, 614–621.

Abraham, J. & Johnson, R.W. (2008) Central inhibition of interleukin-1beta ameliorates sickness behavior in aged mice. *Brain, Behavior, and Immunity*, **22** (3), 396–401.

Abraham, J. & Johnson, R.W. (2009) Consuming a diet supplemented with resveratrol reduced infection-related neuroinflammation and deficits in working memory in aged mice. *Rejuvenation Research*, **12**, 445–453.

Abutbul, S., Shapiro, J., Szaingurten-Solodkin, I. *et al.* (2012) TGF-beta signaling through SMAD2/3 induces the quiescent microglial phenotype within the CNS environment. *Glia*, **60**, 1160–1171.

Ajami, B., Bennett, J.L., Krieger, C., Tetzlaff, W. & Rossi, F.M. (2007) Local self-renewal can sustain CNS microglia maintenance and function throughout adult life. *Nature Neuroscience*, **10**, 1538–1543.

Arfanakis, K., Fleischman, D.A., Grisot, G. *et al.* (2013) Systemic inflammation in non-demented elderly human subjects: brain microstructure and cognition. *PLoS ONE*, **8**, e73107.

Bachstetter, A.D., Morganti, J.M., Jernberg, J. *et al.* (2011) Fractalkine and CX 3 CR1 regulate hippocampal neurogenesis in adult and aged rats. *Neurobiology of Aging*, **32**, 2030–2044.

Barbul, A. (2008) Proline precursors to sustain mammalian collagen synthesis. *Journal of Nutrition*, **138**, 2021S–2024S.

Barrientos, R.M., Frank, M.G., Hein, A.M. *et al.* (2009a) Time course of hippocampal IL-1 beta and memory consolidation impairments in aging rats following peripheral infection. *Brain, Behavior, and Immunity*, **23**, 46–54.

Barrientos, R.M., Higgins, E.A., Biedenkapp, J.C. *et al.* (2006) Peripheral infection and aging interact to impair hippocampal memory consolidation. *Neurobiology of Aging*, **27**, 723–732.

Barrientos, R.M., Watkins, L.R., Rudy, J.W. & Maier, S.F. (2009b) Characterization of the sickness response in young and aging rats following E. coli infection. *Brain, Behavior, and Immunity*, **23**, 450–454.

Bernheim, H.A. & Kluger, M.J. (1976) Fever: effect of drug-induced antipyresis on survival. *Science*, **193**, 237–239.

Biber, K., Neumann, H., Inoue, K. & Boddeke, H.W. (2007) Neuronal 'On' and 'Off' signals control microglia. *Trends in Neurosciences*, **30**, 596–602.

Bluthe, R.M., Castanon, N., Pousset, F. *et al.* (1999) Central injection of IL-10 antagonizes the behavioural effects of lipopolysaccharide in rats. *Psychoneuroendocrinology*, **24**, 301–311.

Broderick, C., Hoek, R.M., Forrester, J.V., Liversidge, J., Sedgwick, J.D. & Dick, A.D. (2002) Constitutive retinal CD200 expression regulates resident microglia and activation state of inflammatory cells during experimental autoimmune uveoretinitis. *American Journal of Pathology*, **161**, 1669–1677.

Butovsky, O., Jedrychowski, M.P., Moore, C.S. *et al.* (2014) Identification of a unique TGF-beta-dependent molecular and functional signature in microglia. *Nature Neuroscience*, **17**, 131–143.

Cagnin, A., Brooks, D.J., Kennedy, A.M. *et al.* (2001) In-vivo measurement of activated microglia in dementia. *Lancet*, **358**, 461.

Cai, D., Deng, K., Mellado, W., Lee, J., Ratan, R.R. & Filbin, M.T. (2002) Arginase I and polyamines act downstream from cyclic AMP in overcoming inhibition of axonal growth MAG and myelin in vitro. *Neuron*, **35**, 711.

Cardona, A.E., Pioro, E.P., Sasse, M.E. *et al.* (2006) Control of microglial neurotoxicity by the fractalkine receptor. *Nature Neuroscience*, **9**, 917–924.

Chen, J., Buchanan, J.B., Sparkman, N.L., Godbout, J.P., Freund, G.G. & Johnson, R.W. (2008) Neuroinflammation and disruption in working memory in aged mice after acute stimulation of the peripheral innate immune system. *Brain, Behavior, and Immunity*, **22**, 301–311.

Cheng, L.C., Pastrana, E., Tavazoie, M. & Doetsch, F. (2009) miR-124 regulates adult neurogenesis in the subventricular zone stem cell niche. *Nature Neuroscience*, **12**, 399–408.

Corona, A.W., Huang, Y., O'Connor, J.C. *et al.* (2010) Fractalkine receptor (CX3CR1) deficiency sensitizes mice to the behavioral changes induced by lipopolysaccharide. *Journal of Neuroinflammation*, **7**, 93.

Cortese, G.P., Barrientos, R.M., Maier, S.F. & Patterson, S.L. (2011) Aging and a peripheral immune challenge interact to reduce mature brain-derived neurotrophic factor and activation of TrkB, PLCgamma1, and ERK in hippocampal synaptoneurosomes. *Journal of Neuroscience*, **31**, 4274–4279.

Costello, D.A., Lyons, A., Denieffe, S., Browne, T.C., Cox, F.F. & Lynch, M.A. (2011) Long term potentiation is impaired in membrane glycoprotein CD200-deficient mice: a role for Toll-like receptor activation. *Journal of Biological Chemistry*, **286**, 34722–34732.

Cowley, T.R., O'Sullivan, J., Blau, C. *et al.* (2012) Rosiglitazone attenuates the age-related changes in astrocytosis and the deficit in LTP. *Neurobiology of Aging*, **33**, 162–175.

Cox, F.F., Carney, D., Miller, A.M. & Lynch, M.A. (2011) CD200 fusion protein decreases microglial activation in the hippocampus of aged rats. *Brain, Behavior, and Immunity*, **26** (5), 789–796.

Craig, D., Mirakhur, A., Hart, D.J., McIlroy, S.P. & Passmore, A.P. (2005) A cross-sectional study of neuropsychiatric symptoms in 435 patients with Alzheimer's disease. *American Journal of Geriatric Psychiatry*, **13**, 460–468.

Cunningham, C., Campion, S., Lunnon, K. *et al.* (2009) Systemic inflammation induces acute behavioral and cognitive changes and accelerates neurodegenerative disease. *Biological Psychiatry*, **65**, 304.

Cunningham, A.J., Murray, C.A., O'Neill, L.A., Lynch, M.A. & O'Connor, J.J. (1996) Interleukin-1 beta (IL-1 beta) and tumour necrosis factor (TNF) inhibit long-term potentiation in the rat dentate gyrus in vitro. *Neuroscience Letters*, **203**, 17–20.

Dantzer, R., O'Connor, J.C., Freund, G.G., Johnson, R.W. & Kelley, K.W. (2008) From inflammation to sickness and depression: when the immune system subjugates the brain. *Nature Reviews Neuroscience*, **9**, 46–56.

David, S. & Kroner, A. (2011) Repertoire of microglial and macrophage responses after spinal cord injury. *Nature Reviews Neuroscience*, **12**, 388–399.

Deak, F. & Sonntag, W.E. (2012) Aging, synaptic dysfunction, and insulin-like growth factor (IGF)-1. *Journals of Gerontology Series A, Biological Sciences and Medical Sciences*, **67**, 611–625.

Deckert, M., Sedgwick, J.D., Fischer, E. & Schluter, D. (2006) Regulation of microglial cell responses in murine Toxoplasma encephalitis by CD200/CD200 receptor interaction. *Acta Neuropathologica*, **111**, 548–558.

Denieffe, S., Kelly, R.J., McDonald, C., Lyons, A. & Lynch, M.A. (2013) Classical activation of microglia in CD200-deficient mice is a consequence of blood brain barrier permeability and infiltration of peripheral cells. *Brain, Behavior, and Immunity*, **34**, 86–97.

Dentino, A.N., Pieper, C.F., Rao, M.K. *et al.* (1999) Association of interleukin-6 and other biologic variables with depression in older people living in the community. *Journal of the American Geriatrics Society*, **47**, 6–11.

Derecki, N.C., Cardani, A.N., Yang, C.H. *et al.* (2010) Regulation of learning and memory by meningeal immunity: a key role for IL-4. *Journal of Experimental Medicine*, **207**, 1067–1080.

Dickson, D.W., Crystal, H.A., Bevona, C., Honer, W., Vincent, I. & Davies, P. (1995) Correlations of synaptic and pathological markers with cognition of the elderly. *Neurobiology of Aging*, **16**, 285.

Dodge, J.C., Haidet, A.M., Yang, W. *et al.* (2008) Delivery of AAV-IGF-1 to the CNS extends survival in ALS mice through modification of aberrant glial cell activity. *Molecular Therapy*, **16**, 1056–1064.

Downer, E.J., Cowley, T.R., Cox, F. *et al.* (2009) A synthetic NCAM-derived mimetic peptide, FGL, exerts anti-inflammatory properties via IGF-1 and interferon-gamma modulation. *Journal of Neurochemistry*, **109**, 1516–1525.

Downer, E.J., Cowley, T.R., Lyons, A. *et al.* (2010) A novel anti-inflammatory role of NCAM-derived mimetic peptide, FGL. *Neurobiology of Aging*, **31**, 118–128.

Ehlenbach, W.J., Hough, C.L., Crane, P.K. *et al.* (2010) Association between acute care and critical illness hospitalization and cognitive function in older adults. *JAMA*, **303**, 763.

Farina, C., Aloisi, F. & Meinl, E. (2007) Astrocytes are active players in cerebral innate immunity. *Trends in Immunology*, **28**, 138–145.

Fenn, A.M., Henry, C.J., Huang, Y., Dugan, A. & Godbout, J.P. (2012) Lipopolysaccharide-induced interleukin (IL)-4 receptor-alpha expression and corresponding sensitivity to the M2 promoting effects of IL-4 are impaired in microglia of aged mice. *Brain, Behavior, and Immunity*, **26**, 766–777.

Fenn, A.M., Smith, K.M., Lovett-Racke, A.E., Guerau-de-Arellano, M., Whitacre, C.C. & Godbout, J.P. (2013) Increased micro-RNA 29b in the aged brain correlates with the reduction of insulin-like growth factor-1 and fractalkine ligand. *Neurobiology of Aging*, **34**, 2748–2758.

Finch, C.E. & Crimmins, E.M. (2004) Inflammatory exposure and historical changes in human life-spans. *Science*, **305**, 1736–1739.

Flanders, K.C., Ludecke, G., Engels, S. *et al.* (1991) Localization and actions of transforming growth factor-beta s in the embryonic nervous system. *Development*, **113**, 183–191.

Floden, A.M. & Combs, C.K. (2011) Microglia demonstrate age-dependent interaction with amyloid-beta fibrils. *Journal of Alzheimer's Disease*, **25**, 279–293.

Frank, M.G., Barrientos, R.M., Biedenkapp, J.C., Rudy, J.W., Watkins, L.R. & Maier, S.F. (2006) mRNA up-regulation of MHC II and pivotal pro-inflammatory genes in normal brain aging. *Neurobiology of Aging*, **27**, 717–722.

Ginhoux, F., Greter, M., Leboeuf, M. *et al.* (2010) Fate mapping analysis reveals that adult microglia derive from primitive macrophages. *Science*, **330**, 841–845.

Glaser, R., Robles, T.F., Sheridan, J., Malarkey, W.B. & Kiecolt-Glaser, J.K. (2003) Mild depressive symptoms are associated with amplified and prolonged inflammatory responses after influenza virus vaccination in older adults. *Archives of General Psychiatry*, **60**, 1009–1014.

Godbout, J.P., Chen, J., Abraham, J. *et al.* (2005) Exaggerated neuroinflammation and sickness behavior in aged mice following activation of the peripheral innate immune system. *FASEB Journal*, **19**, 1329–1331.

Godbout, J.P. & Johnson, R.W. (2004) Interleukin-6 in the aging brain. *Journal of Neuroimmunology*, **147**, 141–144.

Godbout, J.P., Moreau, M., Lestage, J. *et al.* (2008) Aging exacerbates depressive-like behavior in mice in response to activation of the peripheral innate immune system. *Neuropsychopharmacology*, **33**, 2341–2351.

Guerrero, A., Uchida, K., Nakajima, H. *et al.* (2012) Blockade of interleukin-6 signaling inhibits the classic pathway and promotes an alternative pathway of macrophage activation after spinal cord injury in mice. *Journal of Neuroinflammation*, **9**, 1–16.

Hamby, M.E., Hewett, J.A. & Hewett, S.J. (2010) Smad3-dependent signaling underlies the TGF-beta1-mediated enhancement in astrocytic iNOS expression. *Glia*, **58**, 1282–1291.

Harrison, J.K., Jiang, Y., Chen, S. *et al.* (1998) Role for neuronally derived fractalkine in mediating interactions between neurons and CX3CR1-expressing microglia. *Proceedings of the National Academy of Sciences of the United States of America*, **95**, 10896–10901.

Hebert, S.S., Horre, K., Nicolai, L. *et al.* (2008) Loss of microRNA cluster miR-29a/b-1 in sporadic Alzheimer's disease correlates with increased BACE1/beta-secretase expression. *Proceedings of the National Academy of Sciences of the United States of America*, **105**, 6415–6420.

Hellweg, R., Fischer, W., Hock, C., Gage, F.H., Bjorklund, A. & Thoenen, H (1990) Nerve growth factor levels and choline acetyltransferase activity in the brain of aged rats with spatial memory impairments. *Brain Research*, **537**, 123–130.

Henrich-Noack, P., Prehn, J.H. & Krieglstein, J. (1996) TGF-beta 1 protects hippocampal neurons against degeneration caused by transient global ischemia. Dose-response relationship and potential neuroprotective mechanisms. *Stroke*, **27**, 1609–1614.; discussion 1615

Henry, C.J., Huang, Y., Wynne, A.M. & Godbout, J.P. (2009) Peripheral lipopolysaccharide (LPS) challenge promotes microglial hyperactivity in aged mice that is associated with exaggerated induction of both pro-inflammatory IL-1beta and anti-inflammatory IL-10 cytokines. *Brain, Behavior, and Immunity*, **23**, 309–317.

Hickman, S.E., Kingery, N.D., Ohsumi, T.K. *et al.* (2013) The microglial sensome revealed by direct RNA sequencing. *Nature Neuroscience*, **16**, 1896–1905.

Hoeijmakers, J.H. (2009) DNA damage, aging, and cancer. *New England Journal of Medicine*, **361**, 1475–1485.

Hoek, R.M., Ruuls, S.R., Murphy, C.A. *et al.* (2000) Down-regulation of the macrophage lineage through interaction with OX2 (CD200). *Science*, **290**, 1768–1771.

Inukai, S., de Lencastre, A., Turner, M. & Slack, F. (2012) Novel microRNAs differentially expressed during aging in the mouse brain. *PLoS ONE*, **7**, e40028.

Jiang, T., Yu, J.-T., Zhu, X.-C. & Tan, L. (2013) TREM2 in Alzheimer's disease. *Molecular Neurobiology*, **48**, 180–185.

Jonsson, T., Stefansson, H., Steinberg, S. *et al.* (2013) Variant of TREM2 associated with the risk of Alzheimer's disease. *New England Journal of Medicine*, **368**, 107–116.

Kelley, K.W., O'Connor, J.C., Lawson, M.A., Dantzer, R., Rodriguez-Zas, S.L. & McCusker, R.H. (2013) Aging leads to prolonged duration of inflammation-induced depression-like behavior caused by Bacillus Calmette-Guerin. *Brain, Behavior, and Immunity*, **32**, 63–69.

Kumar, A., Stoica, B.A., Sabirzhanov, B., Burns, M.P., Faden, A.I. & Loane, D.J. (2012) Traumatic brain injury in aged animals increases lesion size and chronically alters microglial/macrophage classical and alternative activation states. *Neurobiology of Aging*, **34**, 1397.

Lagos-Quintana, M., Rauhut, R., Lendeckel, W. & Tuschl, T. (2001) Identification of novel genes coding for small expressed RNAs. *Science*, **294**, 853–858.

Lagos-Quintana, M., Rauhut, R., Yalcin, A., Meyer, J., Lendeckel, W. & Tuschl, T. (2002) Identification of tissue-specific microRNAs from mouse. *Current Biology*, **12**, 735.

Lapchak, P.A., Araujo, D.M., Beck, K.D., Finch, C.E., Johnson, S.A. & Hefti, F. (1993) BDNF and trkB mRNA expression in the hippocampal formation of aging rats. *Neurobiology of Aging*, **14**, 121–126.

Lau, P., Verrier, J.D., Nielsen, J.A., Johnson, K.R., Notterpek, L. & Hudson, L.D. (2008) Identification of dynamically regulated microRNA and mRNA networks in developing oligodendrocytes. *Journal of Neuroscience*, **28**, 11720–11730.

Lee, S.I., Jeong, S.R., Kang, Y.M. *et al.* (2010) Endogenous expression of interleukin-4 regulates macrophage activation and confines cavity formation after traumatic spinal cord injury. *Journal of Neuroscience Research*, **88**, 2409.

Lee, C.K., Klopp, R.G., Weindruch, R. & Prolla, T.A. (1999) Gene expression profile of aging and its retardation by caloric restriction. *Science*, **285**, 1390–1393.

Lee, D.C., Ruiz, C.R., Lebson, L. *et al.* (2013) Aging enhances classical activation but mitigates alternative activation in the central nervous system. *Neurobiology of Aging*, **34**, 1610–1620.

Lichtenwalner, R.J., Forbes, M.E., Bennett, S.A., Lynch, C.D., Sonntag, W.E. & Riddle, D.R. (2001) Intracerebroventricular infusion of insulin-like growth factor-I ameliorates the age-related decline in hippocampal neurogenesis. *Neuroscience*, **107**, 603.

Loane, D.J., Deighan, B.F., Clarke, R.M., Griffin, R.J., Lynch, A.M. & Lynch, M.A. (2009) Interleukin-4 mediates the neuroprotective effects of rosiglitazone in the aged brain. *Neurobiology of Aging*, **30**, 920–931.

Lucin, K.M. & Wyss-Coray, T. (2009) Immune activation in brain aging and neurodegeneration: too much or too little? *Neuron*, **64**, 110–122.

Lull, M.E. & Block, M.L. (2010) Microglial activation and chronic neurodegeneration. *Neurotherapeutics*, **7**, 354–365.

Lynch, M.A. (1998) Analysis of the mechanisms underlying the age-related impairment in long-term potentiation in the rat. *Reviews in the Neurosciences*, **9**, 169–201.

Lynch, A.M., Walsh, C., Delaney, A., Nolan, Y., Campbell, V.A. & Lynch, M.A. (2004) Lipopolysaccharide-induced increase in signalling in hippocampus is abrogated by IL-10--a role for IL-1 beta? *Journal of Neurochemistry*, **88**, 635–646.

Lyons, A., Downer, E.J., Crotty, S., Nolan, Y.M., Mills, K.H. & Lynch, M.A. (2007) CD200 ligand receptor interaction modulates microglial activation in vivo and in vitro: a role for IL-4. *Journal of Neuroscience*, **27**, 8309–8313.

Maher, F.O., Martin, D.S. & Lynch, M.A. (2004) Increased IL-1beta in cortex of aged rats is accompanied by downregulation of ERK and PI-3 kinase. *Neurobiology of Aging*, **25**, 795–806.

Maher, F.O., Nolan, Y. & Lynch, M.A. (2005) Downregulation of IL-4-induced signalling in hippocampus contributes to deficits in LTP in the aged rat. *Neurobiology of Aging*, **26**, 717–728.

Mantovani, A., Sica, A., Sozzani, S., Allavena, P., Vecchi, A. & Locati, M. (2004) The chemokine system in diverse forms of macrophage activation and polarization. *Trends in Immunology*, **25**, 677–686.

Markowska, A.L., Mooney, M. & Sonntag, W.E. (1998) Insulin-like growth factor-1 ameliorates age-related behavioral deficits. *Neuroscience*, **87**, 559–569.

Masocha, W. (2009) Systemic lipopolysaccharide (LPS)-induced microglial activation results in different temporal reduction of CD200 and CD200 receptor gene expression in the brain. *Journal of Neuroimmunology*, **214**, 78–82.

Matheu, A., Maraver, A., Klatt, P. *et al.* (2007) Delayed ageing through damage protection by the Arf/p53 pathway. *Nature*, **448**, 375–379.

Melchior, B., Garcia, A.E., Hsiung, B.K. *et al.* (2010) Dual induction of TREM2 and tolerance-related transcript, Tmem176b, in amyloid transgenic mice: implications for vaccine-based therapies for Alzheimer's disease. *ASN Neuro*, **2**, e00037.

Mosser, D.M. & Edwards, J.P. (2008) Exploring the full spectrum of macrophage activation. *Nature Reviews Immunology*, **8**, 958–969.

Mulsant, B.H. & Ganguli, M. (1999) Epidemiology and diagnosis of depression in late life. *Journal of Clinical Psychiatry*, **60** (Suppl. 20), 9–15.

Murray, P.J. (2006) Understanding and exploiting the endogenous interleukin-10/STAT3-mediated anti-inflammatory response. *Current Opinion in Pharmacology*, **6**, 379–386.

Nolan, Y., Maher, F.O., Martin, D.S. *et al.* (2005) Role of interleukin-4 in regulation of age-related inflammatory changes in the hippocampus. *Journal of Biological Chemistry*, **280**, 9354–9362.

Norden, D.M., Fenn, A.M., Dugan, A. & Godbout, J.P. (2014) TGFbeta produced by IL-10 redirected astrocytes attenuates microglial activation. *Glia*, **62**, 881–895.

Norden, D.M. & Godbout, J.P. (2013) Review: microglia of the aged brain: primed to be activated and resistant to regulation. *Neuropathology and Applied Neurobiology*, **39**, 19–34.

O'Connor, J.C., McCusker, R.H., Strle, K., Johnson, R.W., Dantzer, R. & Kelley, K.W. (2008) Regulation of IGF-I function by proinflammatory cytokines: at the interface of immunology and endocrinology. *Cellular Immunology*, **252**, 91–110.

Ouyang, Y.-B., Xu, L., Lu, Y. *et al.* (2013) Astrocyte-enriched miR-29a targets PUMA and reduces neuronal vulnerability to forebrain ischemia. *Glia*, **61**, 1784.

Pang, P.T. & Lu, B. (2004) Regulation of late-phase LTP and long-term memory in normal and aging hippocampus: role of secreted proteins tPA and BDNF. *Ageing Research Reviews*, **3**, 407.

Penninx, B.W., Kritchevsky, S.B., Yaffe, K. *et al.* (2003) Inflammatory markers and depressed mood in older persons: results from the Health, Aging and Body Composition study. *Biological Psychiatry*, **54**, 566–572.

Peters, A., Sethares, C. & Luebke, J.I. (2008) Synapses are lost during aging in the primate prefrontal cortex. *Neuroscience*, **152**, 970.

Ponomarev, E.D., Veremeyko, T., Barteneva, N., Krichevsky, A.M. & Weiner, H.L. (2011) MicroRNA-124 promotes microglia quiescence and suppresses EAE by deactivating macrophages via the C/EBP-alpha-PU.1 pathway. *Nature Medicine*, **17**, 64–70.

Richwine, A.F., Parkin, A.O., Buchanan, J.B. *et al.* (2008) Architectural changes to CA1 pyramidal neurons in adult and aged mice after peripheral immune stimulation. *Psychoneuroendocrinology*, **33**, 1369–1377.

Richwine, A.F., Sparkman, N.L., Dilger, R.N., Buchanan, J.B. & Johnson, R.W. (2009) Cognitive deficits in interleukin-10-deficient mice after peripheral injection of lipopolysaccharide. *Brain, Behavior, and Immunity*, **23**, 794–802.

Rodier, F., Coppe, J.P., Patil, C.K. *et al.* (2009) Persistent DNA damage signalling triggers senescence-associated inflammatory cytokine secretion. *Nature Cell Biology*, **11**, 973–979.

Rozovsky, I., Finch, C.E. & Morgan, T.E. (1998) Age-related activation of microglia and astrocytes: in vitro studies show persistent phenotypes of aging, increased proliferation, and resistance to down-regulation. *Neurobiology of Aging*, **19**, 97–103.

Shibata, M. (1990) Hypothalamic neuronal responses to cytokines. *Yale Journal of Biology and Medicine*, **63**, 147–156.

Shioya, M., Obayashi, S., Tabunoki, H. *et al.* (2010) Aberrant microRNA expression in the brains of neurodegenerative diseases: miR-29a decreased in Alzheimer disease brains targets neurone navigator 3. *Neuropathology and Applied Neurobiology*, **36**, 320.

Sierra, A., Gottfried-Blackmore, A.C., McEwen, B.S. & Bulloch, K. (2007) Microglia derived from aging mice exhibit an altered inflammatory profile. *Glia*, **55**, 412–424.

Sly, L.M., Krzesicki, R.F., Brashler, J.R. *et al.* (2001) Endogenous brain cytokine mRNA and inflammatory responses to lipopolysaccharide are elevated in the Tg2576 transgenic mouse model of Alzheimer's disease. *Brain Research Bulletin*, **56**, 581–588.

Smith, K.M., Guerau-de-Arellano, M., Costinean, S. *et al.* (2012) miR-29ab1 deficiency identifies a negative feedback loop controlling Th1 bias that is dysregulated in multiple sclerosis. *Journal of Immunology*, **189**, 1567–1576.

Sonntag, W.E., Carter, C.S., Ikeno, Y. *et al.* (2005) Adult-onset growth hormone and insulin-like growth factor I deficiency reduces neoplastic disease, modifies age-related pathology, and increases life span. *Endocrinology*, **146**, 2920–2932.

Stefferl, A., Hopkins, S.J., Rothwell, N.J. & Luheshi, G.N. (1996) The role of TNF-alpha in fever: opposing actions of human and murine TNF-alpha and interactions with IL-beta in the rat. *British Journal of Pharmacology*, **118**, 1919–1924.

Steiner, D.F., Thomas, M.F., Hu, J.K. *et al.* (2011) MicroRNA-29 regulates T-box transcription factors and interferon-gamma production in helper T cells. *Immunity*, **35**, 169–181.

Suberbielle, E., Sanchez, P.E., Kravitz, A.V. *et al.* (2013) Physiologic brain activity causes DNA double-strand breaks in neurons, with exacerbation by amyloid-Î². *Nature Neuroscience*, **16**, 613–621.

Takahashi, K., Rochford, C.D.P. & Neumann, H. (2005) Clearance of apoptotic neurons without inflammation by microglial triggering receptor expressed on myeloid cells-2. *Journal of Experimental Medicine*, **201**, 647–657.

Tarozzo, G., Bortolazzi, S., Crochemore, C. *et al.* (2003) Fractalkine protein localization and gene expression in mouse brain. *Journal of Neuroscience Research*, **73**, 81–88.

Tichauer, J.E., Flores, B., Soler, B., Eugenin-von Bernhardi, L., Ramirez, G. & von Bernhardi, R. (2013) Age-dependent changes on TGFbeta1 Smad3 pathway modify the pattern of microglial cell activation. *Brain, Behavior, and Immunity*, **37**, 187–196.

VanGuilder, H.D., Bixler, G.V., Brucklacher, R.M. *et al.* (2011) Concurrent hippocampal induction of MHC II pathway components and glial activation with advanced aging is not correlated with cognitive impairment. *Journal of Neuroinflammation*, **8**, 138.

VanGuilder, H.D., Yan, H., Farley, J.A., Sonntag, W.E. & Freeman, W.M. (2010) Aging alters the expression of neurotransmission-regulating proteins in the hippocampal synaptoproteome. *Journal of Neurochemistry*, **113**, 1577–1588.

Vereker, E., Campbell, V., Roche, E., McEntee, E. & Lynch, M.A. (2000) Lipopolysaccharide inhibits long term potentiation in the rat dentate gyrus by activating caspase-1. *Journal of Biological Chemistry*, **275**, 26252–26258.

Veremeyko, T., Siddiqui, S., Sotnikov, I., Yung, A. & Ponomarev, E.D. (2013) IL-4/IL-13-dependent and independent expression of miR-124 and its contribution to M2 phenotype of monocytic cells in normal conditions and during allergic inflammation. *PLoS ONE*, **8**, e81774.

Wofford, J.L., Loehr, L.R. & Schwartz, E. (1996) Acute cognitive impairment in elderly ED patients: etiologies and outcomes. *American Journal of Emergency Medicine*, **14**, 649–653.

Wu, G. & Morris, S.M. (1998) Arginine metabolism: nitric oxide and beyond. *Biochemical Journal*, **336** (Pt. 1), 1–17.

Wynne, A.M., Henry, C.J., Huang, Y., Cleland, A. & Godbout, J.P. (2010) Protracted downregulation of CX(3)CR1 on microglia of aged mice after lipopolysaccharide challenge. *Brain, Behavior, and Immunity*, **24**, 1190–1201.

Wyss-Coray, T., Lin, C., Yan, F. *et al.* (2001) TGF-beta1 promotes microglial amyloid-beta clearance and reduces plaque burden in transgenic mice. *Nature Medicine*, **7**, 612–618.

Ye, S.M. & Johnson, R.W. (2001) An age-related decline in interleukin-10 may contribute to the increased expression of interleukin-6 in brain of aged mice. *Neuroimmunomodulation*, **9**, 183–192.

Youm, Y.H., Grant, R.W., McCabe, L.R. *et al.* (2013) Canonical Nlrp3 inflammasome links systemic low-grade inflammation to functional decline in aging. *Cell Metabolism*, **18**, 519–532.

Zamanian, J.L., Xu, L., Foo, L.C. *et al.* (2012) Genomic analysis of reactive astrogliosis. *Journal of Neuroscience*, **32**, 6391–6410.

7 Peripheral and Central Immune Mechanisms in Neuropathic Pain

Ji Zhang

The Alan Edwards Centre for Research on Pain, McGill University, Montreal, Quebec, Canada
Faculty of Dentistry, McGill University, Montreal, Quebec, Canada
Department of Neurology and Neurosurgery, Faculty of Medicine, McGill University, Montreal, Quebec, Canada

Introduction

Damage and/or dysfunction of the nervous system, either peripheral or central, occurs quite frequently in our daily life. It can arise from peripheral nerve damage (e.g., surgery-associated nerve lesion, carpal tunnel syndrome), metabolic endocrine disturbances (e.g., diabetic mellitus), infections (human immunodeficiency virus (HIV), herpes zoster), toxins/drugs (e.g., chemotherapies), cancer, primary autoimmune disorders (e.g., Guillain–Barre syndrome), and injury/disease to the central nervous system (CNS) (e.g., spinal cord injury, multiple sclerosis). Irrespective of the cause, a major consequence of such neuropathies is the development of neuropathic pain. Patients often complain of spontaneous pain (i.e., pain that occurs in the absence of external stimulation), usually perceived as burning, prickling, tingling, or shooting pain. Patients may also experience pain caused by stimuli that are normally nonpainful (allodynia), such as simple touching of the skin or by changes in temperature, as well as exaggerated response to noxious stimuli (hyperalgesia). Neuropathic pain represents a severe problem in clinics because it causes debilitating suffering and is largely resistant to current available analgesics, including opioids. Even with an abundance of new research, there has been only a limited improvement in the treatment of neuropathic pain. A large proportion of patients with neuropathic pain are left with insufficient pain relief, which urgently calls for other more effective treatment options to target chronic neuropathic pain.

In physiological conditions, pain is an alarm that alerts us to external stimuli, such as pinprick or excessive heat, and internal stimuli, such as myocardial ischemia in patients with coronary artery disease. Nociceptive pain that is mediated by high threshold unmyelinated C or thinly myelinated Aδ primary sensory neurons feeding into CNS nociceptive pathways (Woolf and Ma, 2007) is a protective response. However, neuropathic pain, resulting from malfunction of

Neuroinflammation: New Insights into Beneficial and Detrimental Functions, First Edition. Edited by Samuel David.
© 2015 John Wiley & Sons, Inc. Published 2015 by John Wiley & Sons, Inc.

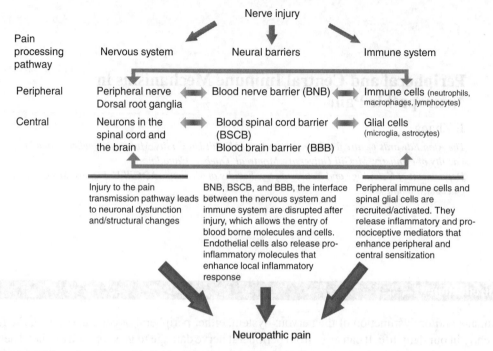

Figure 7.1 Schematic summary of the involvement of neuronal and non-neuronal cells in the generation of neuropathic pain. The importance of the neuroimmune interactions is detailed in the text.

somatosensory pathways, is a disease in its own right (Costigan *et al.*, 2009a). Although clinical features might be distinct in neuropathic pain triggered by various conditions, some major mechanisms are in common, including generation and transduction of ectopic impulses, recruitment of low-threshold myelinated Aβ fibers, central sensitization and disinhibition, as well as some structural changes (Campbell and Meyer, 2006). Nevertheless, neurons are not isolated from their neighbors; they exist in a dynamic environment, surrounded by non-neuronal cells including glial, immune cells, and endothelial cells. When neurons "sense pain, their neighbours feel it too." One of the most important developments in the pain research field over the past two decades is the realization that neurons are not the only cell type involved in the processing of abnormal pain responses. It is now appreciated that immune cells (macrophages, neutrophils, and lymphocytes), glial cells (microglia and astrocytes), and endothelial cells are important players in pain biology, both in the periphery and in the CNS (Fig. 7.1) (Scholz and Woolf, 2007). Indeed, neuropathic pain also involves the immune system. The critical roles of neuro–immune interactions in the pathogenesis of neuropathic pain have been well recognized.

Inflammation in Neuropathic Pain

Inflammation is a reaction by which organism responds to infection and tissue injury. Following an injury or a disease to the nervous system, an inflammatory process occurs, which is an attempt to remove pathogens, clear damaged cell debris, and restore local homeostasis. Various non-neuronal cells including Schwann cells, fibroblasts, resident macrophages, microglia, astrocytes, and endothelial cells in the microvasculature are engaged in this inflammatory reaction (Olsson, 1990). They become activated or damaged by the insults, thus releasing a number of inflammatory mediators. Some of these molecules guide and promote a large influx of blood-borne leukocytes into the parenchyma of the nervous system. A wide range of chemical mediators derived from these recruited cells, including cytokines, chemokines, trophic factors, proteolytic enzymes, and lipid mediators are able to modulate neuronal pain transmission pathways at different levels of the sensory neuraxis (Ellis and Bennett, 2013). In addition to sensitizing and stimulating nociceptors, they promote long-term deleterious plastic changes, thus contributing to persistent pain states (Calvo et al., 2012).

Chronic inflammation has been reported in patients with neuropathic pain. High levels of proinflammatory and low levels of anti-inflammatory cytokines have been detected in the blood and/or cerebrospinal fluid (CSF) of patients with distal painful polyneuropathy, posttraumatic neuralgia, complex regional pain syndrome, and painful diabetic neuropathy (Alexander et al., 2005; Uceyler et al., 2007; Backonja et al., 2008). An imbalance of pro- and anti-inflammatory cytokines appears to be clinically correlated with pain intensity (visual analog scale rating) (Backonja et al., 2008). Although direct evidence of CNS glial cells or peripheral immune cells in the generation of neuropathic pain in humans is sparse, inflammation mediated by peripheral immune cells, CNS glial cells, and endothelial cells is known to play a major role in neuropathic pain in animal models. In this chapter, I will primarily focus on the evidence generated from animal models of nerve-injury-triggered neuropathic pain to highlight inflammatory reactions along the pain pathway (from damaged nerve to the spinal cord) and the critical roles of these reactions in the development and maintenance of neuropathic pain. I will also discuss the current progress and challenges of translating inflammation-related new targets into therapeutics.

Contribution of Peripheral Immune Cells to the Pathogenesis of Neuropathic Pain

Peripheral nerve injury triggers not only the activation of Schwann's cells and resident immune cells, but also the recruitment of circulating inflammatory cells. As the first cells migrating toward damaged sites, neutrophils release mediators capable of sensitizing nociceptors and recruiting macrophages and T cells to the injury site (Kumar and Sharma, 2010). Although the presence of neutrophils in the injured nerves is transient (peak between days 1 and 3 after injury), neutrophil-mediated early immune response is necessary in the development of neuropathic pain. Depletion of circulating neutrophils with an antineutrophil antibody at the time of injury significantly attenuated subsequent hypersensitivity (Perkins and Tracey, 2000; Nadeau et al., 2011).

While neutrophils act as primary sensors of the damage, macrophages play important and persistent roles during the degeneration/regeneration process and the development/maintenance of neuropathic pain. It is well known that an injury to the peripheral nerve triggers the activation of resident macrophages and the recruitment of blood-derived macrophages. Resident macrophages that make up about 2–9% of nucleated cells within the uninjured peripheral nerve respond early to the insults (Vass et al., 1993). They proliferate and express certain inflammatory molecules. Invading hematogenous macrophages supplement and largely out-number the resident macrophage population. Macrophages have incontestable roles in innate immune response. They are key phagocytic cells removing degenerating axons and myelin debris in the process of Wallerian degeneration, which enables a reorganization of Schwann cells and facilitates the regrowth of injured axons (Kiefer et al., 2001). Macrophages are also the major contributors in establishing the cytokine/chemokine network, which is not only critical in orchestrating immune cells trafficking, but also involved directly in the pathogenesis of neuropathic pain following nerve injury (Clark et al., 2013). However, it is not yet clear if the cellular and molecular changes involved in Wallerian degeneration are simultaneously involved in the induction and maintenance of neuropathic pain. Mice with genetically delayed influx of macrophages (Wld^s mice) developed reduced thermal or mechanical hypersensitivity compared to wild-type mice following nerve injury (Myers et al., 1996). However, studies using macrophage depletion with liposome-encapsulated clodronate yielded some controversial results. Some reported slight alleviation of thermal hyperalgesia in nerve-injury-associated neuropathic pain model (Liu et al., 2000) and partially attenuated mechanical and thermal hypersensitivity in diabetic animals (Mert et al., 2009). Others showed that treatment with liposome-encapsulated clodronate reduces established hyperalgesia, albeit with limited effect on mechanical allodynia (Rutkowski et al., 2000). It is worthwhile to note that macrophages are not a homogeneous population. Experiments with manipulation on the entire macrophage population might give rise to misleading conclusion. Macrophage heterogeneity reflects the remarkable plasticity of these cells, as their physiological characteristics can be switched in response to different environmental cues. Macrophages have a spectrum of activation states/phenotypes, which have been categorized as classically activated M1 and alternatively activated M2 macrophages (Mosser and Edwards, 2008). Our recent studies identified two major subsets of macrophages coexisting in injured nerves (Lee and Zhang, 2012). Round-shaped, monocyte-like CD11b (MAC1)$^+$ macrophages are found clustered around the sites of injury, but mainly at the early stage. They are cytokine/chemokine-expressing cells, but do not express MHC II antigens. CD68 (ED1)$^+$ macrophages are abundantly distributed among the damaged nerve fibers and persist for at least 3 months after injury. They are powerful phagocytic cells, expressing MHC II, but their capability to secret cytokine/chemokine is low. When partially ligated sciatic nerve was exposed to an anti-inflammatory cytokine, transforming growth factor beta 1 (TGF-β1), the number of CD11b (MAC1)$^+$ cytokine/chemokine secreting macrophages was significantly reduced, while CD68 (ED1)$^+$ phagocytic macrophages were not affected. Coincidentally, a significant decrease of cytokine and chemokine production was detected. As a consequence, one single intraneural injection of TGF-β1 delayed and attenuated the development of neuropathic pain following injury to the nerve (Echeverry et al., 2013). This provides strong evidence that a subset (or some subsets) of macrophages contributes to the initiation of neuropathic pain through releasing inflammatory mediators. Whether, how, and to what extent phagocytic macrophages found in damaged nerves at chronic stage are required for the maintenance of persistent pain behavior need further investigation.

Following nerve injury, T cells were detected in the damages nerves (Kim and Moalem-Taylor, 2011; Echeverry et al., 2013). The contribution of lymphocytes to neuropathic pain has been investigated in animals genetically deficient in T cells. Athymic nude rats lacking mature T lymphocytes have reduced mechanical and thermal hypersensitivity after peripheral nerve injury

(Moalem *et al.*, 2004). The decreased sensitivity can be reversed by intraperitoneal injection of type I T helper cells (Th1), suggesting a proinflammatory cytokine-mediated enhancement of pain (Moalem *et al.*, 2004). In contrast, injection of type 2 T helper cells (Th2), which secrete anti-inflammatory cytokines, mildly, but significantly, reduces hypersensitivity in wild-type animals (Moalem *et al.*, 2004). Impaired neuropathic pain behavior has also been reported in RAG-1 knockout (KO) (Kleinschnitz *et al.*, 2006), CD4-KO (Cao and DeLeo, 2008), and severe combined immunodeficiency (SCID) mice (Labuz *et al.*, 2010), but these effects were usually moderate and did not appear to be solely attributable to the lack of T cells. However, all of the above-mentioned evidence is derived from genetic approaches by removing (or replacing) T cell population in the blood. With such systemic manipulation, it is difficult to conclude whether behavioral outcomes result from T-cell-mediated systemic inflammatory response or local peripheral or central (i.e., CNS) sensitization of T cells as they migrate into damaged nerve (Kim and Moalem-Taylor, 2011) and the spinal cord (Costigan *et al.*, 2009b) after nerve injury.

Critical Roles of Spinal Glial Activation in Neuropathic Pain

Within the CNS, microglia and astrocytes represent two highly reactive intraparenchymal cell populations. Microglia (resident macrophages in the CNS) are quiescent in normal conditions, fulfilling a constitutive surveillance function (Hanisch and Kettenmann, 2007). They become activated early in response to injury, infections, ischemia, brain tumors, or neurodegeneration. Activated microglia are characterized by an amoeboid morphology, proliferation, increased expression of cell surface markers or receptors, and changes in functional activities, such as migration to areas of damage, phagocytosis, and the production and release of proinflammatory substances or cell-signaling mediators (Gehrmann *et al.*, 1995). Astrocytes also respond to different types of insult, and this activation is characterized by morphological changes, increased production of intermediate filaments such as glial fibrillary acidic protein (GFAP), increased production of signalling molecules, and alterations in homeostatic activity (Maragakis and Rothstein, 2006). Both microglial and astrocytic activation are multidimensional. There are many different activation states, with various components expressed with different time-courses and intensities that are dependent on the stimulus that triggers activation. Functional and morphological changes are not time-locked; one can be detected in the absence of the other (Raivich *et al.*, 1999).

Nerve lesion not only creates a local inflammatory reaction within the damaged nerve, but also provokes a robust reaction at distance, in the spinal cord where the injured nerve afferents terminate. Major players in the central inflammatory response are spinal glial cells, as peripheral nerve injury can induce spinal microglial and astrocyte activation (Colburn *et al.*, 1999; Zhang *et al.*, 2003). The involvement of activated glial cells in chronic pain has been validated substantially by the prevention and reversal of abnormal pain behavior with molecules that have glia-inhibitory properties (Milligan *et al.*, 2003; Tsuda *et al.*, 2003; Hua *et al.*, 2005). This suggests that glial alteration may be a crucial mechanism accounting for the persistence of hypersensitivity.

The events triggering microglial activation as well as the signals resulting from this activation producing pain hypersensitivity consist of a neuron–glia–neuron signaling mechanism. Of special interest is the discovery of the critical role of chemokines released by damaged neurons, such as monocyte chemoattractant protein (MCP-1) also known as CCL2 (Abbadie *et al.*, 2003; Zhang *et al.*, 2007), and fractalkine (CX3CL1) (Verge *et al.*, 2004; Clark *et al.*, 2009), which serve as mediators in neuron–glia communication. Peripheral nerve injury induces not only upregulation of MCP-1 in injured sensory neurons and its receptor CCR2 in microglia (Abbadie *et al.*, 2003; Zhang and De Koninck, 2006), but also activation and proliferation of spinal microglia and recruitment of bone-marrow-derived microglia (Zhang *et al.*, 2007; Echeverry *et al.*, 2008). Furthermore, blockade of MCP-1/CCR2 signaling prevents the infiltration of blood-borne monocytes into the spinal cord (Zhang *et al.*, 2007). Microgliosis in the spinal cord is abolished by intrathecal injection of MCP-1 neutralizing antibody or in mice lacking CCR2 (Zhang *et al.*, 2007). Not only is MCP-1 a necessary mediator for spinal microglial activation, but also it is necessary for the development of mechanical allodynia. It has been demonstrated that mice lacking CCR2 have impairment of the nociceptive response typically associated with neuropathy (Abbadie *et al.*, 2003; Zhang *et al.*, 2007). Interestingly, although total CCR2 knockout mice did not develop mechanical allodynia, CCR2 expression either in resident microglia or in the periphery was sufficient for the development of full mechanical allodynia (Zhang *et al.*, 2007). Thus, to effectively relieve nerve-injury-induced mechanical allodynia, it appears that both CNS resident microglia and blood-borne microglia need to be targeted. In the same family of CC chemokines, MIP-1α, MIP-1β, or RANTES (also known as CCL3, CCL4, CCL5) also induce microglial activation through crosstalk with their cognate receptor CCR5 on activated microglia in nerve injury models (Gamo *et al.*, 2008). The involvement of CCR5 receptor in the pathogenesis of neuropathic pain has been documented with both pharmacological and genetic approaches (Padi *et al.*, 2012; Matsushita *et al.*, 2014). Dual targeting of CCR2 and CCR5 yielded a synergetic effect in reducing neuropathic pain (Padi *et al.*, 2012). Fractalkine is tethered to the extracellular surface of neurons and can be cleaved to form a diffusible signal (Chapman *et al.*, 2000) by lysosomal cysteine protease cathepsin S (CatS) expressed on activated spinal microglia (Clark *et al.*, 2007). While neurons are the source of fractalkine signaling to CX3CR1 on microglia, the initiating signal appears to be microglial CatS. Thus, activated microglia may be signaling to other microglia via the cleavage of fractalkine on neurons. The concurrent increase in CatS expression by microglia and fractalkine by neurons could serve as a mechanism of amplification and coincidence detection. Inhibition of CatS enzymatic activity and neutralization of the CX3CR1 receptor reversed the hypersensitivity in animal models of neuropathic pain with nerve injury (Milligan *et al.*, 2004; Clark *et al.*, 2007). Another well-established trigger in inducing spinal microglia activation is adenosine triphosphate (ATP) (Tsuda and Inoue, 2007). On stimulation or disease conditions, ATP can be released from various types of cells, including primary afferent terminals (Salter *et al.*, 1993), several purinergic receptors, for example, P2X4 (Tsuda *et al.*, 2003), P2X7 (Clark *et al.*, 2010; Kobayashi *et al.*, 2011), and P2Y12 (Haynes *et al.*, 2006; Katagiri *et al.*, 2012) were found in activated microglia. Genetic deletion and pharmacological antagonism of these purinergic receptors suppressed the phosphorylation of p38 mitogen-activated protein kinase (MAPK) in spinal microglia in animals that had undergone nerve lesion and the development of pain behavior (Tsuda *et al.*, 2003; Kobayashi *et al.*, 2008). Therefore, activation of purinergic receptors by released ATP stimulates the MAPK signaling pathway and plays a role in the pathogenesis of neuropathic pain.

How microglia enhance excitability within the dorsal horn of the spinal cords has also been under intense investigation. Activated microglia release pro-nociceptive substances such as proinflammatory cytokines, ATP, brain-derived neurotrophic factor (BDNF), excitatory amino acids, nitric oxide, and prostaglandins (Watkins *et al.*, 2003). These substances are likely to excite spinal nociceptive neurons, either directly or indirectly, and promote the release of other transmitters that can act on nociceptive neurons. Tumor necrosis factor alpha (TNF-α) enhances the amplitude of glutamate-induced excitatory currents; interleukin (IL)-1β increases excitatory synaptic transmission and reduces inhibitory transmission (Kawasaki *et al.*, 2008a). BDNF reverses the polarity of currents activated by gamma-aminobutyric acid (GABA), which switches from an inhibitory to an excitatory neurotransmission (Coull *et al.*, 2005). In addition, pain transmission at spinal levels is under strong descending control from the brainstem, more specifically the rostral ventromedial medulla (RVM). Following nerve injury, microglia within RVM become activated and contribute to descending facilitation and enhanced pain related to nerve injury (Wei *et al.*, 2008).

Compared to the ample evidence for microglial regulation of pain hypersensitivity, much less is known about the importance of astrocytes in chronic pain. A correlation between persistent activation of spinal astrocytes, often evidenced by increased expression of GFAP, and pain hypersensitivity has been observed in different animal models of chronic pain involving peripheral nerve injury (Zhang and De Koninck, 2006), spinal cord injury (Nesic *et al.*, 2005), and bone cancer (Mantyh *et al.*, 2002). Compared to nerve-injury-induced microglial activation, which is robust at acute phase and significant diminished at chronic period, astrocyte activation is characterized by a delayed, moderate, long-lasting GFAP upregulation for several months in models of persistent pain hypersensitivity (Zhang and De Koninck, 2006). Mice deficient in GFAP develop normal pain behavior following nerve injury, but it was shorter-lasting than that observed in wild-type mice (Kim *et al.*, 2009). GFAP antisense treatment reversed established injury-induced hypersensitivity (Kim *et al.*, 2009). Basic fibroblast growth factor, a primary "activator" of astrocytes, appears to be required for producing chronic pain (Madiai *et al.*, 2005). Although the signals that trigger and sustain astrocyte activation are not fully established, it is intriguing to speculate that the astrocyte response occurs secondary to microglial activation, probably through proinflammatory substances released by activated microglia. One prime example demonstrated that microglial IL-18 signaling via its cognate receptor on astrocytes enhanced neuropathic pain following nerve injury (Miyoshi *et al.*, 2008). Accumulating evidence shows that persistent changes in spinal astrocytes in different chronic pain conditions often outlast microglial changes (Zhuang *et al.*, 2005; Zhang and De Koninck, 2006). Consistent with these findings, the activation of extracellular-signal-regulated kinase (ERK) in the spinal cord started in activated microglia (2 days after injury) and then shifted to reactive astrocytes (3 weeks after injury) (Zhuang *et al.*, 2006). Following nerve injury, matrix metalloproteinase (MMP)-9 was induced in dorsal root ganglia (DRG) sensory neurons within hours and returned to baseline 3 days after injury, whereas MMP-2 was induced in DRG satellite cells and in spinal astrocytes at later times (from several days to weeks after injury). Although cellular distribution and temporal profile are different, both MMPs require a common molecular player, the cytokine IL-1β. MMP-9 induces neuropathic pain through IL-1β cleavage and microglia activation at early time points, whereas MMP-2 maintains neuropathic pain through IL-1β cleavage and astrocyte activation at later time points (Kawasaki *et al.*, 2008b). Contribution of astrocytes to the chronic pain status has been attributed to the release of some cytokines/chemokines (Gao *et al.*, 2009), the accumulation of extra amounts of glutamate due to the downregulation of glutamate transporters (GLT1) (Nicholson et al., 2014), and alteration of gap junction connexion 43 (Yoon et al., 2013) leading to enhanced communications in the astrocytic network.

Beyond the glial changes taking place in the spinal cord, marked modifications also occur in various brain regions. These include thalamic microglial activation to nociceptive spinal cord injury (Hains and Waxman, 2006; Zhao et al., 2007), microglia/astrocytic activation in the cingulate cortex following sciatic nerve ligation (Narita et al., 2006; Kuzumaki et al., 2007) and in the nucleus of the tractus solitari following colonic inflammation (Sun et al., 2005). Importantly, the glial reaction observed in these regions may not be directly involved in nociception. Indeed, changes in limbic circuitry (such as the prefrontal cortex) suggest that glia may contribute to the regulation of the affective component of pain.

Significance of Neural Barriers in Inflammatory Response along Pain Transmission Pathway

The stability of another important non-neuronal cell type, in both CNS and peripheral nervous system (PNS) affected by nerve injury is the vascular endothelial cell. The immediate consequence of injury is the disruption of the blood–brain barrier (BBB), the blood–spinal cord barrier (BSCB), and the blood–nerve barrier (BNB), which are the interface between the immune system and the nervous system.

The BSCB constitutes a physical/biochemical barrier between the CNS and the systemic circulation, which serves to protect the microenvironment of the spinal cord. Several studies (Gordh et al., 2006; Beggs et al., 2010; Echeverry et al., 2011) have reported that an injury to the peripheral nerve can increase permeability of the BSCB, a process mediated by local inflammatory response (Echeverry et al., 2011). In turn, the compromised BSCB allows penetration of inflammatory molecules (e.g., cytokine IL-1β) and immune cells (monocytes/macrophages, lymphocytes) into the spinal cords, which further promotes central inflammation and central sensitization that are critical events in the development of neuropathic pain (Echeverry et al., 2011).

Beyond the CNS, peripheral nerve is the second most impermeable tissue in our body. Under physiological conditions, peripheral axons and supporting cells are protected by the BNB, which has a similar structure as the BBB and the BSCB, with the exception of lacking the glia limitans formed by astrocyte end feet (Kanda, 2011). Opening of the BNB has been reported in animals having various types of nerve injury (Omura et al., 2004; Lim et al., 2014). The long-lasting breakdown of the BNB was found concomitant with Wallerian degeneration and behavioral impairment (Lim et al., 2014). Serum from nerve-injured animals or plasma proteins (e.g., fibrinogen) injected intraneurally to bypass the BNB produced a decrease in the thresholds of mechanical allodynia in naïve animals (Lim et al., 2014). This study proposed a novel mechanism for the generation of chronic pain, giving rise to the possibility that one source of generation of neuropathic pain may be the entrance of molecules from the blood, which pass through a defective BNB to act within the nerve.

In addition to the impairment of these barriers, endothelial cells have the capability to secrete immune mediators and express a series of cell surface proteins, such as adhesion molecules and chemokine receptors, to modulate the entrance of immune cells, which have an impact on pain hypersensitivity.

Imbalance of Pro- and Anti-inflammatory Responses in Neuropathic Pain

The problem with inflammation is not only how often it starts, but also how often it fails to subside. In the context of neuropathic pain, shortly after the nerve injury, a robust inflammatory response has been found at almost every level of the somatosensory pathway. The immune system response to nervous system damage is controlled by a highly complex and intricate network of regulatory mechanisms. Resolution of inflammation is indeed an active process, not merely the cessation of proinflammatory stimuli (Serhan *et al.*, 2007). Under physiological conditions, many endogenous anti-inflammatory molecules (IL-4, IL-10, IL-13, TGF-β, resolvins, and cannabinoids) limit the potential damaging effects of excessive inflammatory reactions. Pathological conditions such as chronic pain may arise when these regulatory mechanisms are insufficient to control the proinflammatory response. For example, endogenous TGF-β1 was believed to be masked by the BMP and activin membrane-bound inhibitor homolog (BAMBI). In BAMBI$^{-/-}$ mice in which endogenous TGF-β1 signalling is systemically increased, acute pain behavior and hypersensitivity in a model of neuropathy are attenuated (Tramullas *et al.*, 2010). The absence of IL-10 expression accelerates the kinetics of expansion of spinal cord lesions, peripheral immune response to spinal cord injury, as well as the onset of pain behavior (Abraham *et al.*, 2004). Another regulatory mechanism is the endocannabinoid system. CB2 receptors are expressed in many different types of cells, including activated microglia (Zhang *et al.*, 2003). Endocannabinoid levels are also increased after peripheral nerve injury, and their action through CB2 receptors reduces hypersensitivity and microgliosis (Romero-Sandoval *et al.*, 2008). Pharmacological intervention to enhance endogenous mechanisms by providing exogenous IL-10, TGF-β, and cannabinoid agonists reduces pain behavior in various animal models of neuropathic pain (Soderquist *et al.*, 2010; Echeverry *et al.*, 2013).

To summarize, many molecules in the inflammatory loops (cytokines, chemokines, trophic factors, and signalling events such as p38 MARK) and effector cells (peripheral neutrophils, macrophages, lymphocytes, CNS glial cells, and endothelial cells) have been identified and validated for their involvement in neuropathic pain. Targeting these molecules and/or cells can prevent and/or reverse neuropathic pain. Taken together, the evidence from animal studies clearly demonstrated that there is a maladaptive immune response, imbalanced between pro-inflammation and anti-inflammation, which is not a bystander phenomenon but actively contributes to persistent pain. This immune response might even be a player in the transition from acute to chronic pain.

Challenges in Translating Anti-inflammatory Therapeutic Strategies for the Relief of Neuropathic Pain

Neuropathic pain represents heterogeneous conditions, which can be explained neither by a single cause nor by a specific anatomical lesion. The involvement of inflammation as pain modulators, as highlighted in this chapter, challenges conventional approaches in drug discovery. Therapeutic agents targeting inflammation mediated through neuroimmune interaction could be an exciting prospect. However, activation of different immune/glial cells occurs along complex temporal patterns. In addition, the contribution of each cell population to the modulation of nociceptive processing in pathological conditions follows a well-organized sequence of reciprocal communication between neurons and non-neuronal cells and among glial or immune cells themselves. To date, translation of such knowledge into clinical use for humans has been largely underexplored. Only a few clinical studies have tested immunosuppressive drugs or drugs interfering with glial functions for neuropathic pain. In a double-blind crossover small trial (43 patients completed the study), the p38 MAPK inhibitor SB-6813223 was efficacious for the primary endpoint of improvement in the daily pain score in patients with nerve-injury-triggered neuropathic pain (Anand et al., 2011). However, a randomized controlled trial (180 patients) with propentofylline (NCT00813826), a glial inhibitor, failed to show efficacy in the treatment of post-herpetic neuralgia (Landry et al., 2012). AZD2423, a highly selective antagonist for CCR2, did not show significant effects in a posttraumatic neuralgia trial, despite a trend toward reduction in some sensory components of pain such as paroxysmal pain and paresthesia and dysesthesia (Kalliomaki et al., 2013).

In the past decade, development of novel pain therapeutics, including targeting inflammation has been disappointing. The failures could be the result of multiple factors. Firstly, it is very important to point out that majority of evidence showing inflammation in neuropathic pain was generated from animal models at acute phase, for example, 1–2 weeks after nerve injury. The effect of anti-inflammation therapy on pain behavior was also tested at the acute induction phase of neuropathic pain. Whether and to what extent inflammation persists have not been fully answered, as only a few groups investigated the chronicity of inflammation in conditions of neuropathic pain (Coyle, 1998; Zhang and De Koninck, 2006). Our recent observations (unpublished findings) revealed that although less intense at the late stages (3 months after injury) compared to the early ones (2 weeks after injury), microglial activation in the spinal cord and infiltration of immune cells in the damaged nerves are still noticeable and significantly higher in the ipsilateral side than contralateral to the injury. Furthermore, these glial and/or immune cells at the chronic phase are required for the maintenance of long-lasting hypersensitivity. Our data suggest that nonresolving inflammation contributes significantly to the maintenance of chronic hypersensitivity. Further investigation is necessary, as signaling mechanisms might be different at acute and chronic phases. Different strategies should also be considered for treating pain at early and late phases. Such information is directly relevant to clinical settings and could potentially require new therapeutic targets for relieving chronic pain.

Secondly, the biological complexity of inflammation and our limited understanding of it make the development of anti-inflammatory therapy particularly difficult. One challenge is that immune cells involved in the pathogenesis of neuropathic pain exhibit frequently heterogeneity and plasticity. They are multifunctional at different stages. While detrimental effects of neuroimmune interactions lead to the enhancement of neuropathic pain, macrophages and lymphocytes can also stimulate the nerve regeneration, tissue repair, or motor function recovery after peripheral nerve injury or spinal cord injury, which is mainly attributed to the removal of tissue debris and the production of neurotrophins (Kiefer et al., 2001). Immune cells are also a source of opioid peptides, which are endogenous counterparts of morphine and related compounds, the most powerful pain killers. Flow cytometry using CD45 antibody recognizing hematopoietic cells revealed that 30–40% CD45$^+$ cells in injured nerve express opioid peptides, while μ-, δ-, and κ-opioid receptors were detected in sensory fibers of the injured nerves (Labuz et al., 2009). Thence, attenuation of neuropathic pain by general anti-inflammatory strategies might delay nerve regeneration and tissue repair and hinder the analgesic actions of leukocyte-derived opioids. Immune responses accompanying nerve injury are not exclusively maladaptive; their favorable actions need to be taken into consideration. We are facing a challenge even more demanding than just suppressing inflammation and reducing pain. We need to alleviate pain, but we should also promote functional recovery. Better understanding the diversity of immune response will help to target selectively specific cell populations for effective treatment of neuropathic pain. Another challenge is the redundancy in cytokine and chemokine signalling and their pleiotropic effects; thus drug efficacy might be difficult to achieve if only one is targeted. Whether a strategy aimed at trying to drive the overall response from proinflammatory to anti-inflammatory could be helpful remains to be answered.

Overall, current research suggests that finely tuned strategies to modulate certain aspects of the inflammatory response will be required for the treatment of neuropathic pain. The aim will be to reduce pain while also permitting tissue repair and functional recovery.

Acknowledgment

The author acknowledges financial support from the Canadian Institute of Health Research (CIHR), the Fonds de la recherche en sante du Quebec (FRSQ), and the Louise and Alan Edwards foundation.

References

Abbadie, C., Lindia, J.A., Cumiskey, A.M. *et al.* (2003) Impaired neuropathic pain responses in mice lacking the chemokine receptor CCR2. *Proceedings of the National Academy of Sciences of the United States of America*, **100**, 7947–7952.

Abraham, K.E., McMillen, D. & Brewer, K.L. (2004) The effects of endogenous interleukin-10 on gray matter damage and the development of pain behaviors following excitotoxic spinal cord injury in the mouse. *Neuroscience*, **124**, 945–952.

Alexander, G.M., van Rijn, M.A., van Hilten, J.J., Perreault, M.J. & Schwartzman, R.J. (2005) Changes in cerebrospinal fluid levels of pro-inflammatory cytokines in CRPS. *Pain*, **116**, 213–219.

Anand, P., Shenoy, R., Palmer, J.E. *et al.* (2011) Clinical trial of the p38 MAP kinase inhibitor dilmapimod in neuropathic pain following nerve injury. *European Journal of Pain*, **15**, 1040–1048.

Backonja, M.M., Coe, C.L., Muller, D.A. & Schell, K. (2008) Altered cytokine levels in the blood and cerebrospinal fluid of chronic pain patients. *Journal of Neuroimmunology*, **195**, 157–163.

Beggs, S., Liu, X.J., Kwan, C. & Salter, M.W. (2010) Peripheral nerve injury and TRPV1-expressing primary afferent C-fibers cause opening of the blood–brain barrier. *Molecular Pain*, **6**, 74.

Calvo, M., Dawes, J.M. & Bennett, D.L. (2012) The role of the immune system in the generation of neuropathic pain. *Lancet Neurology*, **11**, 629–642.

Campbell, J.N. & Meyer, R.A. (2006) Mechanisms of neuropathic pain. *Neuron*, **52**, 77–92.

Cao, L. & DeLeo, J.A. (2008) CNS-infiltrating CD4+ T lymphocytes contribute to murine spinal nerve transection-induced neuropathic pain. *European Journal of Immunology*, **38**, 448–458.

Chapman, G.A., Moores, K., Harrison, D., Campbell, C.A., Stewart, B.R. & Strijbos, P.J. (2000) Fractalkine cleavage from neuronal membranes represents an acute event in the inflammatory response to excitotoxic brain damage. *Journal of Neuroscience*, **20**, RC87.

Clark, A.K., Yip, P.K. & Malcangio, M. (2009) The liberation of fractalkine in the dorsal horn requires microglial cathepsin S. *Journal of Neuroscience*, **29**, 6945–6954.

Clark, A.K., Old, E.A. & Malcangio, M. (2013) Neuropathic pain and cytokines: current perspectives. *Journal of Pain Research*, **6**, 803–814.

Clark, A.K., Staniland, A.A., Marchand, F., Kaan, T.K., McMahon, S.B. & Malcangio, M. (2010) P2X7-dependent release of interleukin-1beta and nociception in the spinal cord following lipopolysaccharide. *Journal of Neuroscience*, **30**, 573–582.

Clark, A.K., Yip, P.K., Grist, J. *et al.* (2007) Inhibition of spinal microglial cathepsin S for the reversal of neuropathic pain. *Proceedings of the National Academy of Sciences of the United States of America*, **104**, 10655–10660.

Colburn, R.W., Rickman, A.J. & DeLeo, J.A. (1999) The effect of site and type of nerve injury on spinal glial activation and neuropathic pain behavior. *Experimental Neurology*, **157**, 289–304.

Costigan, M., Scholz, J. & Woolf, C.J. (2009a) Neuropathic pain: A maladaptive response of the nervous system to damage. *Annual Review of Neuroscience*, **32**, 1–32.

Costigan, M., Moss, A., Latremoliere, A. *et al.* (2009b) T-cell infiltration and signaling in the adult dorsal spinal cord is a major contributor to neuropathic pain-like hypersensitivity. *Journal of Neuroscience*, **29**, 14415–14422.

Coull, J.A., Beggs, S., Boudreau, D. *et al.* (2005) BDNF from microglia causes the shift in neuronal anion gradient underlying neuropathic pain. *Nature*, **438**, 1017–1021.

Coyle, D.E. (1998) Partial peripheral nerve injury leads to activation of astroglia and microglia which parallels the development of allodynic behavior. *Glia*, **23**, 75–83.

Echeverry, S., Shi, X.Q. & Zhang, J. (2008) Characterization of cell proliferation in rat spinal cord following peripheral nerve injury and the relationship with neuropathic pain. *Pain*, **135**, 37–47.

Echeverry, S., Wu, Y. & Zhang, J. (2013) Selectively reducing cytokine/chemokine expressing macrophages in injured nerves impairs the development of neuropathic pain. *Experimental Neurology*, **240**, 205–218.

Echeverry, S., Shi, X.Q., Rivest, S. & Zhang, J. (2011) Peripheral nerve injury alters blood-spinal cord barrier functional and molecular integrity through a selective inflammatory pathway. *Journal of Neuroscience*, **31**, 10819–10828.

Ellis, A. & Bennett, D.L. (2013) Neuroinflammation and the generation of neuropathic pain. *British Journal of Anaesthesia*, **111**, 26–37.

Gamo, K., Kiryu-Seo, S., Konishi, H. *et al.* (2008) G-protein-coupled receptor screen reveals a role for chemokine receptor CCR5 in suppressing microglial neurotoxicity. *Journal of Neuroscience*, **28**, 11980–11988.

Gao, Y.J., Zhang, L., Samad, O.A. *et al.* (2009) JNK-induced MCP-1 production in spinal cord astrocytes contributes to central sensitization and neuropathic pain. *Journal of Neuroscience*, **29**, 4096–4108.

Gehrmann, J., Matsumoto, Y. & Kreutzberg, G.W. (1995) Microglia: Intrinsic immuneffector cell of the brain. *Brain Research Brain Research Reviews*, **20**, 269–287.

Gordh, T., Chu, H. & Sharma, H.S. (2006) Spinal nerve lesion alters blood-spinal cord barrier function and activates astrocytes in the rat. *Pain*, **124**, 211–221.

Hains, B.C. & Waxman, S.G. (2006) Activated microglia contribute to the maintenance of chronic pain after spinal cord injury. *Journal of Neuroscience*, **26**, 4308–4317.

Hanisch, U.K. & Kettenmann, H. (2007) Microglia: active sensor and versatile effector cells in the normal and pathologic brain. *Nature Neuroscience*, **10**, 1387–1394.

Haynes, S.E., Hollopeter, G., Yang, G. *et al.* (2006) The P2Y12 receptor regulates microglial activation by extracellular nucleotides. *Nature Neuroscience*, **9**, 1512–1519.

Hua, X.Y., Svensson, C.I., Matsui, T., Fitzsimmons, B., Yaksh, T.L. & Webb, M. (2005) Intrathecal minocycline attenuates peripheral inflammation-induced hyperalgesia by inhibiting p38 MAPK in spinal microglia. *European Journal of Neuroscience*, **22**, 2431–2440.

Kalliomaki, J., Attal, N., Jonzon, B. *et al.* (2013) A randomized, double-blind, placebo-controlled trial of a chemokine receptor 2 (CCR2) antagonist in posttraumatic neuralgia. *Pain*, **154**, 761–767.

Kanda, T. (2011) Blood-nerve barrier: Structure and function. *Brain and Nerve (Shinkei kenkyu no shinpo)*, **63**, 557–569.

Katagiri, A., Shinoda, M., Honda, K., Toyofuku, A., Sessle, B.J. & Iwata, K. (2012) Satellite glial cell P2Y12 receptor in the trigeminal ganglion is involved in lingual neuropathic pain mechanisms in rats. *Molecular Pain*, **8**, 23.

Kawasaki, Y., Zhang, L., Cheng, J.K. & Ji, R.R. (2008a) Cytokine mechanisms of central sensitization: Distinct and overlapping role of interleukin-1beta, interleukin-6, and tumor necrosis factor-alpha in regulating synaptic and neuronal activity in the superficial spinal cord. *Journal of Neuroscience*, **28**, 5189–5194.

Kawasaki, Y., Xu, Z.Z., Wang, X. *et al.* (2008b) Distinct roles of matrix metalloproteases in the early- and late-phase development of neuropathic pain. *Nature Medicine*, **14**, 331–336.

Kiefer, R., Kieseier, B.C., Stoll, G. & Hartung, H.P. (2001) The role of macrophages in immune-mediated damage to the peripheral nervous system. *Progress in Neurobiology*, **64**, 109–127.

Kim, C.F. & Moalem-Taylor, G. (2011) Detailed characterization of neuro-immune responses following neuropathic injury in mice. *Brain Research*, **1405**, 95–108.

Kim, D.S., Figueroa, K.W., Li, K.W., Boroujerdi, A., Yolo, T. & Luo, Z.D. (2009) Profiling of dynamically changed gene expression in dorsal root ganglia post peripheral nerve injury and a critical role of injury-induced glial fibrillary acidic protein in maintenance of pain behaviors [corrected]. *Pain*, **143**, 114–122.

Kleinschnitz, C., Hofstetter, H.H., Meuth, S.G., Braeuninger, S., Sommer, C. & Stoll, G. (2006) T cell infiltration after chronic constriction injury of mouse sciatic nerve is associated with interleukin-17 expression. *Experimental Neurology*, **200**, 480–485.

Kobayashi, K., Takahashi, E., Miyagawa, Y., Yamanaka, H. & Noguchi, K. (2011) Induction of the P2X7 receptor in spinal microglia in a neuropathic pain model. *Neuroscience Letters*, **504**, 57–61.

Kobayashi, K., Yamanaka, H., Fukuoka, T., Dai, Y., Obata, K. & Noguchi, K. (2008) P2Y12 receptor upregulation in activated microglia is a gateway of p38 signaling and neuropathic pain. *Journal of Neuroscience*, **28**, 2892–2902.

Kumar, V. & Sharma, A. (2010) Neutrophils: Cinderella of innate immune system. *International Immunopharmacology*, **10**, 1325–1334.

Kuzumaki, N., Narita, M., Hareyama, N. *et al.* (2007) Chronic pain-induced astrocyte activation in the cingulate cortex with no change in neural or glial differentiation from neural stem cells in mice. *Neuroscience Letters*, **415**, 22–27.

Labuz, D., Schreiter, A., Schmidt, Y., Brack, A. & Machelska, H. (2010) T lymphocytes containing beta-endorphin ameliorate mechanical hypersensitivity following nerve injury. *Brain, Behavior, and Immunity*, **24**, 1045–1053.

Labuz, D., Schmidt, Y., Schreiter, A., Rittner, H.L., Mousa, S.A. & Machelska, H. (2009) Immune cell-derived opioids protect against neuropathic pain in mice. *Journal of Clinical Investigation*, **119**, 278–286.

Landry, R.P., Jacobs, V.L., Romero-Sandoval, E.A. & DeLeo, J.A. (2012) Propentofylline, a CNS glial modulator does not decrease pain in post-herpetic neuralgia patients: In vitro evidence for differential responses in human and rodent microglia and macrophages. *Experimental Neurology*, **234**, 340–350.

Lee, S. & Zhang, J. (2012) Heterogeneity of macrophages in injured trigeminal nerves: cytokine/chemokine expressing vs. phagocytic macrophages. *Brain, Behavior, and Immunity*, **26**, 891–903.

Lim, T.K., Shi, X.Q., Martin, H.C., Huang, H., Luheshi, G. & Rivest, S. (2014) *Zhang J*. Blood-nerve barrier dysfunction contributes to the generation of neuropathic pain and allows targeting of injured nerves for pain relief, Pain.

Liu, T., van Rooijen, N. & Tracey, D.J. (2000) Depletion of macrophages reduces axonal degeneration and hyperalgesia following nerve injury. *Pain*, **86**, 25–32.

Madiai, F., Goettl, V.M., Hussain, S.R., Clairmont, A.R., Stephens, R.L. Jr. & Hackshaw, K.V. (2005) Anti-fibroblast growth factor-2 antibodies attenuate mechanical allodynia in a rat model of neuropathic pain. *Journal of Molecular Neuroscience*, **27**, 315–324.

Mantyh, P.W., Clohisy, D.R., Koltzenburg, M. & Hunt, S.P. (2002) Molecular mechanisms of cancer pain. *Nature Reviews Cancer*, **2**, 201–209.

Maragakis, N.J. & Rothstein, J.D. (2006) Mechanisms of disease: Astrocytes in neurodegenerative disease. *Nature Clinical Practice Neurology*, **2**, 679–689.

Matsushita, K., Tozaki-Saitoh, H., Kojima, C. *et al.* (2014) Chemokine (C-C motif) receptor 5 is an important pathological regulator in the development and maintenance of neuropathic pain. *Anesthesiology*, **120**, 1491–1503.

Mert, T., Gunay, I., Ocal, I. *et al.* (2009) Macrophage depletion delays progression of neuropathic pain in diabetic animals. *Naunyn-Schmiedeberg's Archives of Pharmacology*, **379**, 445–452.

Milligan, E.D., Twining, C., Chacur, M. *et al.* (2003) Spinal glia and proinflammatory cytokines mediate mirror-image neuropathic pain in rats. *Journal of Neuroscience*, **23**, 1026–1040.

Milligan, E.D., Zapata, V., Chacur, M. *et al.* (2004) Evidence that exogenous and endogenous fractalkine can induce spinal nociceptive facilitation in rats. *European Journal of Neuroscience*, **20**, 2294–2302.

Miyoshi, K., Obata, K., Kondo, T., Okamura, H. & Noguchi, K. (2008) Interleukin-18-mediated microglia/astrocyte interaction in the spinal cord enhances neuropathic pain processing after nerve injury. *Journal of Neuroscience*, **28**, 12775–12787.

Moalem, G., Xu, K. & Yu, L. (2004) T lymphocytes play a role in neuropathic pain following peripheral nerve injury in rats. *Neuroscience*, **129**, 767–777.

Mosser, D.M. & Edwards, J.P. (2008) Exploring the full spectrum of macrophage activation. *Nature Reviews Immunology*, **8**, 958–969.

Myers, R.R., Heckman, H.M. & Rodriguez, M. (1996) Reduced hyperalgesia in nerve-injured WLD mice: Relationship to nerve fiber phagocytosis, axonal degeneration, and regeneration in normal mice. *Experimental Neurology*, **141**, 94–101.

Nadeau, S., Filali, M., Zhang, J. *et al.* (2011) Functional recovery after peripheral nerve injury is dependent on the pro-inflammatory cytokines IL-1beta and TNF: Implications for neuropathic pain. *Journal of Neuroscience*, **31**, 12533–12542.

Narita, M., Kuzumaki, N., Kaneko, C. *et al.* (2006) Chronic pain-induced emotional dysfunction is associated with astrogliosis due to cortical delta-opioid receptor dysfunction. *Journal of Neurochemistry*, **97**, 1369–1378.

Nesic, O., Lee, J., Johnson, K.M. *et al.* (2005) Transcriptional profiling of spinal cord injury-induced central neuropathic pain. *Journal of Neurochemistry*, **95**, 998–1014.

Nicholson, K.J., Gilliland, T.M. & Winkelstein, B.A. (2014) Upregulation of GLT-1 by treatment with ceftriaxone alleviates radicular pain by reducing spinal astrocyte activation and neuronal hyperexcitability. *Journal of Neuroscience Research*, **92**, 116–129.

Olsson, Y. (1990) Microenvironment of the peripheral nervous system under normal and pathological conditions. *Critical Reviews in Neurobiology*, **5**, 265–311.

Omura, K., Ohbayashi, M., Sano, M., Omura, T., Hasegawa, T. & Nagano, A. (2004) The recovery of blood-nerve barrier in crush nerve injury – A quantitative analysis utilizing immunohistochemistry. *Brain Research*, **1001**, 13–21.

Padi, S.S., Shi, X.Q., Zhao, Y.Q. *et al.* (2012) Attenuation of rodent neuropathic pain by an orally active peptide, RAP-103, which potently blocks CCR2- and CCR5-mediated monocyte chemotaxis and inflammation. *Pain*, **153**, 95–106.

Perkins, N.M. & Tracey, D.J. (2000) Hyperalgesia due to nerve injury: Role of neutrophils. *Neuroscience*, **101**, 745–757.

Raivich, G., Bohatschek, M., Kloss, C.U., Werner, A., Jones, L.L. & Kreutzberg, G.W. (1999) Neuroglial activation repertoire in the injured brain: Graded response, molecular mechanisms and cues to physiological function. *Brain Research Brain Research Reviews*, **30**, 77–105.

Romero-Sandoval, A., Nutile-McMenemy, N. & DeLeo, J.A. (2008) Spinal microglial and perivascular cell cannabinoid receptor type 2 activation reduces behavioral hypersensitivity without tolerance after peripheral nerve injury. *Anesthesiology*, **108**, 722–734.

Rutkowski, M.D., Pahl, J.L., Sweitzer, S., van Rooijen, N. & DeLeo, J.A. (2000) Limited role of macrophages in generation of nerve injury-induced mechanical allodynia. *Physiology & Behavior*, **71**, 225–235.

Salter, M.W., De Koninck, Y. & Henry, J.L. (1993) Physiological roles for adenosine and ATP in synaptic transmission in the spinal dorsal horn. *Progress in Neurobiology*, **41**, 125–156.

Scholz, J. & Woolf, C.J. (2007) The neuropathic pain triad: Neurons, immune cells and glia. *Nature Neuroscience*, **10**, 1361–1368.

Serhan, C.N., Brain, S.D., Buckley, C.D. *et al.* (2007) Resolution of inflammation: State of the art, definitions and terms. *FASEB Journal*, **21**, 325–332.

Soderquist, R.G., Sloane, E.M., Loram, L.C. *et al.* (2010) Release of plasmid DNA-encoding IL-10 from PLGA microparticles facilitates long-term reversal of neuropathic pain following a single intrathecal administration. *Pharmaceutical Research*, **27**, 841–854.

Sun, Y.N., Luo, J.Y., Rao, Z.R., Lan, L. & Duan, L. (2005) GFAP and Fos immunoreactivity in lumbo-sacral spinal cord and medulla oblongata after chronic colonic inflammation in rats. *World Journal of Gastroenterology*, **11**, 4827–4832.

Tramullas, M., Lantero, A., Diaz, A. *et al.* (2010) BAMBI (bone morphogenetic protein and activin membrane-bound inhibitor) reveals the involvement of the transforming growth factor-beta family in pain modulation. *Journal of Neuroscience*, **30**, 1502–1511.

Tsuda, M. & Inoue, K. (2007) Neuropathic pain and ATP receptors in spinal microglia. *Brain and Nerve (Shinkei kenkyu no shinpo)*, **59**, 953–959.

Tsuda, M., Shigemoto-Mogami, Y., Koizumi, S. *et al.* (2003) P2X4 receptors induced in spinal microglia gate tactile allodynia after nerve injury. *Nature*, **424**, 778–783.

Uceyler, N., Rogausch, J.P., Toyka, K.V. & Sommer, C. (2007) Differential expression of cytokines in painful and painless neuropathies. *Neurology*, **69**, 42–49.

Vass, K., Hickey, W.F., Schmidt, R.E. & Lassmann, H. (1993) Bone marrow-derived elements in the peripheral nervous system. An immunohistochemical and ultrastructural investigation in chimeric rats. *Laboratory Investigation*, **69**, 275–282.

Verge, G.M., Milligan, E.D., Maier, S.F., Watkins, L.R., Naeve, G.S. & Foster, A.C. (2004) Fractalkine (CX3CL1) and fractalkine receptor (CX3CR1) distribution in spinal cord and dorsal root ganglia under basal and neuropathic pain conditions. *European Journal of Neuroscience*, **20**, 1150–1160.

Watkins, L.R., Milligan, E.D. & Maier, S.F. (2003) Glial proinflammatory cytokines mediate exaggerated pain states: Implications for clinical pain. *Advances in Experimental Medicine and Biology*, **521**, 1–21.

Wei, F., Guo, W., Zou, S., Ren, K. & Dubner, R. (2008) Supraspinal glial-neuronal interactions contribute to descending pain facilitation. *Journal of Neuroscience*, **28**, 10482–10495.

Woolf, C.J. & Ma, Q. (2007) Nociceptors--noxious stimulus detectors. *Neuron*, **55**, 353–364.

Yoon, S.Y., Robinson, C.R., Zhang, H. & Dougherty, P.M. (2013) Spinal astrocyte gap junctions contribute to oxaliplatin-induced mechanical hypersensitivity. *Journal of Pain*, **14**, 205–214.

Zhang, J. & De Koninck, Y. (2006) Spatial and temporal relationship between monocyte chemoattractant protein-1 expression and spinal glial activation following peripheral nerve injury. *Journal of Neurochemistry*, **97**, 772–783.

Zhang, J., Hoffert, C., Vu, H.K., Groblewski, T., Ahmad, S. & O'Donnell, D. (2003) Induction of CB2 receptor expression in the rat spinal cord of neuropathic but not inflammatory chronic pain models. *European Journal of Neuroscience*, **17**, 2750–2754.

Zhang, J., Shi, X.Q., Echeverry, S., Mogil, J.S., De Koninck, Y. & Rivest, S. (2007) Expression of CCR2 in both resident and bone marrow-derived microglia plays a critical role in neuropathic pain. *Journal of Neuroscience*, **27**, 12396–12406.

Zhao, P., Waxman, S.G. & Hains, B.C. (2007) Modulation of thalamic nociceptive processing after spinal cord injury through remote activation of thalamic microglia by cysteine cysteine chemokine ligand 21. *Journal of Neuroscience*, **27**, 8893–8902.

Zhuang, Z.Y., Gerner, P., Woolf, C.J. & Ji, R.R. (2005) ERK is sequentially activated in neurons, microglia, and astrocytes by spinal nerve ligation and contributes to mechanical allodynia in this neuropathic pain model. *Pain*, **114**, 149–159.

Zhuang, Z.Y., Wen, Y.R., Zhang, D.R. *et al.* (2006) A peptide c-Jun N-terminal kinase (JNK) inhibitor blocks mechanical allodynia after spinal nerve ligation: respective roles of JNK activation in primary sensory neurons and spinal astrocytes for neuropathic pain development and maintenance. *Journal of Neuroscience*, **26**, 3551–3560.

8   Inflammation in the Pathogenesis of Inherited Peripheral Neuropathies

Janos Groh,[1] Dennis Klein,[1] Antje Kroner,[1,2] and Rudolf Martini[1]

[1]*Department of Neurology, Developmental Neurobiology, University of Wuerzburg, Wuerzburg, Germany*
[2]*Centre for Research in Neuroscience, The Research Institute of the McGill University Health Centre, Montreal, Canada*

Inherited Peripheral Neuropathies

Hereditary peripheral neuropathies are commonly assorted by the Charcot–Marie–Tooth (CMT) classification, named after Jean-Martin Charcot, Pierre Marie, and Howard Tooth, who first described the disease in 1886. CMTs are divided into demyelinating and axonal subtypes, with demyelinating types (CMT1 and CMT4) displaying a reduced nerve conduction velocity (<38 m/s; Harding and Thomas, 1980; Shy *et al.*, 2005), while axonal neuropathies (CMT2) do not show strongly reduced conduction velocity. The currently applied classification system incorporates both clinical and genetic insights, accounting for overlapping phenotypes and very rare subtypes (e.g., CMT3).

Clinically, CMT is characterized by an onset in late childhood or early adult age with progressive distal muscle weakness, muscular atrophy, and deformed feet with high arch and claw toes, as well as the typical stepper's gait, often combined with sensory malfunctions. The typical histology of demyelinating CMT shows segmental demyelination, axonal degeneration, and supernumerary Schwann cells (SCs) forming so-called onion bulbs, which possibly develop from consecutive episodes of de- and remyelination (Suter and Scherer, 2003). Disease onset and progression are remarkably variable, and there are no available therapies to date (Patzko and Shy, 2012; Pareyson *et al.*, 2013).

In the last few years, a vast variety of disease-causing genes or chromosomal alterations have been described, and evolving diagnostic tools for the detection of mutations made it possible to discover genetic causes for unclear or atypical cases of CMT (Rossor *et al.*, 2013). The most frequent cause of CMT1 is a duplication within chromosome 17q11.2, an area containing the *peripheral myelin protein 22* (*PMP22*) gene (Reilly *et al.*, 2011). Other causative mutations include point mutations in *PMP22* and *MPZ*, coding for myelin protein zero (P0) in which more than 120

Neuroinflammation: New Insights into Beneficial and Detrimental Functions, First Edition. Edited by Samuel David.
© 2015 John Wiley & Sons, Inc. Published 2015 by John Wiley & Sons, Inc.

mutations have been described (Shy *et al.*, 2004). The X-chromosomal subtype of CMT, CMT1X, is caused by mutations in the gene coding for the gap junction channel protein connexin 32, *GJB1*. More than 300 causative mutations have been described in this gene (Reilly *et al.*, 2011).

CMT4, similarly to CMT1, a demyelinating subtype, clinically resembles the former, but is often characterized by a childhood onset. Again, various mutations can be causative, among these mutations in genes encoding the Myotubularin-related protein (MTMR2; Bolino *et al.*, 2000) and EGR2 (KROX20), which plays a role in SC differentiation (Le *et al.*, 2005; Jessen and Mirsky, 2008).

Mutations leading to the axonal subtype, CMT2, are, among others, mutations in the *microtubule kinesin family* gene (*KIF1Bβ*), which reduce axonal transport and in the light chain neurofilament gene *NEFL*, which result in abnormal aggregation of neurofilament. Interestingly, mutations affecting mitochondrial functions and thereby interfering with energy supplies are frequently found to cause CMT2. Examples for this are mutations in *mitofusin 2* (*MFN2*), which is essential for the fusion of the outer membrane of mitochondria and can result in perturbed axonal transport (Chapman *et al.*, 2013) and in *mitochondrially encoded ATP synthase 6* (*MT-ATP6*) (Pitceathly *et al.*, 2012).

Numerous genetically modified rodent models of CMT have been generated (see Fledrich *et al.* (2012) for review). In some of these models, inflammation has been identified to play an important role in the pathogenesis, that is, in mice faithfully mimicking the demyelinating forms CMT1A (most common), CMT1X (second most common), and CMT1B (third most common). These models carry genetic modifications that result in mild overexpression of peripheral myelin protein 22 (PMP22tg mice; strain C61; Huxley *et al.*, 1998), deficiency for connexin 32 (Cx32def mice; Anzini *et al.*, 1997), and heterozygous deficiency for myelin protein zero (P0het mice; Giese *et al.*, 1992; Martini *et al.*, 1995), respectively. In most other models of CMT, inflammation has not yet been carefully investigated.

Although the described modifications in these mice affect distinct proteins and result in some characteristic features in each model, there are remarkable similarities in the ultimate outcome of the disease. These common aspects in the phenotype might be related to activation of similar pathomechanistic cascades comprising the disease-modifying secondary inflammatory reaction that will be detailed in the following section.

Subtype-Specific Molecular Patterns of CMT1

Although inherited peripheral neuropathies of the CMT1 type comprise a genetically heterogeneous group of disorders, they display some similarities in the pathological phenotype, mainly represented by demyelination and axonal perturbation often culminating in muscle atrophy. Nevertheless, some abnormalities in the molecular pattern of myelinating SCs can be detected by comparison of models for the three most frequent subtypes. In a recent study, several developmentally regulated molecules and markers for SC differentiation and dedifferentiation were investigated in CMT1 mutant mice, and a nonuniform expression pattern could be observed when the myelinating SCs were considered as opposed to the uniform supernumerary ones (Klein *et al.*, 2014). Myelinating SCs of PMP22tg mice but not of P0het and Cx32def mutants showed early onset alterations, molecularly represented by a robust expression of the adhesion molecule neural cell adhesion molecule (NCAM). However, myelinating SCs of Cx32def mice showed an upregulation of the transcription factor c-Jun, which might be causally linked to early axonal perturbation and compensatory axonal sprouting. This is comparable to the c-Jun-driven molecular alterations seen in SCs during Wallerian degeneration (Parkinson *et al.*, 2008; Arthur-Farraj *et al.*, 2012; Fontana *et al.*, 2012). Therefore, the molecular pattern of mutant myelinating SCs with distinct genotypes differed at early disease stages, that is, before supernumerary and denervated SCs of uniform patterns emerged (Guenard *et al.*, 1996; Klein *et al.*, 2014). Similar observations could be gained in a severe, early onset model of CMT1B (MpzR98C mutation), where the expression of c-Jun was accompanied by Krox20 expression so that an arrest in SC development was considered (Saporta *et al.*, 2012).

Most interestingly, these molecular alterations are not only limited to animal models, but also visible in patients with CMT1 (Hanemann *et al.*, 1996, 1997; Hutton *et al.*, 2011). These observations demonstrate that the genetically distinct subtypes appear to have specific disease patterns.

Molecular Commonalities of CMT1 Subtypes – a Link to Inflammation

In contrast to the specific molecular patterns, a typical commonality found in different CMT1 mouse models is the increased activation of the extracellular signal-regulated kinase 1/2 (ERK1/2) and its upstream activator MAP kinase/ERK kinase 1/2 (MEK1/2) in mutant myelinating SCs [see Fig. 8.1 and Fischer *et al.* (2008a), Groh *et al.* (2010), and Kohl *et al.* (2010a)]. Interestingly, the MEK-ERK pathway is also strongly activated after nerve injury (Harrisingh *et al.*, 2004).

It is currently not clear which mechanisms lead to MEK/ERK activation in SCs under lesion or mutant conditions. In case of myelin mutations, it is possible that an endoplasmic reticulum

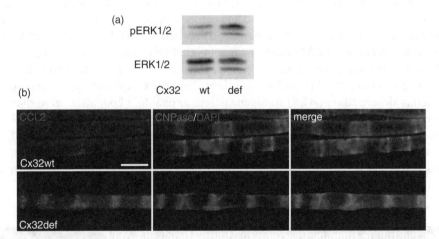

Figure 8.1   Western blot analysis (a) and immunofluorescent labeling of single fiber preparations (b) of femoral quadriceps nerves from age-matched Cx32wt and Cx32def mice. (a) There is increased phosphorylation of ERK in peripheral nerves of Cx32def mice. (b) Mutant myelinating Schwann cells show increased expression of CCL2 (red) in cytoplasmic compartments such as Schmidt–Lanterman incisures which are marked by anti-CNPase reactivity (green). Scale bar: 20 μm. (*See insert for color representation of this figure.*)

(ER)-stress response as identified in distinct P0 mutants (Pennuto *et al.*, 2008; Saporta *et al.*, 2012; Ydens *et al.*, 2013) is linked to increased MEK–ERK activation. It remains to be shown whether ER-stress is indeed linked to the MEK–ERK pathway in myelin mutant mice and whether ER-stress occurs in P0het, Cx32def, and PMP22tg mice.

Another possible cause for increased MEK–ERK activation in mutant SCs might be related to the signaling mechanisms after peripheral nerve injury. Recently, Stassart *et al.* demonstrated an important role for neuregulin 1 type I (NRG1/I) in remyelination after nerve crush (Stassart *et al.*, 2013). They showed that Wallerian degeneration triggered the expression of SC-derived NRG1/I in an autocrine manner and that its overexpression in transgenic mice improved remyelination. Most interestingly, conditional SC-specific NRG1-deficient mice displayed a reduced capacity of myelin regeneration after peripheral nerve injury that was accompanied by an absent ERK1/2 activation in mutant Schwann cells (Stassart *et al.*, 2013). However, if perturbed SC–axon inter- action also occurs in CMT1 mouse models and leads to increased expression of NRG1/I needs to be investigated in further experiments.

Although the upstream mechanisms resulting in increased MEK–ERK signaling are not well understood, a clear link between the MEK/ERK-signaling pathway and inflammation-related factors could be identified in distinct CMT1 mouse models. One of these factors is monocyte chemoattractant protein-1 (MCP-1/CCL2), a chemokine that is elevated in peripheral nerves of myelin mutants in comparison to wild-type mice and expressed by SCs [see Fig. 8.1 and Fischer *et al.* (2008a), Groh *et al.* (2010), and Kohl *et al.* (2010a)]. Pharmacological blockade of the signaling pathway with a specific MEK1/2 inhibitor prevented CCL2 upregulation and thus pro- vided evidence for a direct link between ERK1/2 activation and downstream CCL2 expression (Fischer *et al.*, 2008a; Groh *et al.*, 2010; Kohl *et al.*, 2010a). This link between ERK signaling and inflammation-related cytokines as well as Schwann cell plasticity has also been observed in a reversible *in vivo* model (Napoli *et al.*, 2012). After experimental activation of the MEK–ERK cascade by challenging a transgenic Raf-estrogen receptor fusion protein with tamoxifen, several cytokines including CCL2 were upregulated and caused activation of macrophages and demyeli- nation. However, the similarities and differences between the cytokine milieu expressed after nerve injury and in nerves of CMT models are not completely characterized as yet.

In addition to inflammation-related cytokines, some axonal degeneration pathways are also shared between models of CMT and nerve injury. This is exemplified by the finding that the slow Wallerian degeneration (*Wld^S*) transgene delays axonal loss both after nerve injury and in CMT models (Samsam *et al.*, 2003; Coleman, 2005; Meyer zu Horste *et al.*, 2011). However, the cause of axonal damage and the subsequent regenerative success are certainly different. In addition, inflammation is viewed as a beneficial aspect required for efficient regeneration after nerve injury, whereas several findings have demonstrated a detrimental role of immune reactions in models of CMT.

The Impact of Innate Immune Reactions in Mouse Models of CMT1

Activation of the MEK–ERK-signaling pathway in SCs and upregulation of inflammation-related cytokines in models of inherited peripheral neuropathies have been recognized to result in low-grade innate immune reactions. In several rodent models of different CMT subtypes, an age-dependent increase in the number of endoneurial macrophages has been detected in the peripheral nerves in comparison to wild-type littermates (Schmid *et al.*, 2000; Kobsar *et al.*, 2002, 2005; Berghoff *et al.*, 2005; Ip *et al.*, 2006). Although the numbers of macrophages are already increased early on in PMP22tg mice and only moderately expand during aging (Kobsar *et al.*, 2005; Kohl *et al.*, 2010a), there is a later onset but constant increase of macrophage numbers in Cx32def and P0het mice (Schmid *et al.*, 2000; Kobsar *et al.*, 2002). This kinetics correlates well with the progression of the nerve pathology, as PMP22tg mice also exhibit myelin and Schwann cell alterations at an earlier age compared to the other models (Klein *et al.*, 2014).

The increased recruitment of macrophages appears to be mediated by elevated expression of at least two different cytokines, which control the infiltration, proliferation, and activation of macrophages. Studies on the corresponding CMT1 mouse models demonstrated that the chemokine CCL2 is important for the infiltration of macrophages of hematogeneous origin into the mutant nerves in Cx32def and P0het mice (Fischer *et al.*, 2008b; Groh *et al.*, 2010). This chemokine is also upregulated by SCs after axotomy and causes macrophage influx (Toews *et al.*, 1998; Perrin *et al.*, 2005). In addition, colony-stimulating factor-1 [CSF-1/M-CSF (macrophage colony-stimulating factor)] expression regulates the local proliferation of nerve-resident macrophages in the myelin mutant nerves (Müller *et al.*, 2007). CSF-1 is known to be an important regulator of the survival, activation, and proliferation of macrophages (Chitu and Stanley, 2006) and was shown to be upregulated in peripheral nerves of distinct myelin mutant mice (Fischer *et al.*, 2008b; Groh *et al.*, 2012). Local expression of CSF-1 in the nerve had been suggested previously. Indeed, recent observations could identify endoneurial fibroblasts as the cellular source of CSF-1 (Groh *et al.*, 2012). Intricate cell–cell contacts between CSF-1-producing fibroblasts and macrophages can be observed in the peripheral nerves. This is reminiscent of other systems and diseases and their corresponding models such as osteoclastic bone resorption, Wallerian degeneration, and rheumatoid arthritis (Ohara *et al.*, 1986; Hamilton *et al.*, 1993; Bischof *et al.*, 2000; Teitelbaum, 2000).

In addition to increased numbers, the macrophages in peripheral nerves of myelin mutants also exhibit morphological alterations in comparison to wild-type mice. Macrophages in the mutant mice often have a "foamy" appearance indicating increased phagocytic activity and con-tain myelin debris at varying stages of degradation [see Fig. 8.2 and Carenini *et al.* (2001) and Kobsar *et al.* (2002, 2005)]. Moreover, in the nerves of the mutants, some macrophages can be found within endoneurial tubes contacting myelin or demyelinated axons (Ip *et al.*, 2006). This apposition is suggestive of an active involvement in myelin degradation and is reminiscent of macrophage–myelin interactions in Guillain–Barré syndrome, an acute primary inflammatory disorder of the peripheral nervous system (PNS) (Lampert, 1969; Ho *et al.*, 1998).

As a functional proof that macrophages are actively involved in demyelination in the described mouse models, crossbreeding experiments have been performed to genetically block macrophage recruitment and activation. When P0het and Cx32def mice are crossbred to osteopetrotic (op) mice, spontaneous CSF-1 null mutants, increased macrophage recruitment in the peripheral nerves is prevented, and this is accompanied by a robust and persistent amelioration of neuropathological alterations [see Fig. 8.2 and Carenini *et al.* (2001) and Groh *et al.* (2012)]. This finding clearly demonstrates that macrophages are not just scavengers of myelin debris in the mutant nerve, but are actively involved and amplify the demyelinating abnormalities.

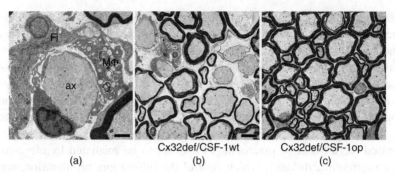

Figure 8.2   Electron micrographs of lumbar ventral roots from age-matched Cx32def/CSF-1wt (a,b) and Cx32def/CSF-1op (c) mice. Foamy macrophages (MΦ) containing myelin debris can be frequently observed in peripheral nerves of Cx32def/CSF-1wt mice (a) and are often associated with endoneurial fibroblasts (Fi) and demyelinated axons (ax). Scale bar: 2 μm. Cx32def/CSF-1op mice (c) exhibit a profound amelioration of the demyelinating phenotype in comparison with Cx32def/CSF-1wt mice (b). Scale bar: 5 μm.

Further evidence for a prominent role of macrophages in the CMT1 models was gained by crossbreeding experiments with CCL2 knockout mice. Heterozygous deficiency in CCL2 resulted in attenuation of macrophage recruitment in P0het, Cx32def, and PMP22tg mice and also significantly ameliorated the demyelinating phenotype (Fischer *et al.*, 2008b; Groh *et al.*, 2010; Kohl *et al.*, 2010a). Interestingly, homozygous deficiency for CCL2 did not attenuate macrophage recruitment in P0het and Cx32def mice, as reduced influx into the nerve was compensated with increased proliferation of resident macrophages and upregulation of CSF-1 expression (Fischer *et al.*, 2008b; Groh *et al.*, 2010). Accordingly, the demyelinating phenotype was also not ameliorated, demonstrating a close correlation between the total numbers of endoneurial macrophages and the severity of the demyelinating phenotype.

While the contribution of macrophages is prominent and well documented in the models of demyelinating neuropathies (P0het, Cx32def mice), less is known about their impact in early onset dysmyelinating conditions. Homozygous P0 knockout mice display defective myelin compaction and myelin degeneration from the outset and a loss of myelinated axons that is most prominent during the first 3 months of life (Giese *et al.*, 1992; Frei *et al.*, 1999; Samsam *et al.*, 2003). Similarly, endoneurial macrophage numbers are elevated early, peak at 3 months of age, and steadily decline afterward (Berghoff *et al.*, 2005). In addition, macrophages are often associated with degenerating axons (Ey *et al.*, 2007). However, the exact impact of these innate immune reactions regarding neuropathological alterations in P0-deficient mice remains to be determined. Of particular interest, PMP22tg mice exhibit both early onset myelination and differentiation defects and an additional demyelinating component without prominent loss of axons (Klein *et al.*, 2014). In this model, a detrimental impact of macrophages has been demonstrated by the reduced pathology in CCL2-deficient double mutants (Kohl *et al.*, 2010a) and is also observed in CSF-1-deficient double mutants (J.G. and R.M., unpublished observations), but the beneficial effects appear less pronounced in comparison to P0het and Cx32def mice.

In general, the exact mechanisms and molecular factors of macrophage-mediated myelin defects and demyelination require further characterization. However, the observation that the innate immune system plays a key role in a demyelinating disease of primarily genetic cause opens novel therapeutic possibilities.

Importantly, the described crossbreeding experiments not only proved a prominent role of macrophages in demyelination, but also revealed their involvement in axonal perturbation. Axonal damage and degeneration and the resulting muscular atrophy are the key determinants of clinical symptoms in patients with CMT1 (Scherer and Wrabetz, 2008). Thus, understanding the mechanisms related to axonal damage in the context of Schwann cell mutations is of critical importance. Although it is conceivable that Schwann cells support axonal integrity (Nave, 2010), it might also be possible that immune reactions directly or indirectly harm axons. Mouse models of CMT1 also display characteristics of axonal perturbation such as formation of periaxonal vacuoles, juxtaparanodal ion channel disturbances, and denervation of distal muscles (Groh et al., 2010, 2012; Kohl et al., 2010a). Similarly to the demyelinating alterations, axonal perturbation is significantly ameliorated when macrophage recruitment or activation is genetically blocked. Heterozygous deficiency for CCL2 or lack of CSF-1 resulted in significantly improved axonal properties in all three models. This amelioration was reflected in preserved juxtaparanodal axonal domains and an attenuation of muscle denervation, ultimately resulting in improved strength (Groh et al., 2010, 2012; Kohl et al., 2010a).

In Wallerian degeneration, macrophages are important for rapid removal of nerve-growth-inhibiting myelin and thus appear to participate in an evolutionary conserved repair program. However, in case of CMT-related glial mutations, this repair program appears to be detrimental to neural integrity when activated under nonlesion conditions (Martini et al., 2013). In line with an inappropriate activation of this repair program, macrophages in Wallerian degeneration (Ydens et al., 2012) and also in CMT1 models (D.K. and R.M., unpublished observations) exhibit an alternative M2 activation, which is supposed to foster regeneration and tissue repair. However, in conditions with primary Schwann cell deficits also alternatively activated, macrophages appear to be harmful to initially healthy axons.

Previous studies in models of Wallerian degeneration have also highlighted that the complement system is involved in the efficient removal of myelin and the recruitment and function of macrophages in this process (Dailey et al., 1998; Liu et al., 1999; Ramaglia et al., 2009). In addition, complement attack of myelinated axons has been described in some polyneuropathies (Ferrari et al., 1998). Therefore, it might be of future interest to investigate reactions of the complement system also in the CMT1 models, which could possibly also provide a link between innate and adaptive immune reactions in models of CMT.

The Impact of Adaptive Immune Reactions in Mouse Models of CMT1

First reports indicating a role of the adaptive immune system in hereditary neuropathies focused on the presence of elevated numbers of lymphocytes and activated lymphocytes in the peripheral blood of patients with CMT (Williams et al., 1987, 1993).

Functional evidence that lymphocytes are crucial contributors to the pathology in CMT1 models was derived from P0het and Cx32def mice. In both mouse models, CD8+ T-lymphocytes accumulated in the peripheral nerves (Shy et al., 1997; Schmid et al., 2000). Crossbreeding of these myelin mutants with mice deficient in *Rag1* (*recombinase activating gene 1*), which leads to the lack of mature T- and B-lymphocytes, resulted in a marked amelioration of the demyelinating and axonopathic phenotype and a reduction of macrophage numbers (Schmid *et al.*, 2000; Kobsar *et al.*, 2003). A similar amelioration of the phenotype was seen in P0het mice on a TCR-α null background, lacking αβ T-cells. Proof that peripheral lymphocytes were indeed responsible for the deterioration of pathological features in this model was derived from the fact that transplantation of wild-type bone marrow into P0het RAG1−/− mice restored the pathological phenotype to a similar level as in genetically immune competent P0het mice (Maurer *et al.*, 2001).

However, the involvement of lymphocytes in the pathology of neuropathies does not appear to be uniform in all models of CMT disease. In PMP22tg mice, the absence of lymphocytes does not influence nerve pathology, while macrophages are crucial players in the development of the pathology (Kohl *et al.*, 2010a, 2010b). Interestingly, P0 null mice that lack mature lymphocytes even show increased axonal damage, but further studies are necessary to understand the mechanisms behind this finding (Berghoff *et al.*, 2005).

Corroborating a pathogenic impact of lymphocytes, P0het mice additionally deficient in programmed cell death-1 (PD-1) showed an aggravation of nerve inflammation and neuropathy (Kroner *et al.*, 2009). PD-1 is a coinhibitory molecule that is expressed on the surface of activated B-cells, T-cells, and macrophages and terminates immune responses by binding its ligand PD-L1, which is expressed by a variety of antigen-presenting cells and in tissues and PD-L2, which is restricted to dendritic cells (Okazaki *et al.*, 2013).

Which lymphocytes are responsible for the disease-amplifying effect in P0het and Cx32def mice is not yet known. In principle, B-lymphocytes might be interesting candidates, as antibodies produced by plasma cells could function as potential recognition signals for phagocytosing macrophages to detect or opsonize their target in the peripheral nerves of CMT1 mouse models. Such a function of endogenous antibodies was recently shown in a peripheral nerve injury model (Vargas *et al.*, 2010). In this study, the authors detected a strong deposition of antibodies along myelinated fibers distal to the lesion site. Furthermore, Vargas *et al.* could prove that this accumulation is necessary for rapid macrophage activation, myelin clearance, and regeneration during Wallerian degeneration by using B-cell-deficient mice that are not able to produce endogenous antibodies (JHD-mice). Most interestingly, a similar antibody deposition could also be detected in affected nerves of CMT1 mouse mutants in contrast to wild-type mice (D.K. and R.M., unpublished observations). However, future studies are needed to clarify the exact function of antibodies in the pathogenesis of CMT1 mutants.

Implications for Putative Therapeutic Approaches

The finding that reactions of the innate and adaptive immune system amplify disease severity in mouse models of CMT1 might have important implications for novel treatment approaches. However, a prerequisite for applying putative immunosuppressive or immunomodulatory therapies is that the observations in the mouse models actually are of relevance for patients and reflect the pathomechanisms in human nerves. Studies on CMT1 patient biopsies regarding the recruitment of immune cells are limited. However, there are observations that similar processes occur as in the mouse models, especially in children with CMT1. Analogous to the mouse models, myelin-laden foamy macrophages within the endoneurial space can occasionally be detected by electron microscopy (Crawford and Griffin, 1991; Carvalho et al., 2005), and this was previously mainly attributed to superimposed inflammation in atypical cases (see the following section). However, the combination of electron microscopy with immunohistochemical approaches revealed not only the presence of macrophages often laden with myelin debris, but also contacts of these cells with fibroblasts that expressed CSF-1 in nerve biopsies of patients with different CMT1 subtypes (Groh et al., 2012). In addition, major histocompatibility complex (MHC) class II-positive macrophages can often be found integrated into onion bulb formations (Stoll et al., 1998). These findings suggest that similar low-grade inflammatory reactions might occur in the peripheral nerves of patients with CMT1, especially early in pathogenesis. Nevertheless, more extensive studies are necessary to investigate inflammation in biopsies, preferentially at different stages of disease. In addition, thorough treatment studies will have to be performed in the rodent models to find safe and appropriate drugs that can be applied over years, if not lifelong. For such long-term approaches to treat non-life-threatening diseases, mechanism-specific drugs with minimal adverse reactions have to be identified.

Prominent inflammation is described only in an atypical subgroup of patients with CMT with pathological similarities to inflammatory demyelinating polyradiculoneuropathy (Chronic inflammatory demyelinating polyneuropathy, CIDP) (Martini and Toyka, 2004; Desurkar et al., 2009; Cottenie et al., 2013). However, some of these cases appear to react to anti-inflammatory treatment such as intravenous immunoglobulin (IVIG) application (Ginsberg et al., 2004; Martini and Toyka, 2004; Schneider-Gold et al., 2010; Miki et al., 2013).

On the basis of these observations and the fact that immune cells contribute to neural pathology in CMT1 models, the use of potent immune suppressors appears to be a possible therapeutic approach. Tacrolimus (FK506) is frequently used to suppress the immune system in patients receiving organ transplants. However, when used to treat P0het mice, it did not successfully reduce the amount of CD8+ T-lymphocytes in the peripheral nerves of myelin mutants, and it strongly increased demyelination (Ip et al., 2009). This neurotoxic side effect is likely due to a "second hit" in mice with a predisposition. Some substances might have no or mild neurotoxic effects in a healthy nerve but could be counterproductive for CMT models and patients who appear to have a higher susceptibility for additional detrimental effects.

Other possible approaches to inhibit or attenuate the mechanisms related to inflammation have been identified in the mouse models. Pharmacologic inhibition of the MEK–ERK cascade has been performed in three CMT1 mouse models. Short-term treatment approaches using the MEK inhibitor CI-1040 resulted in reduced CCL2 upregulation (Fischer et al., 2008a; Groh et al., 2010; Kohl et al., 2010a). Importantly, in at least one of the models, macrophage recruitment and neuropathology were also reduced in comparison to sham-treated controls (Groh et al., 2010). Therefore, inhibition of the MEK–ERK-signaling cascade might be one approach to block the downstream inflammatory reactions. However, despite being tested for possible clinical applications in severe malignancies (Rusconi et al., 2012), the MEK–ERK pathway is pleiotropically involved in a variety of cell biological processes, and thus side effects have to be expected by long-term inhibition of this pathway.

Another direction for an immunosuppressive treatment approach might emerge by interfering with the CSF-1 signaling pathway, based on the robust and persistent amelioration of neuropathy by CSF-1 deficiency in different CMT1 mouse models (Carenini et al., 2001; Groh et al.,

2012). Recently, Elmore *et al.* could demonstrate that the treatment of wild-type mice with a selective CSF-1 receptor (CSF-1R) kinase inhibitor depleted nearly all microglia, the resident macrophages of the brain, without having negative effects on motor or cognitive behavior during the investigated period (Elmore *et al.*, 2014). Given the fact that not only microglia but also nearly all macrophages in peripheral nerves express the CSF-1R (Carenini *et al.*, 2001; Groh *et al.*, 2012), such inhibitors might be an interesting therapeutic option. Indeed, first preliminary experiments showed a drastic reduction of macrophage numbers in peripheral nerves of wild-type and mutant mice after treatment with a selective CSF-1R inhibitor (D.K. and R.M., unpublished observations). However, the effects of CSF-1Ri-mediated reduction of macrophage numbers on myelin degeneration and axonal damage in CMT1 mouse mutants need to be investigated in further experiments. In addition, similarly to inhibition of pleiotropic signaling pathways, potent immunosuppressive drugs used to treat acute inflammatory conditions are often inappropriate for long-term application. Ideal treatment approaches should have a narrow activity spectrum and specifically inhibit detrimental aspects of the chronic low-grade inflammation present in CMT nerves without disturbing physiological functions of the immune system.

Looking for such alternative approaches to modulate chronic low-grade inflammation in peripheral neuropathies, the potential use of mesenchymal stem cells (MSCs) might come into focus. MSCs are multipotent progenitor cells that can be isolated from several human tissues (i.e., bone marrow or adipose tissue) and possess the potential of self-renewal and differentiation into several cell types (Dominici *et al.*, 2009; Baer and Geiger, 2012). There are several recent

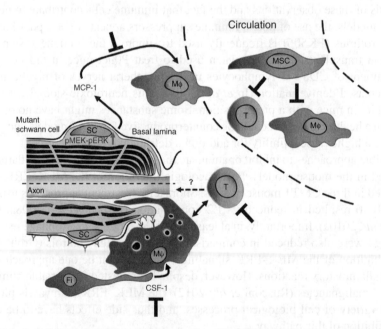

Figure 8.3 Schematic depicting inflammation-related molecular and cellular players involved in CMT pathomechanisms as identified in the mouse models as well as hypothetical targets (**T**) for treatment options. SC, Schwann cell; MΦ, macrophage; Fi, fibroblast; T, T-lymphocyte; Y, antibody; MSC, mesenchymal stem cell. *Source*: Adapted from Martini *et al.* (2013), with permission from Elsevier. (*See insert for color representation of this figure.*)

studies dealing with a direct (systemic) immunomodulatory function of MSCs rather than MSC engraftment and differentiation (Abrams *et al.*, 2009; Gebler *et al.*, 2012). Leal *et al.* already proposed the use of immunomodulatory MSCs as a therapeutic option in CMT1 disorders (Leal *et al.*, 2008). After application, MSCs might systemically attenuate inflammation and thereby foster the regeneration capacity in affected peripheral nerves, making them a promising tool for treatment of CMT1.

Synopsis

Despite being caused by a plethora of mutations in distinct genes, the final clinical presentation of patients with CMT1 shows some common aspects. Rodent models have emerged as important tools to study mechanisms and identify putative treatment approaches. A growing body of evidence raises hope for feasible approaches by targeting low-grade secondary inflammation of the innate and adaptive immune system to preserve neural integrity in different subtypes (see Fig. 8.3).

Acknowledgments

The studies of the laboratory of RM were supported by the German Research Foundation (SFB581; MA 1053/6-1), Charcot-Marie-Tooth association, Plexxikon Inc., and local funds of the University of Wuerzburg (IZKF). The authors are grateful to previous members of the Martini laboratory who substantially contributed to the concept of peripheral nerve inflammation in inherited neuropathies (alphabetical order): Stefano Carenini, Stefan Fischer, Chi Wang Ip, Igor Kobsar, Bianca Kohl, Mathias Mäurer, and Christoph Schmid. The authors are indebted to Karen Bieback and Steve Scherer for valuable discussions.

References

Abrams, M.B., Dominguez, C., Pernold, K. *et al.* (2009) Multipotent mesenchymal stromal cells attenuate chronic inflammation and injury-induced sensitivity to mechanical stimuli in experimental spinal cord injury. *Restorative Neurology and Neuroscience*, **27**, 307–321.

Anzini, P., Neuberg, D.H., Schachner, M. *et al.* (1997) Structural abnormalities and deficient maintenance of peripheral nerve myelin in mice lacking the gap junction protein connexin 32. *Journal of Neuroscience*, **17**, 4545–4551.

Arthur-Farraj, P.J., Latouche, M., Wilton, D.K. *et al.* (2012) c-Jun reprograms Schwann cells of injured nerves to generate a repair cell essential for regeneration. *Neuron*, **75**, 633–647.

Baer, P.C. & Geiger, H. (2012) Adipose-derived mesenchymal stromal/stem cells: Tissue localization, characterization, and heterogeneity. *Stem Cells International*, **2012**, 812693.

Berghoff, M., Samsam, M., Muller, M. *et al.* (2005) Neuroprotective effect of the immune system in a mouse model of severe dysmyelinating hereditary neuropathy: Enhanced axonal degeneration following disruption of the RAG-1 gene. *Molecular and Cellular Neuroscience*, **28**, 118–127.

Bischof, R.J., Zafiropoulos, D., Hamilton, J.A. & Campbell, I.K. (2000) Exacerbation of acute inflammatory arthritis by the colony-stimulating factors CSF-1 and granulocyte macrophage (GM)-CSF: Evidence of macrophage infiltration and local proliferation. *Clinical and Experimental Immunology*, **119**, 361–367.

Bolino, A., Muglia, M., Conforti, F.L. *et al.* (2000) Charcot-Marie-Tooth type 4B is caused by mutations in the gene encoding myotubularin-related protein-2. *Nature Genetics*, **25**, 17–19.

Carenini, S., Maurer, M., Werner, A. *et al.* (2001) The role of macrophages in demyelinating peripheral nervous system of mice heterozygously deficient in p0. *Journal of Cell Biology*, **152**, 301–308.

Carvalho, A.A., Vital, A., Ferrer, X. *et al.* (2005) Charcot-Marie-Tooth disease type 1A: Clinicopathological correlations in 24 patients. *Journal of the Peripheral Nervous System*, **10**, 85–92.

Chapman, A.L., Bennett, E.J., Ramesh, T.M., De Vos, K.J. & Grierson, A.J. (2013) Axonal transport defects in a mitofusin 2 loss of function model of Charcot-Marie-Tooth disease in zebrafish. *PLoS One*, **8**, e67276.

Chitu, V. & Stanley, E.R. (2006) Colony-stimulating factor-1 in immunity and inflammation. *Current Opinion in Immunology*, **18**, 39–48.

Coleman, M. (2005) Axon degeneration mechanisms: Commonality amid diversity. *Nature Reviews Neuroscience*, **6**, 889–898.

Cottenie, E., Menezes, M.P., Rossor, A.M. *et al.* (2013) Rapidly progressive asymmetrical weakness in Charcot-Marie-Tooth disease type 4J resembles chronic inflammatory demyelinating polyneuropathy. *Neuromuscular Disorders*, **23**, 399–403.

Crawford, T.O. & Griffin, J.W. (1991) Morphometrical and ultrastructural evaluation of the sural nerve in children with Charcot-Marie-Tooth: Implication for pathogenesis and treatment. *Annals of Neurology*, **30**, 500.

Dailey, A.T., Avellino, A.M., Benthem, L., Silver, J. & Kliot, M. (1998) Complement depletion reduces macrophage infiltration and activation during Wallerian degeneration and axonal regeneration. *Journal of Neuroscience*, **18**, 6713–6722.

Desurkar, A., Lin, J.P., Mills, K. *et al.* (2009) Charcot-Marie-Tooth (CMT) disease 1A with superimposed inflammatory polyneuropathy in children. *Neuropediatrics*, **40**, 85–88.

Dominici, M., Paolucci, P., Conte, P. & Horwitz, E.M. (2009) Heterogeneity of multipotent mesenchymal stromal cells: From stromal cells to stem cells and vice versa. *Transplantation*, **87**, S36–42.

Elmore, M.R., Najafi, A.R., Koike, M.A. *et al.* (2014) Colony-stimulating factor 1 receptor signaling is necessary for microglia viability, unmasking a microglia progenitor cell in the adult brain. *Neuron*, **82**, 380–397.

Ey, B., Kobsar, I., Blazyca, H., Kroner, A. & Martini, R. (2007) Visualization of degenerating axons in a dysmyelinating mouse mutant with axonal loss. *Molecular and Cellular Neuroscience*, **35**, 153–160.

Ferrari, S., Morbin, M., Nobile-Orazio, E. *et al.* (1998) Antisulfatide polyneuropathy: Antibody-mediated complement attack on peripheral myelin. *Acta Neuropathologica*, **96**, 569–574.

Fischer, S., Weishaupt, A., Troppmair, J. & Martini, R. (2008a) Increase of MCP-1 (CCL2) in myelin mutant Schwann cells is mediated by MEK-ERK signaling pathway. *Glia*, **56**, 836–843.

Fischer, S., Kleinschnitz, C., Muller, M. *et al.* (2008b) Monocyte chemoattractant protein-1 is a pathogenic component in a model for a hereditary peripheral neuropathy. *Molecular and Cellular Neuroscience*, **37**, 359–366.

Fledrich, R., Stassart, R.M. & Sereda, M.W. (2012) Murine therapeutic models for Charcot-Marie-Tooth (CMT) disease. *British Medical Bulletin*, **102**, 89–113.

Fontana, X., Hristova, M., Da Costa, C. *et al.* (2012) c-Jun in Schwann cells promotes axonal regeneration and motoneuron survival via paracrine signaling. *Journal of Cell Biology*, **198**, 127–141.

Frei, R., Motzing, S., Kinkelin, I., Schachner, M., Koltzenburg, M. & Martini, R. (1999) Loss of distal axons and sensory Merkel cells and features indicative of muscle denervation in hindlimbs of P0-deficient mice. *Journal of Neuroscience*, **19**, 6058–6067.

Gebler, A., Zabel, O. & Seliger, B. (2012) The immunomodulatory capacity of mesenchymal stem cells. *Trends in Molecular Medicine*, **18**, 128–134.

Giese, K.P., Martini, R., Lemke, G., Soriano, P. & Schachner, M. (1992) Mouse P0 gene disruption leads to hypomyelination, abnormal expression of recognition molecules, and degeneration of myelin and axons. *Cell*, **71**, 565–576.

Ginsberg, L., Malik, O., Kenton, A.R. *et al.* (2004) Coexistent hereditary and inflammatory neuropathy. *Brain*, **127**, 193–202.

Groh, J., Weis, J., Zieger, H., Stanley, E.R., Heuer, H. & Martini, R. (2012) Colony-stimulating factor-1 mediates macrophage-related neural damage in a model for Charcot-Marie-Tooth disease type 1X. *Brain*, **135**, 88–104.

Groh, J., Heinl, K., Kohl, B. *et al.* (2010) Attenuation of MCP-1/CCL2 expression ameliorates neuropathy in a mouse model for Charcot-Marie-Tooth 1X. *Human Molecular Genetics*, **19**, 3530–3543.

Guenard, V., Montag, D., Schachner, M. & Martini, R. (1996) Onion bulb cells in mice deficient for myelin genes share molecular properties with immature, differentiated non-myelinating, and denervated Schwann cells. *Glia*, **18**, 27–38.

Hamilton, J.A., Filonzi, E.L. & Ianches, G. (1993) Regulation of macrophage colony-stimulating factor (M-CSF) production in cultured human synovial fibroblasts. *Growth Factors*, **9**, 157–165.

Hanemann, C.O., Gabreels-Fasten, A.A., Muller, H.W. & Stoll, G. (1996) Low affinity NGF receptor expression in CMT1A nerve biopsies of different disease stages. *Brain*, **119** (Pt 5), 1461–1469.

Hanemann, C.O., Gabreels-Festen, A.A., Stoll, G. & Muller, H.W. (1997) Schwann cell differentiation in Charcot-Marie-Tooth disease type 1A (CMT1A): Normal number of myelinating Schwann cells in young CMT1A patients and neural cell adhesion molecule expression in onion bulbs. *Acta Neuropathologica*, **94**, 310–315.

Harding, A.E. & Thomas, P.K. (1980) The clinical features of hereditary motor and sensory neuropathy types I and II. *Brain*, **103**, 259–280.

Harrisingh, M.C., Perez-Nadales, E., Parkinson, D.B., Malcolm, D.S., Mudge, A.W. & Lloyd, A.C. (2004) The Ras/Raf/ERK signalling pathway drives Schwann cell dedifferentiation. *EMBO Journal*, **23**, 3061–3071.

Ho, T.W., McKhann, G.M. & Griffin, J.W. (1998) Human autoimmune neuropathies. *Annual Review of Neuroscience*, **21**, 187–226.

Hutton, E.J., Carty, L., Laura, M. *et al.* (2011) c-Jun expression in human neuropathies: A pilot study. *Journal of the Peripheral Nervous System*, **16**, 295–303.

Huxley, C., Passage, E., Robertson, A.M. *et al.* (1998) Correlation between varying levels of PMP22 expression and the degree of demyelination and reduction in nerve conduction velocity in transgenic mice. *Human Molecular Genetics*, **7**, 449–458.

Ip, C.W., Kroner, A., Kohl, B., Wessig, C. & Martini, R. (2009) Tacrolimus (FK506) causes disease aggravation in models for inherited peripheral myelinopathies. *Neurobiology of Disease*, **33**, 207–212.

Ip, C.W., Kroner, A., Fischer, S. *et al.* (2006) Role of immune cells in animal models for inherited peripheral neuropathies. *NeuroMolecular Medicine*, **8**, 175–190.

Jessen, K.R. & Mirsky, R. (2008) Negative regulation of myelination: Relevance for development, injury, and demyelinating disease. *Glia*, **56**, 1552–1565.

Klein, D., Groh, J., Wettmarshausen, J. & Martini, R. (2014) Nonuniform molecular features of myelinating Schwann cells in models for CMT1: Distinct disease patterns are associated with NCAM and c-Jun upregulation. *Glia*, **62**, 736–750.

Kobsar, I., Maurer, M., Ott, T. & Martini, R. (2002) Macrophage-related demyelination in peripheral nerves of mice deficient in the gap junction protein connexin 32. *Neuroscience Letters*, **320**, 17–20.

Kobsar, I., Hasenpusch-Theil, K., Wessig, C., Muller, H.W. & Martini, R. (2005) Evidence for macrophage-mediated myelin disruption in an animal model for Charcot-Marie-Tooth neuropathy type 1A. *Journal of Neuroscience Research*, **81**, 857–864.

Kobsar, I., Berghoff, M., Samsam, M. *et al.* (2003) Preserved myelin integrity and reduced axonopathy in connexin32-deficient mice lacking the recombination activating gene-1. *Brain*, **126**, 804–813.

Kohl, B., Fischer, S., Groh, J., Wessig, C. & Martini, R. (2010a) MCP-1/CCL2 modifies axon properties in a PMP22-overexpressing mouse model for Charcot-Marie-tooth 1A neuropathy. *American Journal of Pathology*, **176**, 1390–1399.

Kohl, B., Groh, J., Wessig, C., Wiendl, H., Kroner, A. & Martini, R. (2010b) Lack of evidence for a pathogenic role of T-lymphocytes in an animal model for Charcot-Marie-Tooth disease 1A. *Neurobiology of Disease*, **38**, 78–84.

Kroner, A., Schwab, N., Ip, C.W. *et al.* (2009) The co-inhibitory molecule PD-1 modulates disease severity in a model for an inherited, demyelinating neuropathy. *Neurobiology of Disease*, **33**, 96–103.

Lampert, P.W. (1969) Mechanism of demyelination in experimental allergic neuritis. Electron microscopic studies. *Laboratory Investigation*, **20**, 127–138.

Le, N., Nagarajan, R., Wang, J.Y., Araki, T., Schmidt, R.E. & Milbrandt, J. (2005) Analysis of congenital hypomyelinating Egr2Lo/Lo nerves identifies Sox2 as an inhibitor of Schwann cell differentiation and myelination. *Proceedings of the National Academy of Sciences of the United States of America*, **102**, 2596–2601.

Leal, A., Ichim, T.E., Marleau, A.M., Lara, F., Kaushal, S. & Riordan, N.H. (2008) Immune effects of mesenchymal stem cells: Implications for Charcot-Marie-Tooth disease. *Cellular Immunology*, **253**, 11–15.

Liu, L., Lioudyno, M., Tao, R., Eriksson, P., Svensson, M. & Aldskogius, H. (1999) Hereditary absence of complement C5 in adult mice influences Wallerian degeneration, but not retrograde responses, following injury to peripheral nerve. *Journal of the Peripheral Nervous System*, **4**, 123–133.

Martini, R. & Toyka, K.V. (2004) Immune-mediated components of hereditary demyelinating neuropathies: Lessons from animal models and patients. *Lancet Neurology*, **3**, 457–465.

Martini, R., Klein, D. & Groh, J. (2013) Similarities between inherited demyelinating neuropathies and Wallerian degeneration: An old repair program may cause myelin and axon perturbation under nonlesion conditions. *American Journal of Pathology*, **183**, 655–660.

Martini, R., Zielasek, J., Toyka, K.V., Giese, K.P. & Schachner, M. (1995) Protein zero (P0)-deficient mice show myelin degeneration in peripheral nerves characteristic of inherited human neuropathies. *Nature Genetics*, **11**, 281–286.

Maurer, M., Schmid, C.D., Bootz, F. *et al.* (2001) Bone marrow transfer from wild-type mice reverts the beneficial effect of genetically mediated immune deficiency in myelin mutants. *Molecular and Cellular Neuroscience*, **17**, 1094–1101.

Meyer zu Horste, G., Miesbach, T.A., Muller, J.I. *et al.* (2011) The Wlds transgene reduces axon loss in a Charcot-Marie-Tooth disease 1A rat model and nicotinamide delays post-traumatic axonal degeneration. *Neurobiology of Disease*, **42**, 1–8.

Miki, Y., Tomiyama, M., Haga, R. *et al.* (2013) A family with IVIg-responsive Charcot-Marie-Tooth disease. *Journal of Neurology*, **260**, 1147–1151.

Müller, M., Berghoff, M., Kobsar, I., Kiefer, R. & Martini, R. (2007) Macrophage colony stimulating factor is a crucial factor for the intrinsic macrophage response in mice heterozygously deficient for the myelin protein P0. *Experimental Neurology*, **203**, 55–62.

Napoli, I., Noon, L.A., Ribeiro, S. *et al.* (2012) A central role for the ERK-signaling pathway in controlling Schwann cell plasticity and peripheral nerve regeneration in vivo. *Neuron*, **73**, 729–742.

Nave, K.A. (2010) Myelination and support of axonal integrity by glia. *Nature*, **468**, 244–252.

Ohara, S., Takahashi, H. & Ikuta, F. (1986) Specialised contacts of endoneurial fibroblasts with macrophages in Wallerian degeneration. *Journal of Anatomy*, **148**, 77–85.

Okazaki, T., Chikuma, S., Iwai, Y., Fagarasan, S. & Honjo, T. (2013) A rheostat for immune responses: The unique properties of PD-1 and their advantages for clinical application. *Nature Immunology*, **14**, 1212–1218.

Pareyson, D., Marchesi, C. & Salsano, E. (2013) Dominant Charcot–Marie–Tooth syndrome and cognate disorders. *Handbook of Clinical Neurology*, **115**, 817–845.

Parkinson, D.B., Bhaskaran, A., Arthur-Farraj, P. *et al.* (2008) c-Jun is a negative regulator of myelination. *Journal of Cell Biology*, **181**, 625–637.

Patzko, A. & Shy, M.E. (2012) Charcot-Marie-Tooth disease and related genetic neuropathies. *Continuum (Minneap Minn)*, **18**, 39–59.

Pennuto, M., Tinelli, E., Malaguti, M. *et al.* (2008) Ablation of the UPR-mediator CHOP restores motor function and reduces demyelination in Charcot-Marie-Tooth 1B mice. *Neuron*, **57**, 393–405.

Perrin, F.E., Lacroix, S., Aviles-Trigueros, M. & David, S. (2005) Involvement of monocyte chemoattractant protein-1, macrophage inflammatory protein-1alpha and interleukin-1beta in Wallerian degeneration. *Brain*, **128**, 854–866.

Pitceathly, R.D. *et al.* (2012) Genetic dysfunction of MT-ATP6 causes axonal Charcot-Marie-Tooth disease. *Neurology*, **79**, 1145–1154.

Ramaglia, V., King, R.H., Morgan, B.P. & Baas, F. (2009) Deficiency of the complement regulator CD59a exacerbates Wallerian degeneration. *Molecular Immunology*, **46**, 1892–1896.

Reilly, M.M., Murphy, S.M. & Laura, M. (2011) Charcot-Marie-Tooth disease. *Journal of the Peripheral Nervous System*, **16**, 1–14.

Rossor, A.M., Polke, J.M., Houlden, H. & Reilly, M.M. (2013) Clinical implications of genetic advances in Charcot-Marie-Tooth disease. *Nature Reviews Neurology*, **9**, 562–571.

Rusconi, P., Caiola, E. & Broggini, M. (2012) RAS/RAF/MEK inhibitors in oncology. *Current Medicinal Chemistry*, **19**, 1164–1176.

Samsam, M., Mi, W., Wessig, C. *et al.* (2003) The Wlds mutation delays robust loss of motor and sensory axons in a genetic model for myelin-related axonopathy. *Journal of Neuroscience*, **23**, 2833–2839.

Saporta, M.A., Shy, B.R., Patzko, A. *et al.* (2012) MpzR98C arrests Schwann cell development in a mouse model of early-onset Charcot–Marie–Tooth disease type 1B. *Brain*, **135**, 2032–2047.

Scherer, S.S. & Wrabetz, L. (2008) Molecular mechanisms of inherited demyelinating neuropathies. *Glia*, **56**, 1578–1589.

Schmid, C.D., Stienekemeier, M., Oehen, S. *et al.* (2000) Immune deficiency in mouse models for inherited peripheral neuropathies leads to improved myelin maintenance. *Journal of Neuroscience*, **20**, 729–735.

Schneider-Gold, C., Kotting, J., Epplen, J.T., Gold, R. & Gerding, W.M. (2010) Unusual Charcot-Marie-Tooth phenotype due to a mutation within the intracellular domain of myelin protein zero. *Muscle & Nerve*, **41**, 550–554.

Shy, M.E., Arroyo, E., Sladky, J. *et al.* (1997) Heterozygous P0 knockout mice develop a peripheral neuropathy that resembles chronic inflammatory demyelinating polyneuropathy (CIDP). *Journal of Neuropathology and Experimental Neurology*, **56**, 811–821.

Shy, M.E., Blake, J., Krajewski, K. *et al.* (2005) Reliability and validity of the CMT neuropathy score as a measure of disability. *Neurology*, **64**, 1209–1214.

Shy, M.E., Jani, A., Krajewski, K. *et al.* (2004) Phenotypic clustering in MPZ mutations. *Brain*, **127**, 371–384.

Stassart, R.M., Fledrich, R., Velanac, V. *et al.* (2013) A role for Schwann cell-derived neuregulin-1 in remyelination. *Nature Neuroscience*, **16**, 48–54.

Stoll, G., Gabreels-Festen, A.A., Jander, S., Muller, H.W. & Hanemann, C.O. (1998) Major histocompatibility complex class II expression and macrophage responses in genetically proven Charcot-Marie-Tooth type 1 and hereditary neuropathy with liability to pressure palsies. *Muscle & Nerve*, **21**, 1419–1427.

Suter, U. & Scherer, S.S. (2003) Disease mechanisms in inherited neuropathies. *Nature Reviews Neuroscience*, **4**, 714–726.

Teitelbaum, S.L. (2000) Bone resorption by osteoclasts. *Science*, **289**, 1504–1508.

Toews, A.D., Barrett, C. & Morell, P. (1998) Monocyte chemoattractant protein 1 is responsible for macrophage recruitment following injury to sciatic nerve. *Journal of Neuroscience Research*, **53**, 260–267.

Vargas, M.E., Watanabe, J., Singh, S.J., Robinson, W.H. & Barres, B.A. (2010) Endogenous antibodies promote rapid myelin clearance and effective axon regeneration after nerve injury. *Proceedings of the National Academy of Sciences of the United States of America*, **107**, 11993–11998.

Williams, L.L., Shannon, B.T. & Wright, F.S. (1993) Circulating cytotoxic immune components in dominant Charcot-Marie-Tooth syndrome. *Journal of Clinical Immunology*, **13**, 389–396.

Williams, L.L., Shannon, B.T., O'Dougherty, M. & Wright, F.S. (1987) Activated T cells in type I Charcot–Marie–Tooth disease: Evidence for immunologic heterogeneity. *Journal of Neuroimmunology*, **16**, 317–330.

Ydens, E., Lornet, G., Smits, V., Goethals, S., Timmerman, V. & Janssens, S. (2013) The neuroinflammatory role of Schwann cells in disease. *Neurobiology of Disease*, **55**, 95–103.

Ydens, E., Cauwels, A., Asselbergh, B. *et al.* (2012) Acute injury in the peripheral nervous system triggers an alternative macrophage response. *Journal of Neuroinflammation*, **9**, 176.

9   Obesity- and Neuroinflammation-Associated Mood and Cognitive Disorders

Nathalie Castanon,[1,2] Giamal Luheshi,[3] and Sophie Layé[1,2]

[1] Laboratory of "Nutrition and Integrative Neurobiology", INRA UMR 1286, Bordeaux, France
[2] University of Bordeaux, Bordeaux, France
[3] Department of Psychiatry, Douglas Mental Health University Institute, McGill University, Montreal, Quebec, Canada

Introduction

Obesity is fast becoming the disease of the twenty-first century mainly due to its association with secondary disorders, most notably type 2 diabetes and cardiovascular disease, which are collectively known as metabolic syndrome (MetS). While diet and lifestyle are often advanced as the main reason for the development of these conditions in obese individuals, a more recent, mechanistic link indicates a role for inflammation in this process. Morbid obesity is now associated with an underlying increase in the levels of circulating inflammatory mediators, cytokines, some of which are directly connected with the development of MetS. In addition to these "systemic" diseases, obesity has recently also been associated with the development of a number of psychopathologies, including depression, with neuroinflammation being suggested as a direct link (Emery *et al.*, 2007; Capuron *et al.*, 2008, 2010).

In the present chapter, we aim to provide a new perspective on the pathophysiological mechanisms contributing to the development of neuropsychiatric symptoms in the context of obesity/MetS. We propose that mood and cognitive alterations occurring in obese patients may reflect the neural consequences of molecular and cellular events playing a pivotal role in the evolution of the disease and that inflammation may contribute to the development of these behavioral alterations. In addition, we will discuss possible mechanisms that underlie this development on the basis of recent experimental data, particularly from studies using experimental models of obesity/MetS. These studies have produced converging evidence implicating immune mediators in the pathophysiology of various chronic somatic disorders by being able to alter brain functions, even when they are produced in peripheral tissues. The critical role of inflammation in normal

Neuroinflammation: New Insights into Beneficial and Detrimental Functions, First Edition. Edited by Samuel David.

and abnormal brain functioning provides the framework for characterizing its role in the etiology, progression, and treatment of neuropsychiatric symptoms associated with several inflammatory conditions, including obesity.

Neuropsychiatric Comorbidity in Obesity

Chronic obesity is often characterized by hypertension, coronary artery disease, dyslipidemia, and impaired glucose tolerance linked to hyperinsulinemia and insulin resistance, which are collectively defined as MetS. Along with metabolic dysregulations, basal low-grade inflammation increasingly appears as another key component of this condition (Dandona *et al.*, 2005; Marsland *et al.*, 2010). In addition to peripheral organ dysfunction, increasing evidence suggests that obesity/MetS is also a risk factor for neurological disorders such as neuropsychiatric disorders (depression, anxiety, and cognitive impairments), stroke, and Alzheimer's disease (Frisardi *et al.*, 2010; Farooqui *et al.*, 2012).

Neuropsychiatric comorbidity is more frequent in obese patients than in the general age-matched population (Roberts *et al.*, 2010; Pan *et al.*, 2012). The overwhelming influence of metabolic and neuropsychiatric disorders considerably reduces the quality of life of these patients, increases morbidity and mortality rates, and results in incremental costs to health care systems around the world. Moreover, this is amplified (alarmingly) by the fact that neuropsychiatric disorders may reciprocally increase the risk for a pattern of physiological and biochemical dysregulations consistent with being overweight. Higher age-adjusted MetS/obesity rates have been reported among individuals with schizophrenia, or major depressive disorders when compared to unaffected population (McEvoy *et al.*, 2005; Grover *et al.*, 2012). Similarly, lifetime history of neuropsychiatric disorders or stressful life events is a reliable predictor for weight gain and the subsequent development of obesity/MetS in middle-aged women (Goldbacher *et al.*, 2009) or young adults (McIntyre *et al.*, 2012). Altogether, these data point to a bidirectional relationship between neuropsychiatric disorders and obesity/MetS. Understanding the etiology of these disorders therefore represents a major public health challenge. Experimental approaches using animal models of obesity/MetS that also display emotional and cognitive alterations may be particularly appropriate to address this important question.

Animal Models of Obesity and MetS

Using animal models to study complex clinical pathological conditions, particularly those affecting brain and mental functions, often appears limiting and even controversial. However, the development of consistent and reliable models focusing on different core symptoms of the human diseases rather than on the entire disorders *per se* has provided very useful tools to study their respective pathophysiology (Biessels and Gispen, 2005; Varga *et al.*, 2009). For obesity/MetS a large number of complementary rodent models have been developed in the last few decades. These include ones that have been generated by specific environmental manipulations (e.g., exposure to high-fat and high-sucrose diets), genetic manipulations, spontaneous mutations (e.g., *ob/ob* and *db/db* mice, *fa/fa* Zucker rats), or through mechanical interventions including chemical lesions of the ventromedial hypothalamus (Biessels and Gispen, 2005; Varga *et al.*, 2009). The major components of obesity and MetS, such as hypertension, impaired glucose tolerance, and insulin resistance, are found in most of these models. These changes are particularly evident in the genetically [*ob/ob* (deficient for leptin) and *db/db* (deficient for functional leptin receptor)] modified mice, which also display signs of dysfunctions within the brain (Stranahan *et al.*, 2008; Erion *et al.*, 2014), making them perhaps the most complete models for studying the long-term adverse effects of obesity. These mice are also particularly noted for their basal low-grade inflammation and significantly altered immune responses to infection both in the periphery and in the brain (Cani *et al.*, 2009; Rummel *et al.*, 2010; Lawrence *et al.*, 2012; Dinel *et al.*, 2014).

There are now numerous studies demonstrating exacerbated neuroinflammation as a function of obesity. For example, using diet-induced obesity (DIO) models, in particular high-fat-diet-induced obese rats, we demonstrated a clear potentiation of expression of inflammatory markers (interleukin (IL)-1β, IL-6, cyclooxygenase (COX)-2) induced by an acute systemic injection of a potent immunogen, in this case, lipopolysaccharide (LPS) (Pohl *et al.*, 2009). In more recent studies, we showed in DIO models that obese animals also display, after systemic LPS challenge, exacerbated expression of brain cytokines [IL-1β, tumor necrosis factor alpha (TNF-α)], in particular in the hippocampus (André *et al.*, 2014; Boitard *et al.*, 2014). In addition, this time using a different model, namely *db/db* mice, we demonstrated that peripheral inflammation is associated with increased hippocampus cytokine expression (IL-1β, IL-6, TNF-α) in unstimulated conditions (Dinel *et al.*, 2011) and exacerbated hippocampal inflammation after LPS challenge (Dinel *et al.*, 2014). In these studies, the exacerbated neuroinflammation was associated with altered, brain-orchestrated sickness-type behaviors mediated by inflammatory mediators such as IL-1β acting on specific brain nuclei (Konsman *et al.*, 2002). Our studies to date suggest therefore that these experimental models of obesity/MetS are very useful for studying behavioral alterations associated with obesity and MetS. Our latest studies in particular (Dinel *et al.*, 2011; André *et al.*, 2014) suggest that these models are especially suited for investigating changes in cognitive and emotional behaviors reported in chronically obese individuals (Evans *et al.*, 2005; Roberts *et al.*, 2010; Lin *et al.*, 2013).

Clinical studies have reported that obesity and/or MetS adversely impairs cognition but that not all cognitive domains are equally affected (Roberts *et al.*, 2010). Similarly, experimental obesity/MetS is associated with a wide array of cognitive abnormalities. For example, DIO and associated metabolic alterations decrease both spatial learning performances (André *et al.*, 2014; Boitard *et al.*, 2014) and hippocampal plasticity in rodents (Molteni *et al.*, 2002; Boitard *et al.*, 2014). Impaired hippocampus-dependent spatial memory performances and synaptic plasticity are also displayed by *db/db* mice (Stranahan *et al.*, 2008, 2009; Erion *et al.*, 2014). On the contrary, acquisition of a conditioned taste aversion learning task (Ohta *et al.*, 2003), as well as working memory performances tested in a hippocampus-independent task, is preserved in *db/db* mice (Dinel *et al.*, 2011). Altogether, these data point to the importance of the hippocampus as a key brain area for mediating cognitive impairments linked to obesity/MetS.

Interestingly, experimental obesity also impairs emotional reactivity, although with a different time-course of development than cognition. For example, we recently showed that DIO in mice alters first spatial memory, then anxiety-like behavior, whereas depressive-like behavior remains unchanged unless the inflammatory system is challenged (André *et al.*, 2014). Similarly, *db/db* mice display impaired spatial memory and increased anxiety-like behavior without any effect on depressive-like behavior (Dinel *et al.*, 2011). Of note, depressive-like behaviors mostly increase under challenging conditions such as stress exposure (Lu *et al.*, 2008) or immune stimulation (Frenois *et al.*, 2007; Moreau *et al.*, 2008). In obesity/MetS models, depressive-like behaviors are also increased compared to lean animals when experimental conditions are particularly stressful (e.g., sustained and/or repeated exposure to the test, successive exposures to different behavioral tests over short periods of time), as reported in *ob/ob* mice (Collin *et al.*, 2000). By tightly controlling these stressful factors in our study, we showed that both *db/db* and *db/+* mice display similar levels of depressive-like behavior (Dinel *et al.*, 2011). These results strongly suggest an important role for the inflammatory system and/or the hypothalamo-pituitary-adrenal (HPA) axis, which are functionally related (Raison and Miller, 2003), in underlying emotional alterations associated with obesity/MetS. In addition, these results indicate that obesity, in conjunction with environmental conditions, can amplify central nervous system (CNS) dysfunctions and/or their harmful consequences on mood and cognition. In a very recent study, we have demonstrated this association in DIO mice injected systemically with LPS, a study that implicated the exacerbation of the neuroinflammatory response as the underlying mechanisms for the increased depressive-like behaviors in these animals (Aguilar-Valles *et al.*, 2014). Moreover, we also report in another recent study that together with exacerbated neuroinflammation and depressive-like behaviors, LPS-injected DIO mice also display exacerbated HPA axis activation (André *et al.*, 2014). These works are examples of recent studies investigating the interaction between an aggravated peripheral immune response associated with the obesity condition and the activation of psychopathologies. More studies are needed to further delineate the relationship between obesity/MetS and the increased incidence of psychopathologies in these susceptible individuals.

Mechanisms Underlying the Association between Obesity/MetS and Neuropsychiatric Symptoms

Although the impact of metabolic disturbances on the hepatic, endocrine, and cardiovascular systems is well established, there remains a noticeable void in understanding the basis by which the CNS becomes altered in obese individuals or patients with MetS and why this alteration induces neuropsychiatric symptoms. Social and psychological factors are classically put forward to explain the comorbidity of neuropsychiatric disorders with obesity/MetS, especially in situations of poor social support (Goldbacher and Matthews, 2007). This psychological distress leads to a deterioration of positive health behaviors, concomitant with an increase in deleterious behaviors, and poor compliance with treatments. Altogether, these changes impact the functioning of several biological systems and undoubtedly therefore contribute to increased occurrence of neuropsychiatric disorders in obese patients and/or patients with MetS (McIntyre *et al.*, 2012). In fact, psychosocial factors likely precipitate or worsen the pathological consequences that altered key biological components of obesity/MetS may induce on brain function.

Among the main biological components of obesity/MetS able to act within the brain, insulin, leptin, and inflammatory factors are likely candidates to underlie the behavioral alterations associated with this condition. Several reviews already described the potential consequences that insulin- and/or leptin-resistance may have on mood and cognition (Yates *et al.*, 2012). Discussing this topic is beyond the scope of this chapter. However, it is worth noting that these factors may not be, at least in some cases, essential or sufficient to explain neuropsychiatric symptoms in obesity/MetS. It has been recently shown in patients with MetS, for example, that the increased risk of cognitive dysfunction is independent of the presence of diabetes (Muller *et al.*, 2010). In support of this, we recently reported increased emotional behaviors and cognitive impairment in DIO animals in the absence of any significant hyperinsulinemia (André *et al.*, 2014; Boitard *et al.*, 2014). Similarly, spatial cognitive impairment or anxiety-like behavior remains unchanged in *db/db* mice despite normalization of their peripheral hyperglycemia (Stranahan *et al.*, 2008, 2009). Besides, this normalization does not alter brain concentrations of glucose and insulin that are similar in both *db/db* and *db/+*mice (Stranahan *et al.*, 2008). Conversely, behavioral alterations are associated in *db/db* mice with increased expression of inflammatory factors in the hippocampus that are known to influence hippocampal plasticity and behavior (Dinel *et al.*, 2011). In addition, blockade of hippocampal IL-1β expression in *db/db* mice normalizes hippocampal dendritic spine density and prevents synaptic dysfunction and cognitive impairment (Erion *et al.*, 2014). These interesting findings fit with what has been certainly the least easily predicted result in the study of inflammation, namely the discovery of the profound action of cytokines on brain functions and their involvement in neuropsychiatric disorders (Dantzer *et al.*, 2008).

Neuroinflammation, Sickness Behavior, and Neuropsychiatric Symptoms

Inflammation is an active defense reaction against various insults that aims at neutralizing noxious agents. It results from the activation of the innate immune system by specific molecular motifs that are an intrinsic component of microbial pathogens. This activation induces a cascade of intracellular events that ultimately leads to the synthesis and release of inflammatory mediators, including chemokines that permit the local recruitment of phagocytic cells, and inflammatory cytokines. Although inflammation serves a protective function in controlling infection and promoting tissue repair, it can also cause tissue damage. It therefore needs to be tightly controlled particularly thanks to the production of several anti-inflammatory cytokines that are either specific of a given cytokine or exert their inhibitory activity on multiple cytokines at the level of intracellular signaling pathways.

Proinflammatory cytokines that are released at the site of infection by innate immune cells are also able to act systemically on distant organs, including the brain. Peripheral cytokines that are relatively large hydrophilic molecules do not readily cross the blood–brain barrier (BBB). However, several nonexclusive humoral, neural, and cellular pathways allow peripheral immune messages to be transmitted from the periphery to the brain (Fig. 9.1) (Dantzer *et al.*, 2008). Activation of immune-to-brain communication ultimately induces the production of brain cytokines by activated glial cells, particularly microglia. On detection of homeostatic disturbances, microglia are transiently activated and rapidly engaged in brain-adaptive immune responses, mainly due to their ability to produce cytokines, express their receptors, and amplify their signals (Ransohoff and Perry, 2009). If microglia activation normally protects CNS function, uncontrolled or sustained activation of these cells may become neurotoxic.

By altering neurotransmitter function, neuroendocrine activity, neural plasticity, and/or brain circuitry, transient activation of brain cytokine network during an infection ultimately coordinates the behavioral changes that are necessary for infection recovery. These adaptive

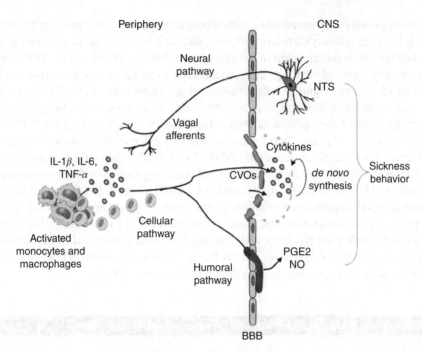

Figure 9.1 Neuroimmune pathways underlying cytokine-induced sickness behavior. Inflammatory cytokines (IL-1β, IL-6, TNF-α) released at the periphery by activated monocytes and macrophages can reach the brain by several nonexclusive humoral, neural, and cellular pathways. In the humoral pathway, circulating cytokines reach the brain at the level of the circumventricular organs (CVOs) that are devoid of functional blood–brain barrier (BBB). Within the brain parenchyma, activated endothelial cells are responsible for the subsequent release of second messengers such as prostaglandins (PGE₂) or nitric oxide (NO). The neural pathway involves activation of the primary afferent nerves such as the vagal afferents by peripherally produced cytokines. The information is then relayed to the brain through the nucleus of the tractus solitaries (NTS). Lastly, a direct entry into the brain parenchyma of peripherally activated monocytes can be detected in response to monocyte-chemoattractant proteins released by activated microglia (cellular pathway). All these pathways ultimately induce *de novo* synthesis of brain cytokines by activated glial cells.

behavioral changes (including weakness, listlessness, malaise, anorexia, fatigue and transient cognition, and mood alterations), which are collectively referred to as sickness behavior, are normally fully reversible once microbial pathogens have been cleared and the innate immune system is no longer activated. However, failure to tightly regulate systemic immune activation and/or brain microglial activation leads to significant and prolonged induction of peripheral and brain cytokines. This induction in turn might culminate in medical conditions adversely affecting patient outcomes, including neuropsychiatric symptoms, particularly when microglial overactivation ultimately affect key brain areas, such as the hippocampus, the cortex or the amygdala (Dantzer *et al.*, 2008). Although both inflammation-related sickness behavior and neuropsychiatric symptoms share some common components, they differ by their duration, intensity, and respective underlying mechanisms.

Converging animal (Frenois *et al.*, 2007; Moreau *et al.*, 2008; Salazar *et al.*, 2012) and clinical findings (Raison *et al.*, 2010; Capuron and Miller, 2011) support a main role for cytokines in mood disorders and cognitive decline through processes related to neuroinflammation, neurodegeneration, and structural remodeling (Noble *et al.*, 2007; Hein *et al.*, 2010). Interestingly, development of neuropsychiatric symptoms in medically ill patients chronically treated with interferon alpha (IFN-α) (Raison *et al.*, 2010), elderly patients (Capuron *et al.*, 2011), or patients with Alzheimer's disease (Gulaj *et al.*, 2010) is associated with reduced circulating tryptophan levels and concomitant increase of one of its main metabolite, kynurenine. Similarly, neuropsychiatric symptoms correlate in some instances with increase in serum kynurenine/tryptophan ratio (Forrest *et al.*, 2011; Gold *et al.*, 2011). These clinical findings suggested a possible link between cytokine-induced activation of the indoleamine 2,3-dioxygenase (IDO), which is the first and rate-limiting enzyme that degrades tryptophan along the kynurenine pathway, and neuropsychiatric symptoms. We and others have experimentally confirmed this assumption by showing, for example, that peripheral administration of kynurenine dose-dependently induces depressive-like behaviors, anxiety-like behaviors, and cognitive impairment in mice (Chess *et al.*, 2009; O'Connor *et al.*, 2009c; Alexander *et al.*, 2012; Salazar *et al.*, 2012). Concurrently, pharmacological or genetic inhibition of brain IDO activation prevents induction of depressive-like and anxiety-like behaviors by systemic immune challenges (Henry *et al.*, 2009; O'Connor *et al.*, 2009a, 2009b, 2009c; Salazar *et al.*, 2012). Interestingly, further studies shed light on the hippocampus as important brain area for cytokine and IDO activation in those conditions (Frenois *et al.*, 2007; André *et al.*, 2008; Corona *et al.*, 2010; Fu *et al.*, 2010) and on the link between dysregulated activation of hippocampal microglia, sustained IDO activity, and protracted depressive-like behavior (Corona *et al.*, 2010). Taken together, these results clearly point to a pivotal role of IDO activation, particularly in the hippocampus, in mediating cytokine-induced mood and cognitive alterations.

As part of the immune response to infection, increased IDO activity occurring in activated monocytes, macrophages, and brain microglia is usually beneficial to the host (Mellor and Munn, 2008). However, sustained brain IDO activation can also be deleterious because of its negative impact on monoaminergic neurotransmission, particularly serotonin neurotransmission, and neuronal survival. As tryptophan is the biosynthetic precursor for the synthesis of serotonin, increased degradation of tryptophan by IDO has been postulated to reduce serotonin production. Concurrently, increased brain kynurenine levels resulting from IDO activation can be further metabolized to produce several neuroactive glutamatergic compounds, including 3-hydroxykynurenine (3-HKyn) and quinolinic acid (QA), which play a key role in neuronal death and neurodegenerative diseases by stimulating N-methyl-D-aspartate (NMDA) receptors and promoting oxidative stress (Fig. 9.2) (Stone *et al.*, 2012). On the other hand, kynurenine can also be metabolized in kynurenic acid (KA) that rather displays neuroprotective properties. However, these apparently antagonistic pathways are compartmentalized in the brain, with microglia preferentially producing QA, whereas astrocytes produce KA. Immune activation therefore tips the scale in favor of neurotoxicity. Increased brain or cerebrospinal fluid (CSF) concentrations of kynurenine and its neurotoxic metabolites have been reported in patients with major depression (Myint *et al.*, 2007), schizophrenia (Schwarcz *et al.*, 2001), or neurodegenerative diseases (Stone *et al.*, 2012). Moreover, increased concentrations of these neurotoxic metabolites have been related with the stretch of brain damages and with mood and cognitive impairments (Chess *et al.*, 2009; Stone *et al.*, 2012), suggesting that IDO activation may lead to both functional and structural alterations in the brain. In line with these findings, emotional alterations linked to hippocampus IDO activation

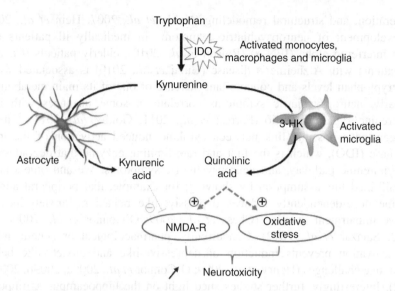

Figure 9.2   Tryptophan metabolism through the kynurenine pathway. Increased indoleamine 2,3-dioxygenase (IDO) activity occurring in activated monocytes, macrophages, and brain microglia in conditions of immune activation catabolizes tryptophan in kynurenine. This compound can then be metabolized into different neuroactive glutamatergic metabolites, including 3-hydroxykynurenine (3-HKyn) and quinolinic acid that are produced by activated microglia, and kynurenic acid produced by astrocytes. Elevated levels of quinolinic acid have been shown to be neurotoxic by activating glutamatergic NMDA receptors and promoting oxidative stress.

by an immune challenge is associated with reduced hippocampal expression of the brain-derived neurotrophic factor (BDNF) (Gibney *et al.*, 2013). This neurotrophin contributes to mood regulation and memory function, including in conditions of immune activation (Barrientos *et al.*, 2004), by supporting synaptic plasticity and neuronal excitability in the hippocampus (Yamada and Nabeshima, 2003; Martinowich *et al.*, 2007). Of note, brain IDO activation did not result in these studies in a detectable reduction of the serotonin concentrations (O'Connor *et al.*, 2009c; Gibney *et al.*, 2013). On the other hand, NMDA receptor blockade abrogates cytokine-induced depressive-like behavior in mice (Walker *et al.*, 2013). Altogether, although these results do not exclude the possible role of impaired serotonin synthesis in inflammation-induced neuropsychiatric symptoms, they clearly support a key role for the neuroactive kynurenine metabolites resulting from activation of the kynurenine pathway initiated by IDO.

Role of Neuroinflammation in Neuropsychiatric Symptoms Associated with Obesity and MetS

In light of the present knowledge on the mechanisms leading to the development of neuropsychiatric symptoms in conditions of elevated inflammation (e.g., chronic infection, immunotherapy, and chronic inflammatory diseases), an important question arises as to whether the same mechanisms may take place in conditions of chronic low-grade inflammation such as obesity/MetS. We will present in this case some data suggesting that neuroinflammation indeed contributes to obesity/MetS-related mood and cognitive alterations.

It is now widely accepted that basal systemic low-grade inflammation is one of the key components of obesity/MetS (Dandona *et al.*, 2005; Marsland *et al.*, 2010) that is characterized by elevated levels of circulating inflammatory cytokines, accumulation of leukocytes within adipose tissue and other organs, activation of macrophages in liver and fat, and activation of proinflammatory signaling pathways in multiple organs (Cancello and Clement, 2006; Gregor and Hotamisligil, 2011). Part of systemic inflammation originates from adipose tissue that secretes adipokines, and in which macrophages accumulate and potently secrete inflammatory cytokines (Cancello and Clement, 2006; Gregor and Hotamisligil, 2011). Moreover, an additional role for T cells in the development of adiposity-related inflammation is supported by several recent studies (Zeyda *et al.*, 2011; Lasselin *et al.*, 2013). Alternatively, inflammation can be triggered by pathogens, as there is now evidence of gut microbiota alterations associated with inflammatory processes in obesity (Ley *et al.*, 2005; Cani *et al.*, 2007). In obese animals, gut microbial population is altered independently of diet characteristics (Ley *et al.*, 2005), although high-fat diet causes a state of chronic low-grade endotoxemia believed to contribute to obesity-induced inflammation (Cani *et al.*, 2007). Changes in gut microbiota have also been shown to control inflammation in *ob/ob* and *db/db* mice (Cani *et al.*, 2009; Geurts *et al.*, 2011). Similarly, recent clinical data in obese individuals indicate significant associations between gut microbiota modifications and markers of local and systemic inflammation (Verdam *et al.*, 2013) and document improvement in the intestinal microbiota profile following weight loss (Furet *et al.*, 2010; Aron-Wisnewsky *et al.*, 2012). Whatever the mechanisms triggering systemic inflammation in obesity/MetS, it is now clear that this inflammatory state contributes to metabolic dysregulations characterizing this condition, as illustrated by the role of TNF-α in the pathogenesis of insulin resistance and type 2 diabetes (Lann and LeRoith, 2007). Interestingly, inflammatory factors also modulate energy balance, and this is mainly due to their actions on the hypothalamus (Cai and Liu, 2012). Actually, mounting evidence converges to show signs of enhanced cytokine expression and activation of inflammatory processes in the hypothalamus of different obesity/MetS models (De Souza *et al.*, 2005; Cai and Liu, 2012). However, neuroinflammation is not restricted to the areas involved in physiological homeostasis. For instance, *db/db* mice or DIO models also display increased expression of cytokines in the hippocampus (Dinel *et al.*, 2011; Kanoski and Davidson, 2011), suggesting a potential role of hippocampal cytokines in promoting obesity-associated behavioral alterations.

Recent experimental findings clearly support a relevance of neuroinflammation for the emotional and cognitive alterations reported in rodent models of obesity/MetS. Blocking hippocampal IL-1β expression in *db/db* mice prevents their cognitive impairment by normalizing dendritic spine density and synaptic dysfunction in the hippocampus (Erion *et al.*, 2014). Moreover, cognitive impairment and emotional alterations reported in DIO and genetic models of obesity are linked to increased inflammation and reduced BDNF levels in the cortex (Pistell *et al.*, 2010) and the hippocampus (Dinel *et al.*, 2011, 2014). Reciprocally, anti-inflammatory interventions in DIO mice reduce body weight, normalize hippocampal levels of BDNF, and prevent hippocampus-mediated cognitive impairments (Moy and McNay, 2012). Given the present knowledge on the consequences of dysregulated hippocampal cytokines and neurotrophins expression, and impaired synaptic function on mood, learning, and memory (Yamada and Nabeshima, 2003; Martinowich *et al.*, 2007; Dantzer *et al.*, 2008), these results, on the whole, point to a link between increased hippocampal and cortical inflammation, impaired neurogenesis/synaptic plasticity, and behavioral alterations in animal models of obesity/MetS.

Interestingly, mounting clinical reports converge to support this assumption. For example, associations have been documented between inflammatory status and cognitive performance/decline among overweight and obese women (Sweat et al., 2008) and elderly with MetS (Yaffe, 2007). Moreover, cognitive impairments have been shown more likely associated with obesity/MetS in the presence of marked systemic inflammation (Yaffe, 2007; Roberts et al., 2010). Other clinical reports point to elevated circulating levels of IL-6 as important determinant of mood symptoms (Capuron et al., 2008, 2010) and cognitive decline (Roberts et al., 2010) associated with obesity/MetS, with higher inflammation predicting worse neuropsychiatric symptoms. Conversely, surgery-induced weight loss is associated with reduced inflammation (Cancello and Clement, 2006) and significant improvement in emotional status (Emery et al., 2007; Capuron et al., 2010). Of note, body weight loss induced by lifestyle intervention program in young patients with MetS also normalizes plasma levels of BDNF (Corripio et al., 2012).

Another important mechanism potentially linking inflammation with neuropsychiatric symptoms in obesity/MetS involves IDO activation. This activation has already been reported in several neurological disorders such as major depression (Myint et al., 2007; Gulaj et al., 2010), Alzheimer's disease (Gulaj et al., 2010), Huntington's disease (Stone et al., 2012), or schizophrenia (Schwarcz et al., 2001), all of which have been linked with obesity/MetS. Interestingly, it has been reported that severely obese individuals display reduced plasma tryptophan levels and increased peripheral IDO activity, as assessed by the kynurenine/tryptophan ratio (Brandacher et al., 2006, 2007; Mangge et al., 2013). Consistent with these clinical findings, we recently reported that DIO in mice exacerbates lung IDO activation in response to an immune challenge (André et al., 2014). More importantly, obese mice also display in those conditions exacerbated brain IDO activation and related depressive-like behavior (André et al., 2014). Similarly, a direct relationship has been recently reported by our group between inflammation-related brain IDO activation and the development of depressive-like behavior in db/db mice (Dinel et al., 2014). In addition, exacerbated activation of brain IDO displayed by obese mice challenged with LPS induces a huge increase of brain kynurenine concentrations compared to lean mice, but similar impairment of brain serotonin levels (André et al., 2014). Although we still need to assess the production of the neurotoxic kynurenine metabolites in obesity/MetS models, these data suggest that increased neurotoxicity resulting from enhanced IDO activity may contribute to the onset of neuropsychiatric symptoms in the context of obesity, as reported in other inflammatory conditions (André et al., 2008; O'Connor et al., 2009c; Raison et al., 2010).

Conclusions

Altogether, evidence provided in this chapter shows that brain dysfunctions related with neuroinflammation, particularly when they occur in key brain areas for mood, learning, and memory such as the hippocampus, may contribute to the increased prevalence of neuropsychiatric symptoms reported in chronically obese/MetS patients. A well balanced relationship between neurogenesis and neuronal death allows normal hippocampal functioning. On the contrary, unbalanced ratio initiates neuronal dysfunction and reduces synaptic plasticity that contributes to impairment of learning, memory, and mood. Exacerbation of this phenomenon can ultimately culminate in real neurodegenerative disorders. By enhancing either neuroprotection or neurotoxicity, microglia

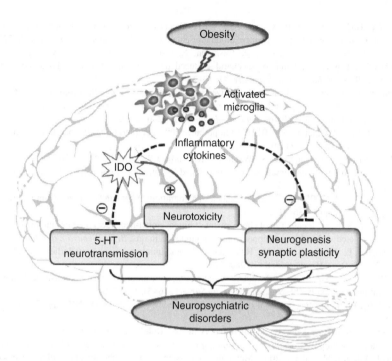

Figure 9.3 Proposed role of neuroinflammation in obesity-associated neuropsychiatric disorders. By sustaining neuroinflammation, as manifested by chronic activation of microglia, indoleamine 2,3-dioxygenase (IDO), and brain production of inflammatory cytokines, obesity may promote neurotoxicity. Increased neurotoxicity, associated with impaired serotonin (5-hydroxytryptamine, 5-HT) neurotransmission, neurogenesis, and synaptic plasticity, may then contribute to induce neuropsychiatric disorders in obese patients.

and the inflammatory cytokines they produce are a double-edged sword in terms of neurogenesis (Ekdahl *et al.*, 2009; Gemma *et al.*, 2010). On the basis of these findings, it can be proposed that in obesity, uncontrolled microglia activation as manifested by sustained cytokine production and IDO activity, together with increased production of neurotoxic compounds and impaired neurogenesis, may alter serotonin neurotransmission and promote neuronal death (Fig. 9.3). Neuroinflammation is therefore the cornerstone of the different mechanisms contributing to induce neuropsychiatric symptoms in obesity/MetS. Given the increasing prevalence of the obesity condition in modern societies, and its role as risk factor for many other diseases, developing methods for preventing inflammation-related neuropsychiatric disturbances needs to be prioritized. Such strategies may help to improve the quality of life and life expectancy of obese patients, and may avoid, or at least delay, the development of others serious neurological disorders such as depression, Alzheimer's disease, and many others.

References

Aguilar-Valles, A., Kim, J., Jung, S., Woodside, B. & Luheshi, G.N. (2014) Role of brain transmigrating neutrophils in depression-like behavior during systemic infection. *Molecular Psychiatry*, **19** (5), 599–606.

Alexander, K.S., Wu, H.Q., Schwarcz, R. & Bruno, J.P. (2012) Acute elevations of brain kynurenic acid impair cognitive flexibility: Normalization by the alpha7 positive modulator galantamine. *Psychopharmacology (Berl)*, **220** (3), 627–637.

André, C., Dinel, A.L., Ferreira, G., Laye, S. & Castanon, N. (2014) Diet-induced obesity progressively alters cognition, anxiety-like behavior and lipopolysaccharide-induced depressive-like behavior: Focus on brain indoleamine 2,3-dioxygenase. *Brain, Behavior, and Immunity*, **41**, 10–21.

André, C., O'Connor, J.C., Kelley, K.W., Lestage, J., Dantzer, R. & Castanon, N. (2008) Spatio-temporal differences in the profile of murine brain expression of proinflammatory cytokines and indoleamine 2,3-dioxygenase in response to peripheral lipopolysaccharide administration. *Journal of Neuroimmunology*, **200** (1–2), 90–99.

Aron-Wisnewsky, J., Dore, J. & Clement, K. (2012) The importance of the gut microbiota after bariatric surgery. *Nature Reviews Gastroenterology & Hepatology*, **9** (10), 590–598.

Barrientos, R.M., Sprunger, D.B., Campeau, S., Watkins, L.R., Rudy, J.W. & Maier, S.F. (2004) BDNF mRNA expression in rat hippocampus following contextual learning is blocked by intrahippocampal IL-1beta administration. *Journal of Neuroimmunology*, **155** (1–2), 119–126.

Biessels, G.J. & Gispen, W.H. (2005) The impact of diabetes on cognition: What can be learned from rodent models? *Neurobiology of Aging*, **26** (Suppl 1), 36–41.

Boitard, C., Cavaroc, A., Sauvant, J. *et al.* (2014) Impairment of hippocampal-dependent memory induced by juvenile high-fat diet intake is associated with enhanced hippocampal inflammation in rats. *Brain, Behavior, and Immunity*, **40**, 9–17.

Brandacher, G., Hoeller, E., Fuchs, D. & Weiss, H.G. (2007) Chronic immune activation underlies morbid obesity: Is IDO a key player? *Current Drug Metabolism*, **8** (3), 289–295.

Brandacher, G., Winkler, C., Aigner, F. *et al.* (2006) Bariatric surgery cannot prevent tryptophan depletion due to chronic immune activation in morbidly obese patients. *Obesity Surgery*, **16** (5), 541–548.

Cai, D. & Liu, T. (2012) Inflammatory cause of metabolic syndrome via brain stress and NF-kappaB. *Aging (Albany NY)*, **4** (2), 98–115.

Cancello, R. & Clement, K. (2006) Is obesity an inflammatory illness? Role of low-grade inflammation and macrophage infiltration in human white adipose tissue. *British Journal of Obstetrics and Gynaecology*, **113** (10), 1141–1147.

Cani, P.D., Amar, J., Iglesias, M.A. *et al.* (2007) Metabolic endotoxemia initiates obesity and insulin resistance. *Diabetes*, **56** (7), 1761–1772.

Cani, P.D., Possemiers, S., Van de Wiele, T. *et al.* (2009) Changes in gut microbiota control inflammation in obese mice through a mechanism involving GLP-2-driven improvement of gut permeability. *Gut*, **58** (8), 1091–1103.

Capuron, L. & Miller, A.H. (2011) Immune system to brain signaling: Neuropsychopharmacological implications. *Pharmacology & Therapeutics*, **130** (2), 226–238.

Capuron, L., Poitou, C., Machaux-Tholliez, D. *et al.* (2010) Relationship between adiposity, emotional status and eating behaviour in obese women: Role of inflammation. *Psychological Medicine*, **41** (7), 1517–1528.

Capuron, L., Schroecksnadel, S., Feart, C. *et al.* (2011) Chronic low-grade inflammation in elderly persons is associated with altered tryptophan and tyrosine metabolism: Role in neuropsychiatric symptoms. *Biological Psychiatry*, **70** (2), 175–182.

Capuron, L., Su, S., Miller, A.H. *et al.* (2008) Depressive symptoms and metabolic syndrome: Is inflammation the underlying link? *Biological Psychiatry*, **64** (10), 896–900.

Chess, A.C., Landers, A.M. & Bucci, D.J. (2009) L-kynurenine treatment alters contextual fear conditioning and context discrimination but not cue-specific fear conditioning. *Behavioural Brain Research*, **201** (2), 325–331.

Collin, M., Hakansson-Ovesjo, M.L., Misane, I., Ogren, S.O. & Meister, B. (2000) Decreased 5-HT transporter mRNA in neurons of the dorsal raphe nucleus and behavioral depression in the obese leptin-deficient ob/ob mouse. *Brain Research Molecular Brain Research*, **81** (1–2), 51–61.

Corona, A.W., Huang, Y., O'Connor, J.C. *et al.* (2010) Fractalkine receptor (CX3CR1) deficiency sensitizes mice to the behavioral changes induced by lipopolysaccharide. *Journal of Neuroinflammation*, **7**, 93.

Corripio, R., Gonzalez-Clemente, J.M., Jacobo, P.S. *et al.* (2012) Plasma brain-derived neurotrophic factor in prepubertal obese children. Results from a 2-year lifestyle intervention programme. *Clinical Endocrinology*, **77** (5), 715–720.

Dandona, P., Aljada, A., Chaudhuri, A., Mohanty, P. & Garg, R. (2005) Metabolic syndrome: A comprehensive perspective based on interactions between obesity, diabetes, and inflammation. *Circulation*, **111** (11), 1448–1454.

Dantzer, R., O'Connor, J.C., Freund, G.G., Johnson, R.W. & Kelley, K.W. (2008) From inflammation to sickness and depression: When the immune system subjugates the brain. *Nature Reviews Neuroscience*, **9** (1), 46–56.

De Souza, C.T., Araujo, E.P., Bordin, S. *et al.* (2005) Consumption of a fat-rich diet activates a proinflammatory response and induces insulin resistance in the hypothalamus. *Endocrinology*, **146** (10), 4192–4199.

Dinel, A.L., Andre, C., Aubert, A., Ferreira, G., Laye, S. & Castanon, N. (2011) Cognitive and emotional alterations are related to hippocampal inflammation in a mouse model of metabolic syndrome. *PLoS One*, **6** (9), e24325.

Dinel, A.L., Andre, C., Aubert, A., Ferreira, G., Laye, S. & Castanon, N. (2014) Lipopolysaccharide-induced brain activation of the indoleamine 2,3-dioxygenase and depressive-like behavior are impaired in a mouse model of metabolic syndrome. *Psychoneuroendocrinology*, **40**, 48–59.

Ekdahl, C.T., Kokaia, Z. & Lindvall, O. (2009) Brain inflammation and adult neurogenesis: The dual role of microglia. *Neuroscience*, **158** (3), 1021–1029.

Emery, C.F., Fondow, M.D., Schneider, C.M. *et al.* (2007) Gastric bypass surgery is associated with reduced inflammation and less depression: A preliminary investigation. *Obesity Surgery*, **17** (6), 759–763.

Erion, J.R., Wosiski-Kuhn, M., Dey, A. *et al.* (2014) Obesity elicits interleukin 1-mediated deficits in hippocampal synaptic plasticity. *Journal of Neuroscience*, **34** (7), 2618–2631.

Evans, D.L., Charney, D.S., Lewis, L. *et al.* (2005) Mood disorders in the medically ill: Scientific review and recommendations. *Biological Psychiatry*, **58** (3), 175–189.

Farooqui, A.A., Farooqui, T., Panza, F. & Frisardi, V. (2012) Metabolic syndrome as a risk factor for neurological disorders. *Cellular and Molecular Life Sciences*, **69** (5), 741–762.

Forrest, C.M., Mackay, G.M., Oxford, L. *et al.* (2011) Kynurenine metabolism predicts cognitive function in patients following cardiac bypass and thoracic surgery. *Journal of Neurochemistry*, **119** (1), 136–152.

Frenois, F., Moreau, M., O'Connor, J. *et al.* (2007) Lipopolysaccharide induces delayed FosB/DeltaFosB immunostaining within the mouse extended amygdala, hippocampus and hypothalamus, that parallel the expression of depressive-like behavior. *Psychoneuroendocrinology*, **32** (5), 516–531.

Frisardi, V., Solfrizzi, V., Seripa, D. *et al.* (2010) Metabolic-cognitive syndrome: A cross-talk between metabolic syndrome and Alzheimer's disease. *Ageing Research Reviews*, **9** (4), 399–417.

Fu, X., Zunich, S.M., O'Connor, J.C., Kavelaars, A., Dantzer, R. & Kelley, K.W. (2010) Central administration of lipopolysaccharide induces depressive-like behavior in vivo and activates brain indoleamine 2,3 dioxygenase in murine organotypic hippocampal slice cultures. *Journal of Neuroinflammation*, **7**, 43.

Furet, J.P., Kong, L.C., Tap, J. *et al.* (2010) Differential adaptation of human gut microbiota to bariatric surgery-induced weight loss: Links with metabolic and low-grade inflammation markers. *Diabetes*, **59** (12), 3049–3057.

Gemma, C., Bachstetter, A.D. & Bickford, P.C. (2010) Neuron-microglia dialogue and hippocampal neurogenesis in the aged brain. *Aging & Disease*, **1** (3), 232–244.

Geurts, L., Lazarevic, V., Derrien, M. *et al.* (2011) Altered gut microbiota and endocannabinoid system tone in obese and diabetic leptin-resistant mice: Impact on apelin regulation in adipose tissue. *Frontiers in Microbiology*, **2**, 149.

Gibney, S.M., McGuinness, B., Prendergast, C., Harkin, A. & Connor, T.J. (2013) Poly I:C-induced activation of the immune response is accompanied by depression and anxiety-like behaviours, kynurenine pathway activation and reduced BDNF expression. *Brain, Behavior, and Immunity*, **28**, 170–181.

Gold, A.B., Herrmann, N., Swardfager, W. *et al.* (2011) The relationship between indoleamine 2,3-dioxygenase activity and post-stroke cognitive impairment. *Journal of Neuroinflammation*, **8**, 17.

Goldbacher, E.M., Bromberger, J. & Matthews, K.A. (2009) Lifetime history of major depression predicts the development of the metabolic syndrome in middle-aged women. *Psychosomatic Medicine*, **71** (3), 266–272.

Goldbacher, E.M. & Matthews, K.A. (2007) Are psychological characteristics related to risk of the metabolic syndrome? A review of the literature. *Annals of Behavioral Medicine*, **34** (3), 240–252.

Gregor, M.F. & Hotamisligil, G.S. (2011) Inflammatory mechanisms in obesity. *Annual Review of Immunology*, **29**, 415–445.

Grover, S., Malhotra, N., Chakrabarti, S. & Kulhara, P. (2012) Metabolic syndrome in bipolar disorders. *Indian Journal of Psychological Medicine*, **34** (2), 110–118.

Gulaj, E., Pawlak, K., Bien, B. & Pawlak, D. (2010) Kynurenine and its metabolites in Alzheimer's disease patients. *Advances in Medical Sciences*, **55** (2), 204–211.

Hein, A.M., Stasko, M.R., Matousek, S.B. *et al.* (2010) Sustained hippocampal IL-1beta overexpression impairs contextual and spatial memory in transgenic mice. *Brain, Behavior, and Immunity*, **24** (2), 243–253.

Henry, C.J., Huang, Y., Wynne, A.M. & Godbout, J.P. (2009) Peripheral lipopolysaccharide (LPS) challenge promotes microglial hyperactivity in aged mice that is associated with exaggerated induction of both pro-inflammatory IL-1beta and anti-inflammatory IL-10 cytokines. *Brain, Behavior, and Immunity*, **23** (3), 309–317.

Kanoski, S.E. & Davidson, T.L. (2011) Western diet consumption and cognitive impairment: Links to hippocampal dysfunction and obesity. *Physiology & Behavior*, **103** (1), 59–68.

Konsman, J.P., Parnet, P. & Dantzer, R. (2002) Cytokine-induced sickness behaviour: Mechanisms and implications. *Trends in Neurosciences*, **25** (3), 154–159.

Lann, D. & LeRoith, D. (2007) Insulin resistance as the underlying cause for the metabolic syndrome. *Medical Clinics of North America*, **91** (6), 1063–1077, viii.

Lasselin, J., Magne, E., Beau, C. *et al.* (2013) Adipose inflammation in obesity: Relationship with circulating levels of inflammatory markers and association with surgery-induced weight loss. *Journal of Clinical Endocrinology and Metabolism*, **99** (1), E53–E61.

Lawrence, C.B., Brough, D. & Knight, E.M. (2012) Obese mice exhibit an altered behavioural and inflammatory response to lipopolysaccharide. *Disease Models & Mechanisms*, **5** (5), 649–659.

Ley, R.E., Backhed, F., Turnbaugh, P., Lozupone, C.A., Knight, R.D. & Gordon, J.I. (2005) Obesity alters gut microbial ecology. *Proceedings of the National Academy of Sciences of the United States of America*, **102** (31), 11070–11075.

Lin, H.Y., Huang, C.K., Tai, C.M. *et al.* (2013) Psychiatric disorders of patients seeking obesity treatment. *BMC Psychiatry*, **13**, 1.

Lu, A., Steiner, M.A., Whittle, N. *et al.* (2008) Conditional mouse mutants highlight mechanisms of corticotropin-releasing hormone effects on stress-coping behavior. *Molecular Psychiatry*, **13** (11), 1028–1042.

Mangge, H., Summers, K.L., Meinitzer, A. *et al.* (2013) Obesity-related dysregulation of the tryptophan-kynurenine metabolism: Role of age and parameters of the metabolic syndrome. *Obesity (Silver Spring)*, **22** (1), 195–201.

Marsland, A.L., McCaffery, J.M., Muldoon, M.F. & Manuck, S.B. (2010) Systemic inflammation and the metabolic syndrome among middle-aged community volunteers. *Metabolism*, **59** (12), 1801–1808.

Martinowich, K., Manji, H. & Lu, B. (2007) New insights into BDNF function in depression and anxiety. *Nature Neuroscience*, **10** (9), 1089–1093.

McEvoy, J.P., Meyer, J.M., Goff, D.C. *et al.* (2005) Prevalence of the metabolic syndrome in patients with schizophrenia: Baseline results from the Clinical Antipsychotic Trials of Intervention Effectiveness (CATIE) schizophrenia trial and comparison with national estimates from NHANES III. *Schizophrenia Research*, **80** (1), 19–32.

McIntyre, R.S., Soczynska, J.K., Liauw, S.S. *et al.* (2012) The association between childhood adversity and components of metabolic syndrome in adults with mood disorders: Results from the international mood disorders collaborative project. *International Journal of Psychiatry in Medicine*, **43** (2), 165–177.

Mellor, A.L. & Munn, D.H. (2008) Creating immune privilege: Active local suppression that benefits friends, but protects foes. *Nature Reviews Immunology*, **8** (1), 74–80.

Molteni, R., Barnard, R.J., Ying, Z., Roberts, C.K. & Gomez-Pinilla, F. (2002) A high-fat, refined sugar diet reduces hippocampal brain-derived neurotrophic factor, neuronal plasticity, and learning. *Neuroscience*, **112** (4), 803–814.

Moreau, M., Andre, C., O'Connor, J.C. *et al.* (2008) Inoculation of Bacillus Calmette-Guerin to mice induces an acute episode of sickness behavior followed by chronic depressive-like behavior. *Brain, Behavior, and Immunity*, **22** (7), 1087–1095.

Moy, G.A. & McNay, E.C. (2012) Caffeine prevents weight gain and cognitive impairment caused by a high-fat diet while elevating hippocampal BDNF. *Physiology & Behavior*, **109**, 69–74.

Muller, M., van Raamt, F., Visseren, F.L. *et al.* (2010) Metabolic syndrome and cognition in patients with manifest atherosclerotic disease: The SMART study. *Neuroepidemiology*, **34** (2), 83–89.

Myint, A.M., Kim, Y.K., Verkerk, R., Scharpe, S., Steinbusch, H. & Leonard, B. (2007) Kynurenine pathway in major depression: Evidence of impaired neuroprotection. *Journal of Affective Disorders*, **98** (1–2), 143–151.

Noble, F., Rubira, E., Boulanouar, M. *et al.* (2007) Acute systemic inflammation induces central mitochondrial damage and mnesic deficit in adult Swiss mice. *Neuroscience Letters*, **424** (2), 106–110.

O'Connor, J.C., Andre, C., Wang, Y. *et al.* (2009a) Interferon-gamma and tumor necrosis factor-alpha mediate the upregulation of indoleamine 2,3-dioxygenase and the induction of depressive-like behavior in mice in response to bacillus Calmette-Guerin. *Journal of Neuroscience*, **29** (13), 4200–4209.

O'Connor, J.C., Lawson, M.A., Andre, C. *et al.* (2009b) Induction of IDO by bacille Calmette-Guerin is responsible for development of murine depressive-like behavior. *Journal of Immunology*, **182** (5), 3202–3212.

O'Connor, J.C., Lawson, M.A., Andre, C. *et al.* (2009c) Lipopolysaccharide-induced depressive-like behavior is mediated by indoleamine 2,3-dioxygenase activation in mice. *Molecular Psychiatry*, **14** (5), 511–522.

Ohta, R., Shigemura, N., Sasamoto, K., Koyano, K. & Ninomiya, Y. (2003) Conditioned taste aversion learning in leptin-receptor-deficient db/db mice. *Neurobiology of Learning and Memory*, **80** (2), 105–112.

Pan, A., Keum, N., Okereke, O.I. *et al.* (2012) Bidirectional association between depression and metabolic syndrome: A systematic review and meta-analysis of epidemiological studies. *Diabetes Care*, **35** (5), 1171–1180.

Pistell, P.J., Morrison, C.D., Gupta, S. *et al.* (2010) Cognitive impairment following high fat diet consumption is associated with brain inflammation. *Journal of Neuroimmunology*, **219** (1–2), 25–32.

Pohl, J., Woodside, B. & Luheshi, G.N. (2009) Changes in hypothalamically mediated acute-phase inflammatory responses to lipopolysaccharide in diet-induced obese rats. *Endocrinology*, **150** (11), 4901–4910.

Raison, C.L., Dantzer, R., Kelley, K.W. *et al.* (2010) CSF concentrations of brain tryptophan and kynurenines during immune stimulation with IFN-alpha: Relationship to CNS immune responses and depression. *Molecular Psychiatry*, **15** (4), 393–403.

Raison, C.L. & Miller, A.H. (2003) When not enough is too much: The role of insufficient glucocorticoid signaling in the pathophysiology of stress-related disorders. *American Journal of Psychiatry*, **160** (9), 1554–1565.

Ransohoff, R.M. & Perry, V.H. (2009) Microglial physiology: Unique stimuli, specialized responses. *Annual Review of Immunology*, **27**, 119–145.

Roberts, R.O., Geda, Y.E., Knopman, D.S. *et al.* (2010) Metabolic syndrome, inflammation, and nonamnestic mild cognitive impairment in older persons: A population-based study. *Alzheimer Disease and Associated Disorders*, **24** (1), 11–18.

Rummel, C., Inoue, W., Poole, S. & Luheshi, G.N. (2010) Leptin regulates leukocyte recruitment into the brain following systemic LPS-induced inflammation. *Molecular Psychiatry*, **15** (5), 523–534.

Salazar, A., Gonzalez-Rivera, B.L., Redus, L., Parrott, J.M. & O'Connor, J.C. (2012) Indoleamine 2,3-dioxygenase mediates anhedonia and anxiety-like behaviors caused by peripheral lipopolysaccharide immune challenge. *Hormones and Behavior*, **62** (3), 202–209.

Schwarcz, R., Rassoulpour, A., Wu, H.Q., Medoff, D., Tamminga, C.A. & Roberts, R.C. (2001) Increased cortical kynurenate content in schizophrenia. *Biological Psychiatry*, **50** (7), 521–530.

Stone, T.W., Forrest, C.M., Stoy, N. & Darlington, L.G. (2012) Involvement of kynurenines in Huntington's disease and stroke-induced brain damage. *Journal of Neural Transmission*, **119** (2), 261–274.

Stranahan, A.M., Arumugam, T.V., Cutler, R.G., Lee, K., Egan, J.M. & Mattson, M.P. (2008) Diabetes impairs hippocampal function through glucocorticoid-mediated effects on new and mature neurons. *Nature Neuroscience*, **11** (3), 309–317.

Stranahan, A.M., Lee, K., Martin, B. *et al.* (2009) Voluntary exercise and caloric restriction enhance hippocampal dendritic spine density and BDNF levels in diabetic mice. *Hippocampus*, **19** (10), 951–961.

Sweat, V., Starr, V., Bruehl, H. *et al.* (2008) C-reactive protein is linked to lower cognitive performance in overweight and obese women. *Inflammation*, **31** (3), 198–207.

Varga, O., Harangi, M., Olsson, I.A. & Hansen, A.K. (2009) Contribution of animal models to the understanding of the metabolic syndrome: A systematic overview. *Obesity Reviews*, **11** (11), 792–807.

Verdam, F.J., Fuentes, S., de Jonge, C. *et al.* (2013) Human intestinal microbiota composition is associated with local and systemic inflammation in obesity. *Obesity (Silver Spring)*, **21** (12), E607–E615.

Walker, A.K., Budac, D.P., Bisulco, S. *et al.* (2013) NMDA receptor blockade by ketamine abrogates lipopolysaccharide-induced depressive-like behavior in C57BL/6J mice. *Neuropsychopharmacology*, **38** (9), 1609–1616.

Yaffe, K. (2007) Metabolic syndrome and cognitive decline. *Current Alzheimer Research*, **4** (2), 123–126.

Yamada, K. & Nabeshima, T. (2003) Brain-derived neurotrophic factor/TrkB signaling in memory processes. *Journal of Pharmacological Sciences*, **91** (4), 267–270.

Yates, K.F., Sweat, V., Yau, P.L., Turchiano, M.M. & Convit, A. (2012) Impact of metabolic syndrome on cognition and brain: A selected review of the literature. *Arteriosclerosis, Thrombosis, and Vascular Biology*, **32** (9), 2060–2067.

Zeyda, M., Wernly, B., Demyanets, S. *et al.* (2011) Severe obesity increases adipose tissue expression of interleukin-33 and its receptor ST2, both predominantly detectable in endothelial cells of human adipose tissue. *International Journal of Obesity*, **37** (5), 658–665.

10 Viral Infections of the Central Nervous System: Pathogenic and Protective Effects of Neuroinflammation

John G. Walsh and Christopher Power

Department of Medicine (Neurology), University of Alberta, Edmonton, Alberta, Canada

Introduction

Viral infections of the central nervous system (CNS) cause substantial rates of morbidity and mortality, both as acute infections, including West Nile virus (WNV), herpes simplex virus (HSV), and rabies virus, and as chronic infections such as human immunodeficiency virus (HIV), human T-lymphotropic virus-1, cytomegalovirus, and John Cunningham (JC) virus in humans (Johnson, 1998). Indeed, there are new emerging viral infections of the CNS worldwide including Nipah, Hendra, Toscana, and Circoviruses as well as resurging viruses such as tick-borne encephalitis virus, all of which carry important implications for human and animal health (Wilson, 2013). There is also a burgeoning appreciation of viruses once thought not to affect (Holman *et al.*, 2010) or infect the CNS that now are recognized as CNS infections; for example, hepatitis C virus (HCV) infects glial cells in the CNS resulting in a chronic encephalopathy and rarely vasculitis (Monaco *et al.*, 2012). Similarly, influenza A and dengue viruses (Carod-Artal *et al.*, 2013) are increasingly recognized as causes of neurological disorders. Furthermore, the spectrum of clinical manifestations of viruses known to infect the CNS is growing, as evidenced by newly recognized syndromes caused by varicella zoster virus (VZV) (Gilden *et al.*, 2011). Both RNA and DNA virus infections of the CNS exhibit diverse clinical and neuropathological phenotypes depending on the individual virus species and strain, infected neural cell type, neuroanatomical site of infection (e.g., brain and spinal cord), together with host factors (age, health status, comorbidity, and genetic background).

CNS viral infections are defined by several properties including *neuroinvasion*, the initial stage during which a virus enters the CNS through the circulation as free virus and/or infected leukocyte infiltration (e.g., HIV) across the blood–brain barrier (or choroid plexus) or retrograde transport from a peripheral tissue (e.g., rabies). On CNS entry, the virus infects one or several cell types, termed *neurotropism*, allowing it to replicate depending on the cell type;

Neuroinflammation: New Insights into Beneficial and Detrimental Functions, First Edition. Edited by Samuel David.
© 2015 John Wiley & Sons, Inc. Published 2015 by John Wiley & Sons, Inc.

for example, HSV-1 infects neurons in the trigeminal ganglion but does not necessarily exhibit signs of brain disease, although it may manifest as a labial lesion ("cold sore"). However, CNS viral infections are usually recognized for their capacity to cause disease, *neurovirulence*, which is often evident as seizures, headache, confusion/psychosis but can also progress to chronic encephalopathy, dementia, or death. The neuropathological correlates of these clinical features can include viral inclusions, leukocyte infiltration, cell injury and death, hemorrhage, gliosis, resulting in "encephalitis," the severity of which is determined by both the individual virus and its specific pathogenic properties, coupled with the extent and profile of host immune response. The development of neurovirulence during viral infections can arise from two principal mechanisms: (i) direct virus-induced cellular injury through the cytotoxic effects of viral replication and protein expression and (ii) off-target inflammatory effects of host immune responses including released cytokines, chemokines, reactive oxygen species (ROS), and proteases (Fig. 10.1). In fact, pathogenic inflammatory responses that occur as part of host antiviral defense strategies are often associated with tissue injury (cell death) and swelling (edema), resulting in increased intracranial pressure and worsened clinical outcomes. Moreover, individual inflammatory responses [e.g., release of cytokines such as interleukin (IL)-1β or tumor necrosis factor (TNF)-α] also exacerbate virus-mediated effects by amplifying viral replication or acting synergistically with viral proteins to cause cellular injury and death. Host factors are key determinants of neurological outcomes, which are collectively described as host *neurosusceptibility* (Patrick *et al.*, 2002). These include

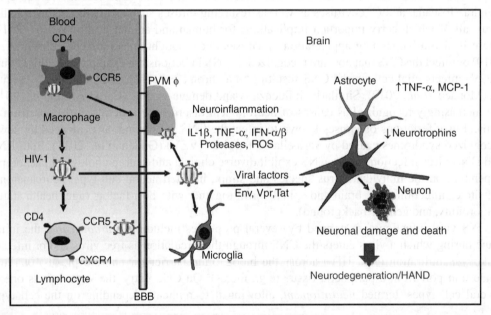

Figure 10.1 HIV neuropathogenesis is defined by multiple stages, including neuroinvasion during which HIV-infected macrophages traverse the blood–brain barrier; neurotropism is evident as infection of microglia and perivascular macrophages (PVMφ); neurovirulence is predicated on neuronal injury and death. Neuroinflammation, evident as TNF-α, IL-1β, protease, and ROS production, and together with viral proteins (Env, Vpr, and Tat) contribute to neuronal injury and eventually HAND, but neuroinflammation also exerts antiviral effects (IFN-α/β).

age (e.g., infants and elderly), health status (e.g., immunosuppression due to transplantation and medications), comorbidities (e.g., diabetes and autoimmune disease), and genetic background (e.g., single nucleotide polymorphisms and inherited immunodeficiency disorders).

A major challenge in the clinical care of a patient with a presumed CNS viral infection lies in the prompt diagnosis of the infection. Accurate diagnosis rests on timely evaluation of demographic and clinical features together with neuroimaging [computed tomography (CT) and magnetic resonance imaging (MRI)] and laboratory investigations of blood and cerebrospinal fluid using both immunological (viral serology) and molecular (polymerase chain reaction) detection tools. Few therapeutic pharmacological options exist for treatment of viral infections of the nervous system; these drugs are largely nucleoside analogues (acyclovir, ribavirin, and ganciclovir), although protease, integrase, and non-nucleoside reverse transcriptase inhibitors are available for HIV and HCV infections (Nath and Tyler, 2013). Other interventions include supportive care by maintaining cardiorespiratory stability, reducing intracranial pressure, preventing coinfections, restoring immune status when possible, and treating associated complications (seizures and psychosis).

Nervous System Infection and Inflammation

Nervous system infections in general are defined by a broad range of host immune responses that include both innate and adaptive immune responses that affect the nervous system locally such as during such parasitic or bacterial infections (e.g., tuberculous abscess) or more diffusely through the brain, spinal cord, and/or peripheral nerves (e.g., cytomegalovirus). The CNS is unique in that there are no resident lymphoid tissues, although lymphocytes provide ongoing surveillance of the CNS and respond accordingly to neural infection or injury as required (Ousman and Kubes, 2012). In contrast, the CNS contains a robust innate immune system that is composed of mononuclear phagocytes (MPs) including resident microglia, parenchymal-infiltrating and meningeal/choroid plexus macrophages, dendritic cells (DCs), as well as astrocytes. Indeed, studies have also implicated neurons in the CNS innate immune response repertoire (Yazdi et al., 2010). Under normal conditions, there are relatively few resident lymphocytes within the brain. The brain's resident immune system is largely composed of specialized mononuclear phagocyte populations, the most prominent of which are the perivascular macrophages (PVMφ) and microglia (Prinz et al., 2011). PVMφ populate the space around blood vessels, while microglia are located within brain parenchyma. Owing to their location around blood vessels and to the fact that they are regularly repopulated from circulating monocytes, PVMφ are the first responders to viral entry into the CNS (Williams et al., 2001; Fischer-Smith et al., 2004). The innate immune response within the CNS is also supplemented by innate immune cells derived from the circulation including neutrophils, γδ-T cells, mast, and natural killer (NK) cells that can be summoned into the CNS depending on the stimulus, often by chemokine release (e.g., infection, trauma, and ischemia), as required. All of these cell types with their individual molecular mechanisms and associated effector molecules can be engaged during CNS viral infections. The host response to a viral infection of the CNS is time dependent in that innate immune responses are immediately activated through well-recognized interactions between pathogen-associated molecular patterns (PAMPs) (e.g., viral envelope or secreted proteins) with pattern recognition receptors (PRRs) such as Toll-like receptors (TLRs), inflammasomes, retinoic-acid-inducible gene 1 (RIG-I), mitochondrial antiviral signaling protein (MAVS), and endoplasmic reticulum (ER) stress. The ensuing immune effector molecules including cytokines, chemokines, ROS, and proteases are rapidly activated and can remain in a state of chronic activation in part due to ongoing PAMP exposure as well as encounters with infiltrating lymphoid cells. Both humoral and cellular adaptive immune responses exert vigorous effects on CNS viral infections; these adaptive responses include antibody targeting and neutralization of viruses as well as cytotoxic (CD8+) lymphocyte-mediated actions on virus-infected cells. The specificity and extent of immune responses are governed by both viral (e.g., antigenicity of individual proteins and replicative capacity) and host factors (age, immune status, genotype, and comorbidities). Importantly, off-target effects of both innate and adaptive immune responses substantially contribute to neurovirulence. In fact, immune responses to a given infectious agent may diverge within versus outside of the nervous system with differential pathogenic outcomes. The disease tempo can also favor distinct immune responses; for example, HIV-1 infection of the CNS results in a chronic subacute encephalopathy affecting a large proportion of infected persons, which is largely defined by innate immune processes. Conversely, WNV infection of the CNS has a comparatively acute onset with a robust adaptive immune response that promotes neurovirulence but affects only a small proportion of WNV-infected individuals.

HIV-1 Infection: Neurological and Neuropathological Features

HIV is a retrolentivirus that currently infects approximately 35 million people globally and is lethal unless treated with combined antiretroviral therapy (CART). Human immunodeficiency virus type 1 (HIV-1) is the predominant virus causing disease globally, while HIV-2 is largely limited to West Africa and is associated with a less severe disease course. HIV replicates at very high levels, which is accompanied by the generation of extraordinary viral molecular diversity causing immunological exhaustion over time, evident as CD4+ T cell depletion, eventually leading to acquired immunodeficiency syndrome (AIDS). Similar to all lentiviruses, including simian immunodeficiency virus (SIV), feline immunodeficiency virus (FIV), bovine immunodeficiency virus (BIV) immunodeficiency viruses and the nonimmunodeficiency lentiviruses (visna-maedi virus, caprine encephalitis-arthritis virus), HIV entry into the brain or neuroinvasion is an early (and recurring) event that affects most, if not all, infected hosts. The leading model of HIV infection into the brain proposes a Trojan horse mechanism by which infected macrophages cross the blood–brain barrier and viral spread occurs through infection of PVMφ and proximal microglia (Jordan et al., 1991; Fischer-Smith et al., 2004). For most infected persons, neuroinvasion occurs in all infected persons and leads to neurotropism, evident as infection of macrophages and microglia, also a signature feature of lentiviruses. Clinically detectable neurological disease, or neurovirulence, is characterized by a constellation of features including neurocognitive (forgetfulness and poor judgment), neurobehavioral (agitation, mania, and apathy), and motor (psychomotor slowing and ataxia) abnormalities, with the most severe form, HIV-associated dementia, affecting 20–40% of infected individuals in the absence of CART (Boisse et al., 2008). The neuropathological hallmarks of untreated HIV-1 infection of the CNS include multinucleated giant (macrophage) cells, microglial nodules, astro- and microgliosis, diffuse myelin pallor, synaptic retraction, neuronal loss with detectable viral antigens (HIV-1 p24) in microglia, and/or PVMφ. The availability of CART, one of the greatest achievements in medicine in the twentieth century, has substantially improved survival with HIV/AIDS and the incidence of HIV-associated-dementia has dropped from 20% to 30% in the pre-CART era to less than 5% currently. However, the total prevalence of neurocognitive impairment (~30%) remains the same, albeit with less severe phenotypes including minor neurocognitive disorder (MND) (5–10%) and asymptomatic neurocognitive impairment (20–30%). This spectrum of neurocognitive disorders, from mild to severe, is now referred to HIV-associated neurocognitive disorders (HAND). Risk factors for the development of HAND include blood CD4+ T cell nadir levels, high baseline viral load, duration of HIV-1 infection, increased age of infected person, together with several host genotypes including polymorphisms in cytokine and chemokine genes, as well as the APOEε4 allele. Importantly, HAND is a virus-mediated syndrome that is evident in patients despite receiving effective CART and is a significant contributor to the morbidity and mortality of these individuals (Ellis *et al.*, 2007; Vivithanaporn *et al.*, 2010; Mothobi and Brew, 2012).

At the cellular and molecular levels, HIV infection in the brain presents all of the current challenges faced by researchers attempting to fully eradicate the systemic infection. The virus is hidden away in nondividing (and inactive) mononuclear phagocytic cells within the notoriously impermeable CNS. Therefore, the brain is one of the most critical viral reservoirs that must be tackled by any viral eradication strategy. HIV infection of the brain not only serves as a key benchmark of eradication efforts, but also provides, through its imperfect ability to hide, a biological/pathological context under which to measure the success of those therapeutic efforts.

HIV Neurotropism is Mediated by Chronically Infected Macrophages/Microglia

Although multiple opportunistic infections of the CNS occur as a result of the immunodeficiency linked to the loss of CD4+ T cells in the periphery, the direct HIV-dependent neuropathology is presumed to result from the infection of MPs within the brain (Burdo *et al.*, 2013). Immunodeficiency and uncontrolled viral replication in the peripheral circulation promote viral infection of the brain, but neurovirulence stems from dysregulated inflammation, triggered by local innate immune responses to the virus. Macrophage/microglia activation within the brain is more predictive of neurocognitive decline compared to actual HIV gene expression (RNA or protein) (Glass *et al.*, 1995; Gelman *et al.*, 2012). The select cell tropism of HIV-1 infection in the brain is further evidenced by the predominance of macrophage-tropic viral strains over lymphocyte-tropic viral strains when virus is specifically isolated from the CNS (Holman *et al.*, 2010). Astrocytes are also infected but do not produce virus, and the significance of this infection *in vivo* is still an area of debate. Neurons and oligodendrocytes are not infected by HIV, and therefore damage to these cell types is indirectly caused by the immunopathological effects of HIV-mediated chronic inflammation. The resulting impact on macrophage/microglia populations provides the defining neuropathological features of HIV-1 infection including extensive microglial activation as well as the appearance of microglial nodules and multinucleated giant cells, which arise through virus-dependent membrane fusion (Glass *et al.*, 1995; Fischer-Smith *et al.*, 2004).

Neuroinflammatory Cascade in Response to HIV Infection

Studies over the past 20 years have identified several inflammatory pathways that contribute to HIV neuropathogenesis and have established the neuroinflammatory nature of HIV infection within the CNS. Particular attention has been paid to the resultant cytokine, chemokine, protease, and free radical responses. The specific cytokines that have been most consistently identified to participate in disease are TNF-α and IL-1β (Tyor *et al.*, 1993; Wesselingh *et al.*, 1997; Xing *et al.*, 2009a, 2009b). These are central regulatory molecules and are largely responsible for driving on the inflammatory response through their effects on immune cell activation and recruitment. Their prominence is indicative of a pathology driven primarily by MP responses. In concert with the cytokine response, HIV infection in the brain is also characterized by a large and complex chemokine response including monocyte chemoattractant protein-1 (MCP-1) (CCL2), macrophage inflammatory protein 1 (MIP-1) (CCL3), stromal cell-derived factor 1a (SDF-1a) (CXCL12), and regulated on activation, normal T cell expressed and secreted (RANTES) (CCL5) among others (Sasseville *et al.*, 1996; Schmidtmayerova *et al.*, 1996; Conant *et al.*, 1998; Kelder *et al.*, 1998; Zhang *et al.*, 2003). In addition to the further recruitment of immune cells into the brain, several of these molecules have been reported to promote neuropathology through effects on local cell types such as astrocytes and neurons (Bezzi *et al.*, 2001; Croitoru-Lamoury *et al.*, 2003; Zhang *et al.*, 2003). The effect on chemokine signaling particularly in astrocytes is a primary example of how the inflammatory response to virus within infected macrophages becomes amplified in the CNS leading to dysregulated homeostasis. Other affected inflammatory pathways include reactive oxygen species and matrix metalloproteases (MMPs) (Bukrinsky *et al.*, 1995; Blond *et al.*, 1998; Johnston *et al.*, 2000; Zhang *et al.*, 2003). There can also be a subsequent convergence of these inflammatory pathways, which serves to escalate local inflammation and accompanying neuronal injury (Vergote *et al.*, 2006).

Neurological Immune Reconstitution Inflammatory Syndrome

Among HIV-1-infected persons with very low CD4+ T cell levels, the initiation of CART occasionally results in deterioration of neurological status, defined by encephalopathy, delirium, seizures, hemiparesis, and ataxia. This paradoxical syndrome is termed neurological immune reconstitution inflammatory syndrome (NeuroIRIS) and usually associated with a concurrent (often unrecognized) CNS infection (cryptococcal meningitis, toxoplasmic encephalitis, CNS tuberculosis, or rarely HAND) (Gray *et al.*, 2005). NeuroIRIS is pathologically defined by a robust T cell infiltration, particularly CD8+ CTLs, accompanied by macrophages and ensuing gliosis that results in clinical deficits. It is widely presumed that potent CART regimens rapidly suppress viral replication, allowing T cells to proliferate and target antigens expressed by infectious agents in a dysregulated manner with extensive off-target effects. However, the specific immune regulatory processes that are interrupted are currently unknown. NeuroIRIS is a significant clinical challenge today for which there are few therapeutic options other than the empiric use of corticosteroids.

Innate Immune Sensing of HIV Infection within the CNS

Despite the characterization of an inflammatory response to HIV-1 CNS infection that is predicated on the sensing of virus by macrophages and microglia, there is relatively little known about the innate immune sensing of virus or virus-infected cells at the molecular level. Current studies on HIV-1's interaction with the innate immune system have focused on the sensing of viral genomic products and activation of antiviral interferon (IFN) responses. In the periphery, HIV elicits strong type 1 IFN-driven responses from plasmacytoid dendritic cells (pDC) (Beignon et al., 2005; Lepelley et al., 2011). In these cells, virus is endocytosed and sensed by the PRRs TLR7 and TLR9, which bind to viral RNA (Beignon et al., 2005). However, in many other cell types such as conventional DCs and certain macrophage subtypes, there is no detectable IFN response despite viral entry into these cells. Importantly, these cell types are often not infected by HIV-1, which underlies their lack of a virus-induced IFN response. Studies have shown that in these cells, multiple host proteins including SAMHD1 and TREX1 prevent the triggering of an IFN response by preventing the formation/accumulation of virus-derived genomic products within the cytoplasm (Yan et al., 2010; Goldstone et al., 2011). Removal of these blocks has revealed the presence of multiple cytosolic DNA sensors. Although type 1 IFN responses have been reported in the context of HIV neurotropism (Polyak et al., 2013), the inflammatory signaling molecules most associated with neuropathology such as TNF-α and IL-1β can arise through a number of other distinct signaling pathways. In fact, unlike type 1 IFN responses, the immunopathological response to viruses in the brain may be independent of the sensing of viral genomic products. For example, the release of both TNF-α and IL-1β in response to whole virus has been replicated using isolated viral proteins such as viral envelope protein gp120/gp160 and HIV trans-activating protein Tat (Merrill et al., 1992; Koka et al., 1995; Nath et al., 1999; Cheung et al., 2008; Jin et al., 2012; Ben Haij et al., 2013).

The specific mechanisms by which viral proteins might trigger cytokine release are not clear, especially with regards to the requirement for specific receptors. It has been recently reported that HIV-1 Tat can directly bind TLR4 and thus activate nuclear factor-κB (NFκB)-associated signaling (Ben Haij et al., 2013). Although cytokine responses are triggered by the HIV-1 envelope (gp120), CD4 binding does not appear to be required, although binding to the viral co-receptor CCR5 has been implicated in at least some studies (Clouse et al., 1991; Merrill et al., 1992; Koka et al., 1995; Cheung et al., 2008). A number of other putative receptors not usually associated with viral entry have been shown to interact with the HIV envelope protein including the integrin, α4β7, and DC-SIGN (dendritic cell-specific intercellular adhesion molecule-3-grabbing non-integrin) (Gringhuis et al., 2007; Arthos et al., 2008). Signaling through DC-SIGN has even been reported to stabilize TLR-initiated NFκB signaling in response to HIV-1 (Gringhuis et al., 2007). Two viral restriction factors, tetherin and tripartite motif-containing protein 5 (TRIM5), have also been reported to signal to NFκB on binding of whole virus or viral capsid proteins respectively (Pertel et al., 2011; Galao et al., 2012).

Activation and release of IL-1β additionally require the formation of a complex termed the inflammasome, which incorporates certain cytosolic PRRs [usually of the NOD-like receptor (NLR) family] and the protease, caspase-1 (Fig. 10.2). Specifically, the NLRP3 inflammasome

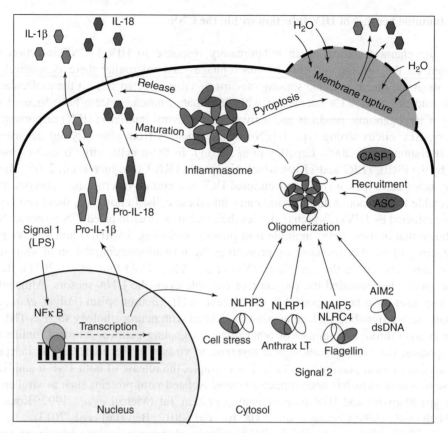

Figure 10.2   Inflammasomes are protein complexes, largely located in macrophage-lineage cells, which act as sensors of infectious or injurious stimuli as well as effectors of innate immune responses, particularly the cleavage and release of IL-1β and IL-18 by caspase-1. Inflammasome activation requires an initial stimulus (Signal 1) to initiate transcription followed by induction of protein assembly by a second stimulus (Signal 2). Multiple inflammasomes are implicated in viral infections including NLRP3 and AIM2. (*See insert for color representation of this figure.*)

has been reported to be activated in a number of neuroinflammatory diseases including multiple sclerosis and Alzheimer's disease [reviewed in Walsh *et al.* (2014a, 2014b)]. Studies from our group have shown that HIV-dependent release of IL-1β from human microglia might also be mediated through the activation of this inflammasome-associated protein (Walsh *et al.*, 2014a, 2014b). The possibility of targeting NLRP3 raises exciting options for future treatment strategies including antagonism of these pathways using novel inhibitors of related pathogenic pathways.

WNV Infection and Neuropathology

WNV is a mosquito-borne flavivirus that has seen significant expansion of its global range in the past 15 years, particularly in North America. The infection is cycled between mosquitoes (*Culex* species) and birds but also regularly infects mammals including humans. Most people who become infected with WNV experience few or no symptoms; 20–40% of infected individuals experiences flu-like symptoms including fever, headache, fatigue, and muscle pain (Kramer *et al.*, 2007). However, a small percentage of individuals (<1%) develops severe neuroinvasive disease such as meningitis, encephalitis, and acute flaccid paralysis with poor outcomes (Kramer *et al.*, 2007). Unlike HIV, WNV is largely observed as an acute infection (2- to 14-day incubation period) and usually completely cleared by the immune system in a relatively short period following infection to ensure host survival.

The risk factors for the development of WNV neuroinvasive disease are poorly understood, although elderly or immunocompromised individuals appear to be more susceptible (Murray *et al.*, 2006, 2009). In addition, genetic risk factors for the development of neuroinvasive disease have been associated with the genes encoding the CCR5 chemokine receptor, interferon response factor 3 (IRF3), MAVS, and the IFN-inducible PRRs of the $2''$-$5'$-oligoadenylate synthase (OAS) family members (Lim *et al.*, 2009, 2010; Bigham *et al.*, 2011). Mice are also permissive to WNV infection, and thus, most pathogenesis studies including those discussed in the following section have used murine models of WNV infection.

Neuroinvasion and Neurotropism of WNV

Unlike HIV-1 infection in which it is established that most infected persons experience some level of viral invasion into the CNS, it is unknown in humans whether WNV neuroinvasion is a common feature of infection or only occurs in those individuals who go on to develop clinically apparent neurologic disease. Following an infected mosquito bite, WNV infects local innate immune cells and is carried to the draining lymph node where it is further amplified and disseminated to the visceral organs (Suthar *et al.*, 2013). In murine models, the expansion of virus in the periphery to sufficient levels has been shown to be an important prerequisite for neuroinvasion (Wang *et al.*, 2003; Bai *et al.*, 2010), suggesting that an effective immune response in the peripheral circulation prevents neuroinvasion in many individuals. Although there is no firm consensus on the primary mechanism by which WNV gains entry into the brain, the disruption of the blood–brain barrier has been consistently observed during infection (Verma *et al.*, 2009; Bai *et al.*, 2010; Roe *et al.*, 2012). Such disruption has been associated with increased expression of inflammatory cytokines and MMPs as well as the infection of microvascular endothelial cells (Wang *et al.*, 2004; Verma *et al.*, 2009; Bai *et al.*, 2010). Increased permeability of the blood–brain barrier could allow for transport of the virus into the CNS or allow infected leukocytes cells to enter the CNS, thereby facilitating a Trojan horse mechanism, similar to HIV-1. In addition, it has been reported that entry might also be mediated through retrograde transport through infected peripheral neurons (Samuel *et al.*, 2007).

The neurotropism of WNV is considerably broader than that of HIV, as WNV readily infects not only local immune cells, but also astrocytes and neurons (Cheeran *et al.*, 2005; van Marle *et al.*, 2007). Importantly, infection of neurons can lead to direct cytopathic effects such as the triggering of programmed cell death, which impacts directly on neurologic function (Parquet *et al.*, 2001; Shrestha *et al.*, 2003). This wide and damaging dissemination of virus within CNS tissues highlights the importance of an effective immune response to remove infected cells and limit viral spread. However, it is also clear from neuropathological studies and from the occurrence of acute meningitis/encephalitis that an inflammation-based immunopathological milieu develops with adverse effects on clinical outcomes (Kelley *et al.*, 2003; van Marle *et al.*, 2007). Therefore, the prognosis in WNV infection depends on an effective early adaptive immune response that clears the virus and avoids prolonged inflammation in the CNS.

Neuroinflammatory Response to WNV

As mentioned previously, the effectiveness of the peripheral immune response to WNV is of foremost importance in avoiding neurologic disease, although, unlike HIV, WNV infection within the CNS can be eliminated by the appropriate neuroinflammatory response. However, because of the brain's particular sensitivity to inflammation, the costs to the host of even a successful response may be significant with regard to morbidities arising due to off-target inflammatory mechanisms. Compared to other sites of infection, inflammation is particularly notable within the CNS (Armah *et al.*, 2007). Studies using mice primarily focus on survival as an endpoint and as such usually report on the beneficial requirement of inflammation, although underlying immunopathologies have also been identified. Regardless, neuroinvasion of WNV is accompanied by infiltration of innate and adaptive immune cells (Kelley *et al.*, 2003). The most prominent immune cells include macrophages and microglia, which can be observed in large numbers around infected neurons and have been described as a feature of lethal WNV infection (Armah *et al.*, 2007; Getts *et al.*, 2008). Macrophages release several proinflammatory cytokines and chemokines in response to WNV, which promote subsequent adaptive immune responses but may also damage neurons (Cheeran *et al.*, 2005; Kumar *et al.*, 2010). Also prominent in the immune response to WNV within the CNS are neutrophils; these cells are found in large numbers in the CSF of both infected humans and mice (Crichlow *et al.*, 2004; Bai *et al.*, 2010), and when mice are depleted of neutrophils after the establishment of a peripheral infection, the neurological outcome is worsened (Bai *et al.*, 2010). However, it is the adaptive immune response and its principal constituents in the form of CD4+/CD8+ T cells and perhaps B cells that are most critical for the elimination of WNV from the CNS. The absence of a CD4+ T cell responses has been reported to result in a protracted infection within the CNS and an increase in lethality (Sitati and Diamond, 2006). Interestingly, the trajectory of infection within the peripheral circulation was much less affected. One of the key targets of CD4+ T cell regulation in WNV-infected mice are cytotoxic CD8+ T cells (Sitati and Diamond, 2006). Several studies have identified the requirement for CD8+ T cells to ultimately stem the infection (Wang *et al.*, 2003; Klein *et al.*, 2005; Brien *et al.*, 2007). However, similar to macrophages and microglia, the beneficial antiviral responses of CD8+ T cells are also accompanied by immunopathology, as suggested by the observation that under some infection paradigms, CD8+ deficiency improves survival of mice (Wang *et al.*, 2003). Likewise, in B-cell-deficient mice, WNV neurovirulence is increased (Chambers *et al.*, 2008), and patients treated with the anti-CD20 humanized monoclonal antibody might be at greater risk of WNV neurovirulence (Levi *et al.*, 2010).

Governing the cellular immune response to WNV infection of the CNS is mediated by a complex milieu of inflammatory cytokines and chemokines. Innate immune cells such as macrophages and microglia are generally considered to be the primary source of these factors, although other cell types such as astrocytes and neurons have also been implicated (Cheeran *et al.*, 2005; Glass *et al.*, 2005; Klein *et al.*, 2005; van Marle *et al.*, 2007; Kumar *et al.*, 2010). Type I IFNs are strongly implicated in WNV infection and essential for the antiviral response systemically (Samuel and Diamond, 2005). In the CNS, type I IFN signaling may also promote neuronal survival independent of any effects on viral replication (Klein *et al.*, 2005). The consequence of signaling from proinflammatory cytokines such as TNF-α and IL-1β can be both protective and pathogenic. TLR3-dependent upregulation of TNF-α has also been implicated in WNV pathogenesis (Wang *et al.*, 2004), and the resistance of MIF-1 knockout mice to WNV infection has been linked to a decrease in proinflammatory cytokine expression in the CNS (Arjona *et al.*, 2007). Both IL-1β and TNF-α have also been reported to exert cytotoxic effects on neurons (Kumar *et al.*, 2010). However, in contradistinction to these latter findings, IL-1β has also been reported to enhance neuronal survival by synergising with type 1 IFNs (Ramos *et al.*, 2012). Chemokines have also been actively studied in the context of WNV including CCL2, CCL5, and CXCL10 (Cheeran *et al.*, 2005; Glass *et al.*, 2005; Klein *et al.*, 2005). As in the response to HIV-1, the cellular sources for these responses include not only macrophages, but also astrocytes and neurons (Cheeran *et al.*, 2005; Klein *et al.*, 2005). The role that chemokines play in promoting the infiltration of immune cells into the CNS appears to be largely beneficial; CCR5 or CXCR10 knockout mice are much more susceptible to WNV infection (Glass *et al.*, 2005; Klein *et al.*, 2005).

Innate Immune Sensing of WNV in the Brain

WNV infection is sensed through a number of distinct PRRs; importantly, these studies have demonstrated not only how the immune response to WNV is mounted, but also how dysregulation between these various pathways could enhance immunopathology. As is the case for most viral infections, the response to WNV is mediated by type 1 IFNs (Klein *et al.*, 2005). The response is primarily dependent on the cytosolic sensors of viral RNA, RIG-I and melanoma differentiation-associated protein 5 (MDA5), and their downstream signaling target IFN-β promoter stimulator-1 (IPS-1) (Fredericksen *et al.*, 2008; Suthar *et al.*, 2010). IPS-1 knockout mice are much more sensitive to WNV dissemination into the CNS (Suthar *et al.*, 2010). However, although in RIG-I/MDA5/IPS-1-deficient cells or mice there was wide spread decrease in IFN-related gene expression, a strong proinflammatory signaling profile remained in place (Fredericksen *et al.*, 2008; Suthar *et al.*, 2010). In IPS-1 knockout mice, this led to an exaggerated inflammatory response concurrent with uncontrolled viral replication (Suthar *et al.*, 2010). Interestingly, deficiency in MyD88 (another adaptor molecule involved in innate immune signaling) also negatively impacted survival following WNV infection but without a reduced type 1 IFN response. Rather, in these animals, a reduction in proinflammatory signaling and the CD8+ T cell response was observed (Szretter *et al.*, 2010). These findings argue for the potential for emergence of immunopathology in response to an imbalance in the strength of innate immune signals derived from several distinct viral sensing pathways.

MyD88 signaling as well as a number of other molecules involved in innate immune sensing of WNV has CNS autonomous roles. For example, MyD88 knockout mice have an increased viral dissemination within the CNS that is independent of the peripheral immune response, and virus replication was increased in MyD88 knockout macrophages and neurons (Szretter *et al.*, 2010). TLR3, which similarly to RIG-I and MDA5, can sense viral RNA and might also be of particular relevance to the sensing of WNV infection within the CNS (Wang *et al.*, 2004; Daffis *et al.*, 2008). Although two independent studies of TLR3 knockout mice reported opposite effects of the knockout on susceptibility to WNV infection, both studies identified relatively little effect of TLR3 knockout on the peripheral immune response as compared to the CNS (Wang *et al.*, 2004; Daffis *et al.*, 2008). In one of these studies, a decreased proinflammatory response in the knockout mice was associated with less neurologic disease (Wang *et al.*, 2004). It has also been reported that increased TLR3 expression by the innate immune cells of elderly individuals might be associated with greater inflammatory response and ensuing immunopathology in response to WNV infection (Kong *et al.*, 2008).

NLRs and inflammasome assembly have also been implicated in sensing of WNV. As described previously, inflammasomes are regulators of IL-1β and -IL-18 maturation and release (Fig. 10.2). Two studies in mice in which components of the NLRP3 inflammasome were deleted [NLRP3 or ASC (apoptosis-associated speck-like protein containing a caspase recruitment domain)] have both reported a protective role for this complex in WNV infection (Ramos *et al.*, 2012; Kumar *et al.*, 2013). Within the CNS, NLRP3 activation was also reported to occur in neurons, and the loss of IL-1R signaling lead to increased viral replication in the brain but not the periphery (Ramos *et al.*, 2012). Although in the ASC knockout mouse, viral replication was increased both inside and outside of the CNS, there were divergent consequences associated with ASC deletion to both locations. Namely, ASC deficiency led to a reduced immune response to WNV in the periphery, while in the CNS, ASC deficiency resulted in a hyperinflammatory phenotype (Kumar *et al.*, 2013). This dichotomy underlines the distinct and often dissociated mechanisms that regulate inflammatory responses within the CNS that differ from the extra-CNS immune processes.

Future Perspectives

Although inflammation is a potent antiviral response, it also represents a potential mechanism for injury to host cells. This dilemma exists for chronic viral infections of the CNS such as HIV in which there is sustained activation of innate immune processes, particularly microglial activation. At the same time, acute viral infections of the CNS are defined by inflammation arising due to antiviral cytotoxic lymphocytes that damage off-target (uninfected) host cells. The underlying molecular pathways vary widely, for example, HIV neuropathogenesis is driven by infection and/or activation of microglia and perivascular macrophages with release of cytotoxic immune molecules and cytotoxic viral proteins, while WNV-infected neurons are targeted by lymphocyte-derived cytotoxic molecules (proteases and cytokines), but their death also promotes local neuroinflammation through the release of proinflammatory molecules including ATP, proteases, and nucleic acids. Several other determinants of neuroinflammation bear further scrutiny, as their contributions remain incompletely understood; molecular diversity within a neurovirulent virus has remarkable capacity to influence neurological disease outcomes as illustrated by some experimental models, although the clinical implications remain unclear (Tucker *et al.*, 1997; Power *et al.*, 1998). Similarly, neuroinflammation in humans might not always reflect the mechanisms recognized in mice for several reasons including genetic redundancy such as the overlap of function for caspase-1 and caspase-11 in mice and the robust expression of endogenized viruses that differs between humans and other species. As the human population continues to grow with greater international travel and transport of goods, evolving social, economic, and scientific milieus, changes in climate and geographical (mining, deforestation, and dams) conditions, together with pervasive poverty, the potential for new viral infections of the CNS to emerge is immense. The therapeutic options for neuroinflammation associated with CNS viral infections are largely restricted to (small molecule) antiviral drugs. However, there are emerging options including the potential to test anti-inflammasome therapies using re-purposed drugs, human monoclonal antibodies targeting viruses (e.g., WNV and rabies), and antisense technologies (e.g., morpholinos) that interrupt gene expression in viruses as well as pathogenic host immune responses.

References

Arjona, A., Foellmer, H.G., Town, T. *et al.* (2007) Abrogation of macrophage migration inhibitory factor decreases West Nile virus lethality by limiting viral neuroinvasion. *Journal of Clinical Investigation*, **117**, 3059–3066.

Armah, H.B., Wang, G., Omalu, B.I. *et al.* (2007) Systemic distribution of West Nile virus infection: Postmortem immunohistochemical study of six cases. *Brain Pathology*, **17**, 354–362.

Arthos, J., Cicala, C., Martinelli, E., Macleod, K., Van Ryk, D., Wei, D., Xiao, Z., Veenstra, T.D., Conrad, T.P., Lempicki, R.A., McLaughlin, S., Pascuccio, M., Gopaul, R., McNally, J., Cruz, C.C., Censoplano, N., Chung, E., Reitano, K.N., Kottilil, S., Goode, D.J. & Fauci, A.S. (2008) HIV-1 envelope protein binds to and signals through integrin alpha4beta7, the gut mucosal homing receptor for peripheral T cells. *Nature Immunology*, **9**, 301–309.

Bai, F., Kong, K.F., Dai, J. *et al.* (2010) A paradoxical role for neutrophils in the pathogenesis of West Nile virus. *Journal of Infectious Diseases*, **202**, 1804–1812.

Beignon, A.S., McKenna, K., Skoberne, M. *et al.* (2005) Endocytosis of HIV-1 activates plasmacytoid dendritic cells via Toll-like receptor-viral RNA interactions. *Journal of Clinical Investigation*, **115**, 3265–3275.

Ben Haij, N., Leghmari, K., Planes, R., Thieblemont, N. & Bahraoui, E. (2013) HIV-1 Tat protein binds to TLR4-MD2 and signals to induce TNF-alpha and IL-10. *Retrovirology*, **10**, 123.

Bezzi, P., Domercq, M., Brambilla, L. *et al.* (2001) CXCR4-activated astrocyte glutamate release via TNFalpha: Amplification by microglia triggers neurotoxicity. *Nature Neuroscience*, **4**, 702–710.

Bigham, A.W., Buckingham, K.J., Husain, S. *et al.* (2011) Host genetic risk factors for West Nile virus infection and disease progression. *PLoS One*, **6**, e24745.

Blond, D., Cheret, A., Raoul, H. *et al.* (1998) Nitric oxide synthesis during acute SIV mac251 infection of macaques. *Research in Virology*, **149**, 75–86.

Boisse, L., Gill, M.J. & Power, C. (2008) HIV infection of the central nervous system: Clinical features and neuropathogenesis. *Neurologic Clinics*, **26**, 799–819.

Brien, J.D., Uhrlaub, J.L. & Nikolich-Zugich, J. (2007) Protective capacity and epitope specificity of CD8(+) T cells responding to lethal West Nile virus infection. *European Journal of Immunology*, **37**, 1855–1863.

Bukrinsky, M.I., Nottet, H.S., Schmidtmayerova, H. *et al.* (1995) Regulation of nitric oxide synthase activity in human immunodeficiency virus type 1 (HIV-1)-infected monocytes: Implications for HIV-associated neurological disease. *Journal of Experimental Medicine*, **181**, 735–745.

Burdo, T.H., Lackner, A. & Williams, K.C. (2013) Monocyte/macrophages and their role in HIV neuropathogenesis. *Immunological Reviews*, **254**, 102–113.

Carod-Artal, F.J., Wichmann, O., Farrar, J. & Gascon, J. (2013) Neurological complications of dengue virus infection. *Lancet Neurology*, **12**, 906–919.

Chambers, T.J., Droll, D.A., Walton, A.H., Schwartz, J., Wold, W.S. & Nickells, J. (2008) West Nile 25A virus infection of B-cell-deficient ((micro)MT) mice: Characterization of neuroinvasiveness and pseudoreversion of the viral envelope protein. *Journal of General Virology*, **89**, 627–635.

Cheeran, M.C., Hu, S., Sheng, W.S., Rashid, A., Peterson, P.K. & Lokensgard, J.R. (2005) Differential responses of human brain cells to West Nile virus infection. *Journal of Neurovirology*, **11**, 512–524.

Cheung, R., Ravyn, V., Wang, L., Ptasznik, A. & Collman, R.G. (2008) Signaling mechanism of HIV-1 gp120 and virion-induced IL-1beta release in primary human macrophages. *Journal of Immunology*, **180**, 6675–6684.

Clouse, K.A., Cosentino, L.M., Weih, K.A. *et al.* (1991) The HIV-1 gp120 envelope protein has the intrinsic capacity to stimulate monokine secretion. *Journal of Immunology*, **147**, 2892–2901.

Conant, K., Garzino-Demo, A., Nath, A. *et al.* (1998) Induction of monocyte chemoattractant protein-1 in HIV-1 Tat-stimulated astrocytes and elevation in AIDS dementia. *Proceedings of the National Academy of Sciences of the United States of America*, **95**, 3117–3121.

Crichlow, R., Bailey, J. & Gardner, C. (2004) Cerebrospinal fluid neutrophilic pleocytosis in hospitalized West Nile virus patients. *Journal of the American Board of Family Practice*, **17**, 470–472.

Croitoru-Lamoury, J., Guillemin, G.J., Boussin, F.D. *et al.* (2003) Expression of chemokines and their receptors in human and simian astrocytes: Evidence for a central role of TNF alpha and IFN gamma in CXCR4 and CCR5 modulation. *Glia*, **41**, 354–370.

Daffis, S., Samuel, M.A., Suthar, M.S., Gale, M. Jr. & Diamond, M.S. (2008) Toll-like receptor 3 has a protective role against West Nile virus infection. *Journal of Virology*, **82**, 10349–10358.

Ellis, R., Langford, D. & Masliah, E. (2007) HIV and antiretroviral therapy in the brain: Neuronal injury and repair. *Nature Reviews Neuroscience*, **8**, 33–44.

Fischer-Smith, T., Croul, S., Adeniyi, A. *et al.* (2004) Macrophage/microglial accumulation and proliferating cell nuclear antigen expression in the central nervous system in human immunodeficiency virus encephalopathy. *American Journal of Pathology*, **164**, 2089–2099.

Fredericksen, B.L., Keller, B.C., Fornek, J., Katze, M.G. & Gale, M. Jr. (2008) Establishment and maintenance of the innate antiviral response to West Nile virus involves both RIG-I and MDA5 signaling through IPS-1. *Journal of Virology*, **82**, 609–616.

Galao, R.P., Le Tortorec, A., Pickering, S., Kueck, T. & Neil, S.J. (2012) Innate sensing of HIV-1 assembly by Tetherin induces NFkappaB-dependent proinflammatory responses. *Cell Host & Microbe*, **12**, 633–644.

Gelman, B.B., Lisinicchia, J.G., Morgello, S. *et al.* (2012) Neurovirological correlation with HIV-associated neurocognitive disorders and encephalitis in a HAART-era cohort. *Journal of Acquired Immune Deficiency Syndromes*, **65**, 487–495.

Getts, D.R., Terry, R.L., Getts, M.T. *et al.* (2008) Ly6c+ "inflammatory monocytes" are microglial precursors recruited in a pathogenic manner in West Nile virus encephalitis. *Journal of Experimental Medicine*, **205**, 2319–2337.

Gilden, D., Mahalingam, R., Nagel, M.A., Pugazhenthi, S. & Cohrs, R.J. (2011) Review: The neurobiology of varicella zoster virus infection. *Neuropathology and Applied Neurobiology*, **37**, 441–463.

Glass, J.D., Fedor, H., Wesselingh, S.L. & McArthur, J.C. (1995) Immunocytochemical quantitation of human immunodeficiency virus in the brain: correlations with dementia. *Annals of Neurology*, **38**, 755–762.

Glass, W.G., Lim, J.K., Cholera, R., Pletnev, A.G., Gao, J.L. & Murphy, P.M. (2005) Chemokine receptor CCR5 promotes leukocyte trafficking to the brain and survival in West Nile virus infection. *Journal of Experimental Medicine*, **202**, 1087–1098.

Goldstone, D.C., Ennis-Adeniran, V., Hedden, J.J. *et al.* (2011) HIV-1 restriction factor SAMHD1 is a deoxynucleoside triphosphate triphosphohydrolase. *Nature*, **480**, 379–382.

Gray, F., Bazille, C., Adle-Biassette, H., Mikol, J., Moulignier, A. & Scaravilli, F. (2005) Central nervous system immune reconstitution disease in acquired immunodeficiency syndrome patients receiving highly active antiretroviral treatment. *Journal of Neurovirology*, **11** (Suppl 3), 16–22.

Gringhuis, S.I., den Dunnen, J., Litjens, M., van Het Hof, B., van Kooyk, Y. & Geijtenbeek, T.B. (2007) C-type lectin DC-SIGN modulates Toll-like receptor signaling via Raf-1 kinase-dependent acetylation of transcription factor NF-kappaB. *Immunity*, **26**, 605–616.

Holman, A.G., Mefford, M.E., O'Connor, N. & Gabuzda, D. (2010) HIVBrainSeqDB: A database of annotated HIV envelope sequences from brain and other anatomical sites. *AIDS Research and Therapy*, **7**, 43.

Jin, J., Lam, L., Sadic, E., Fernandez, F., Tan, J. & Giunta, B. (2012) HIV-1 Tat-induced microglial activation and neuronal damage is inhibited via CD45 modulation: A potential new treatment target for HAND. *American Journal of Translational Research*, **4**, 302–315.

Johnson, R.T. (1998) *Viral infections of the nervous system*, Second edn. Lippincott-Raven, Philadelphia.

Johnston, J.B., Jiang, Y., van Marle, G. *et al.* (2000) Lentiviral infection in the brain induce matrix metalloproteinase expression: The role of envelope diversity. *Journal of Virology*, **74**, 7211–7220.

Jordan, C.A., Watkins, B.A., Kufta, C. & Dubois-Dalcq, M. (1991) Infection of brain microglial cells by human immunodeficiency virus type 1 is CD4 dependent. *Journal of Virology*, **65**, 736–742.

Kelder, W., McArthur, J.C., Nance-Sproson, T., McClernon, D. & Griffin, D.E. (1998) Beta-chemokines MCP-1 and RANTES are selectively increased in cerebrospinal fluid of patients with human immunodeficiency virus- associated dementia. *Annals of Neurology*, **44**, 831–835.

Kelley, T.W., Prayson, R.A., Ruiz, A.I., Isada, C.M. & Gordon, S.M. (2003) The neuropathology of West Nile virus menin-goencephalitis. A report of two cases and review of the literature. *American Journal of Clinical Pathology*, **119**, 749–753.

Klein, R.S., Lin, E., Zhang, B. *et al.* (2005) Neuronal CXCL10 directs CD8+ T-cell recruitment and control of West Nile virus encephalitis. *Journal of Virology*, **79**, 11457–11466.

Koka, P., He, K., Zack, J.A. *et al.* (1995) Human immunodeficiency virus 1 envelope proteins induce interleukin 1, tumor necrosis factor alpha, and nitric oxide in glial cultures derived from fetal, neonatal, and adult human brain. *Journal of Experimental Medicine*, **182**, 941–951.

Kong, K.F., Delroux, K., Wang, X. *et al.* (2008) Dysregulation of TLR3 impairs the innate immune response to West Nile virus in the elderly. *Journal of Virology*, **82**, 7613–7623.

Kramer, L.D., Li, J. & Shi, P.Y. (2007) West Nile virus. *Lancet Neurology*, **6**, 171–181.

Kumar, M., Verma, S. & Nerurkar, V.R. (2010) Pro-inflammatory cytokines derived from West Nile virus (WNV)-infected SK-N-SH cells mediate neuroinflammatory markers and neuronal death. *Journal of Neuroinflammation*, **7**, 73.

Kumar, M., Roe, K., Orillo, B. *et al.* (2013) Inflammasome adaptor protein apoptosis-associated speck-like protein containing CARD (ASC) is critical for the immune response and survival in West Nile virus encephalitis. *Journal of Virology*, **87**, 3655–3667.

Lepelley, A., Louis, S., Sourisseau, M. *et al.* (2011) Innate sensing of HIV-infected cells. *PLoS Pathogens*, **7**, e1001284.

Levi, M.E., Quan, D., Ho, J.T., Kleinschmidt-Demasters, B.K., Tyler, K.L. & Grazia, T.J. (2010) Impact of rituximab-associated B-cell defects on West Nile virus meningoencephalitis in solid organ transplant recipients. *Clinical Transplantation*, **24**, 223–228.

Lim, J.K., McDermott, D.H., Lisco, A. *et al.* (2010) CCR5 deficiency is a risk factor for early clinical manifestations of West Nile virus infection but not for viral transmission. *Journal of Infectious Diseases*, **201**, 178–185.

Lim, J.K., Lisco, A., McDermott, D.H. *et al.* (2009) Genetic variation in OAS1 is a risk factor for initial infection with West Nile virus in man. *PLoS Pathogens*, **5**, e1000321.

Merrill, J.E., Koyanagi, Y., Zack, J., Thomas, L., Martin, F. & Chen, I.S. (1992) Induction of interleukin-1 and tumor necrosis factor alpha in brain cultures by human immunodeficiency virus type 1. *Journal of Virology*, **66**, 2217–2225.

Monaco, S., Ferrari, S., Gajofatto, A., Zanusso, G. & Mariotto, S. (2012) HCV-related nervous system disorders. *Clinical & Developmental Immunology*, **2012**, 236148.

Mothobi, N.Z. & Brew, B.J. (2012) Neurocognitive dysfunction in the highly active antiretroviral therapy era. *Current Opinion in Infectious Diseases*, **25**, 4–9.

Murray, K., Baraniuk, S., Resnick, M. *et al.* (2006) Risk factors for encephalitis and death from West Nile virus infection. *Epidemiology and Infection*, **134**, 1325–1332.

Murray, K.O., Koers, E., Baraniuk, S. *et al.* (2009) Risk factors for encephalitis from West Nile virus: A matched case-control study using hospitalized controls. *Zoonoses and Public Health*, **56**, 370–375.

Nath, A. & Tyler, K.L. (2013) Novel approaches and challenges to treatment of central nervous system viral infections. *Annals of neurology*, **74**, 412–422.

Nath, A., Conant, K., Chen, P., Scott, C. & Major, E.O. (1999) Transient exposure to HIV-1 Tat protein results in cytokine production in macrophages and astrocytes. A hit and run phenomenon. *Journal of Biological Chemistry*, **274**, 17098–17102.

Ousman, S.S. & Kubes, P. (2012) Immune surveillance in the central nervous system. *Nature Neuroscience*, **15**, 1096–1101.

Parquet, M.C., Kumatori, A., Hasebe, F., Morita, K. & Igarashi, A. (2001) West Nile virus-induced bax-dependent apoptosis. *FEBS Letters*, **500**, 17–24.

Patrick, M.K., Johnston, J.B. & Power, C. (2002) Lentiviral neuropathogenesis: Comparative neuroinvasion, neurotropism, neurovirulence and host neurosusceptibility. *Journal of Virology*, **76**, 7923–7931.

Pertel, T., Hausmann, S., Morger, D. *et al.* (2011) TRIM5 is an innate immune sensor for the retrovirus capsid lattice. *Nature*, **472**, 361–365.

Polyak, M.J., Vivithanaporn, P., Maingat, F.G. *et al.* (2013) Differential type 1 interferon-regulated gene expression in the brain during AIDS: Interactions with viral diversity and neurovirulence. *FASEB Journal*, **27**, 2829–2844.

Power, C., Buist, R., Johnston, J.B. *et al.* (1998) Neurovirulence in feline immunodeficiency virus-infected neonatal cats is viral strain specific and dependent on systemic immune suppression. *Journal of Virology*, **72**, 9109–9115.

Prinz, M., Priller, J., Sisodia, S.S. & Ransohoff, R.M. (2011) Heterogeneity of CNS myeloid cells and their roles in neurodegeneration. *Nature Neuroscience*, **14**, 1227–1235.

Ramos, H.J., Lanteri, M.C., Blahnik, G. *et al.* (2012) IL-1beta signaling promotes CNS-intrinsic immune control of West Nile virus infection. *PLoS Pathogens*, **8**, e1003039.

Roe, K., Kumar, M., Lum, S., Orillo, B., Nerurkar, V.R. & Verma, S. (2012) West Nile virus-induced disruption of the blood-brain barrier in mice is characterized by the degradation of the junctional complex proteins and increase in multiple matrix metalloproteinases. *Journal of General Virology*, **93**, 1193–1203.

Samuel, M.A. & Diamond, M.S. (2005) Alpha/beta interferon protects against lethal West Nile virus infection by restricting cellular tropism and enhancing neuronal survival. *Journal of Virology*, **79**, 13350–13361.

Samuel, M.A., Wang, H., Siddharthan, V., Morrey, J.D. & Diamond, M.S. (2007) Axonal transport mediates West Nile virus entry into the central nervous system and induces acute flaccid paralysis. *Proceedings of the National Academy of Sciences of the United States of America*, **104**, 17140–17145.

Sasseville, V.G., Smith, M.M., Mackay, C.R. *et al.* (1996) Chemokine expression in simian immunodeficiency virus-induced AIDS encephalitis. *American Journal of Pathology*, **149**, 1459–1467.

Schmidtmayerova, H., Nottet, H.S., Nuovo, G. *et al.* (1996) Human immunodeficiency virus type 1 infection alters chemokine beta peptide expression in human monocytes: Implications for recruitment of leukocytes into brain and lymph nodes. *Proceedings of the National Academy of Sciences of the United States of America*, **93**, 700–704.

Shrestha, B., Gottlieb, D. & Diamond, M.S. (2003) Infection and injury of neurons by West Nile encephalitis virus. *Journal of Virology*, **77**, 13203–13213.

Sitati, E.M. & Diamond, M.S. (2006) CD4+ T-cell responses are required for clearance of West Nile virus from the central nervous system. *Journal of Virology*, **80**, 12060–12069.

Suthar, M.S., Diamond, M.S. & Gale, M. Jr. (2013) West Nile virus infection and immunity. *Nature Reviews Microbiology*, **11**, 115–128.

Suthar, M.S., Ma, D.Y., Thomas, S. *et al.* (2010) IPS-1 is essential for the control of West Nile virus infection and immunity. *PLoS Pathogens*, **6**, e1000757.

Szretter, K.J., Daffis, S., Patel, J. *et al.* (2010) The innate immune adaptor molecule MyD88 restricts West Nile virus replication and spread in neurons of the central nervous system. *Journal of Virology*, **84**, 12125–12138.

Tucker, P.C., Lee, S.H., Bui, N., Martinie, D. & Griffin, D.E. (1997) Amino acid changes in the Sindbis virus E2 glycoprotein that increase neurovirulence improve entry into neuroblastoma cells. *Journal of Virology*, **71**, 6106–6112.

Tyor, W.R., Glass, J.D., Baumrind, N. *et al.* (1993) Cytokine expression of macrophages in HIV-1-associated vacuolar myelopathy. *Neurology*, **43**, 1002–1009.

van Marle, G., Antony, J., Ostermann, H. *et al.* (2007) West Nile virus-induced neuroinflammation: Glial infection and capsid protein-mediated neurovirulence. *Journal of Virology*, **81**, 10933–10949.

Vergote, D., Butler, G.S., Ooms, M. *et al.* (2006) Proteolytic processing of SDF-1alpha reveals a change in receptor specificity mediating HIV-associated neurodegeneration. *Proceedings of the National Academy of Sciences of the United States of America*, **103**, 19182–19187.

Verma, S., Lo, Y., Chapagain, M. *et al.* (2009) West Nile virus infection modulates human brain microvascular endothelial cells tight junction proteins and cell adhesion molecules: Transmigration across the in vitro blood-brain barrier. *Virology*, **385**, 425–433.

Vivithanaporn, P., Heo, G., Gamble, J. *et al.* (2010) Neurologic disease burden in treated HIV/AIDS predicts survival: A population-based study. *Neurology*, **75**, 1150–1158.

Walsh, J.G., Reinke, S.N., Mamik, M.K. *et al.* (2014a) Rapid inflammasome activation in microglia contributes to brain disease in HIV/AIDS. *Retrovirology*, **11**, 35.

Walsh, J.W., Muruve, D.A. & Power, C. (2014b) Inflammasomes in the central nervous system. *Nature Reviews Neuroscience*, **15**, 84–97.

Wang, T., Town, T., Alexopoulou, L., Anderson, J.F., Fikrig, E. & Flavell, R.A. (2004) Toll-like receptor 3 mediates West Nile virus entry into the brain causing lethal encephalitis. *Nature Medicine*, **10**, 1366–1373.

Wang, Y., Lobigs, M., Lee, E. & Mullbacher, A. (2003) CD8+ T cells mediate recovery and immunopathology in West Nile virus encephalitis. *Journal of Virology*, **77**, 13323–13334.

Wesselingh, S.L., Takahashi, K., Glass, J.D., McArthur, J.C., Griffin, J.W. & Griffin, D.E. (1997) Cellular localization of tumor necrosis factor mRNA in neurological tissue from HIV-infected patients by combined reverse transcriptase/polymerase chain reaction in situ hybridization and immunohistochemistry. *Journal of Neuroimmunology*, **74**, 1–8.

Williams, K.C., Corey, S., Westmoreland, S.V. *et al.* (2001) Perivascular macrophages are the primary cell type productively infected by simian immunodeficiency virus in the brains of macaques: Implications for the neuropathogenesis of AIDS. *Journal of Experimental Medicine*, **193**, 905–915.

Wilson, M.R. (2013) Emerging viral infections. *Current Opinion in Neurology*, **26**, 301–306.

Xing, H.Q., Moritoyo, T., Mori, K., Sugimoto, C., Ono, F. & Izumo, S. (2009a) Expression of proinflammatory cytokines and its relationship with virus infection in the brain of macaques inoculated with macrophage-tropic simian immunodeficiency virus. *Neuropathology*, **29**, 13–19.

Xing, H.Q., Hayakawa, H., Izumo, K. *et al.* (2009b) In vivo expression of proinflammatory cytokines in HIV encephalitis: An analysis of 11 autopsy cases. *Neuropathology*, **29**, 433–442.

Yan, N., Regalado-Magdos, A.D., Stiggelbout, B., Lee-Kirsch, M.A. & Lieberman, J. (2010) The cytosolic exonuclease TREX1 inhibits the innate immune response to human immunodeficiency virus type 1. *Nature Immunology*, **11**, 1005–1013.

Yazdi, A.S., Drexler, S.K. & Tschopp, J. (2010) The role of the inflammasome in nonmyeloid cells. *Journal of Clinical Immunology*, **30**, 623–627.

Zhang, K., McQuibban, G.A., Silva, C. *et al.* (2003) HIV-induced metalloproteinase processing of the chemokine stromal cell derived factor-1 causes neurodegeneration. *Nature Neuroscience*, **6**, 1064–1071.

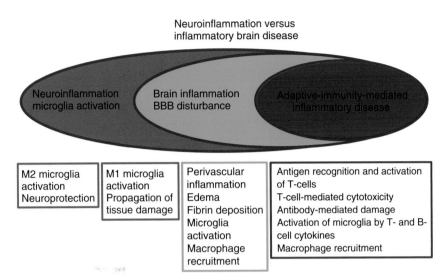

Figure 1.1 Inflammation of the CNS comprises a broad spectrum of tissue alterations including microglia activation, vascular inflammation with blood–brain barrier damage, and inflammation mediated by adaptive immunity.

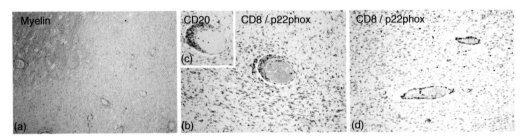

Figure 1.2 Inflammation in multiple sclerosis. (a) Inflammation in active multiple sclerosis lesions is associated with demyelination, reflected by the loss of blue myelin staining in the lesion. (b, c) Infiltration of the tissue with CD8+ T-lymphocytes (b) and CD20+ B-lymphocytes (c) (black cells) in the active lesion edge. The zone of initial demyelination at the lesions edge shows profound microglia activation with intense expression of NADPH oxidase (brown cells; p22phox). (d) CD8+ T-lymphocytes are also present in the lesion center (black cells). Most inflammatory cells are macrophages with low expression of NADPH oxidase (brown cells).

Neuroinflammation: New Insights into Beneficial and Detrimental Functions, First Edition. Edited by Samuel David.
© 2015 John Wiley & Sons, Inc. Published 2015 by John Wiley & Sons, Inc.

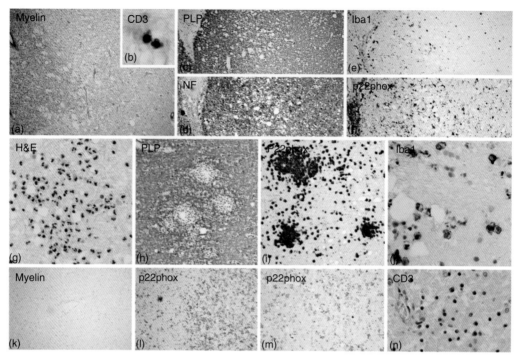

Figure 1.3 Inflammation in stroke. (a–f) Initial white matter stroke lesions (24 h after disease onset) with reduced intensity of staining for conventional myelin markers (a), but preservation of immune reactivity for the (c) myelin protein proteolipid protein (PLP) and (d) neurofilament (NF); such lesions contain single T-cells (b), microglia, which express the pan microglia marker Iba1 (e); NADPH oxidase (brown; p22phox; f) is expressed in microglia at the lesion edge but largely lost from the lesion center. (g–j) Some initial/early stroke lesions (in this example 48 h after disease onset), in which PLP (h) is still preserved, show profound infiltration with granulocytes (g), which intensely express NADPH oxidase (brown cells; p22phox; i), but they reveal very little infiltration of macrophages or microglia activation stained for the microglia and macrophage marker Iba1 (j). (k–n) Advanced stroke lesions, in which myelin and other tissue components are already destroyed (k), reveal profound macrophage activation at the edge (l), macrophages with little NADPH oxidase expression in the lesion center (m), and perivascular or diffuse T-cell infiltrates (n).

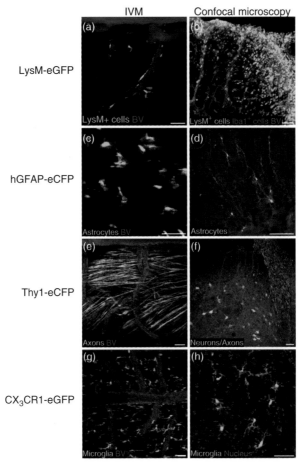

Figure 2.1 Two-photon intravital microscopy and confocal immunofluorescence in transgenic mice in which cell-specific promoters drive GFP or CFP expression. (a, c, e, and g) Two-photon intravital microscopy (2P-IVM) imaging of LysM-positive (+) cells (green in a), astrocytes (cyan in c), axons (cyan in e), and microglia (green in g) in the spinal cord of promoter-specific transgenic mice. Blood vessels (BV) were labeled through tail vein injection of either Texas red-dextran or Qdot705 (red color). Note that eGFP is not expressed in microglia in the CNS of LysM-eGFP mice (a). (b, d, f, and h) Confocal images of spinal cord sections obtained from the transgenic mice mentioned previously. (b) Infiltration of blood-derived LysM[+] cells (green) in the inflamed (EAE) CNS of a LysM-eGFP mouse. Macrophages/microglia and blood vessels were immunostained with antibodies directed against Iba1 (red) and CD31 (blue), respectively. The absence of colocalization between the LysM and Iba1 signals reinforces the idea that the LysM-eGFP mouse line can be used to track hematogenous myeloid cells specifically, as recently suggested by the Debakan laboratory (Mawhinney *et al.*, 2012). (d and f) Confocal imaging of astrocytes (d) and neurons/axons (f) expressing eCFP in the spinal cord of hGFAP-eCFP and Thy1-eCFP-23 transgenic mice, respectively. (h) Confocal imaging of microglia expressing eGFP in the spinal cord of CX_3CR1-eGFP mice. The blue signal in H shows counterstaining with the nuclear dye DAPI. Scale bars: 50 μm.

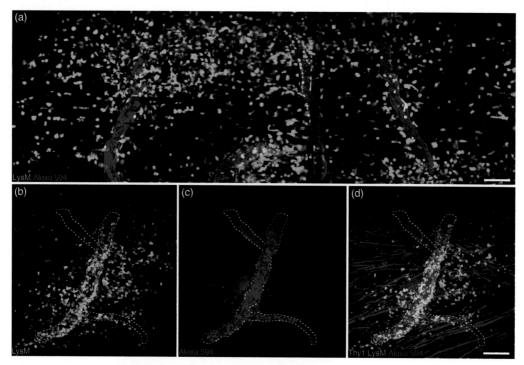

Figure 2.2 Two-photon intravital microscopy in mice shows massive recruitment of blood-derived immune cells and blood–spinal cord barrier (BSCB) leakage during EAE. (a) Peripheral LysM$^+$ cells, which are mainly composed of neutrophils, rapidly infiltrate the spinal cord at EAE onset and are primarily localized along blood vessels. Blood vessels were labeled through tail vein injection of the fluorescent tracer Alexa-594 (Alexa Fluor$^®$ 594 hydrazide, sodium salt; in red) before imaging session. (b–d) *In vivo* permeability of the BSCB to the low molecular weight (760 Da) tracer Alexa-594 indicates that BSCB disruption and leakage coincide with the infiltration of LysM$^+$ cells at EAE onset. Note the high colocalization between LysM$^+$ cell infiltration (b) and Alexa-594 egress (c) outside of blood vessels (defined by the white dashed lines). (d) Merge of LysM (green) and Alexa-594 (red) channels with CFP-labeled axons (cyan/blue) imaged in the spinal cord of an LysM-eGFP; Thy1-eCFP-23 mouse. Scale bars, 50 μm.

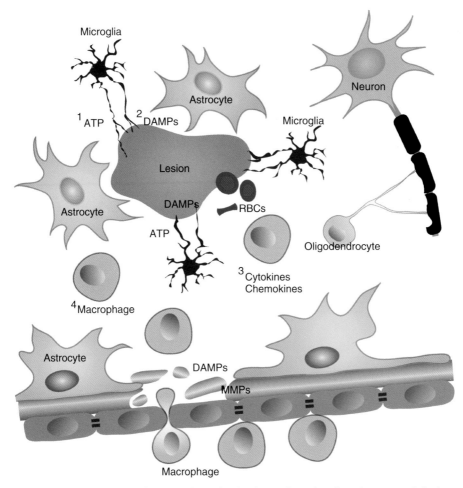

Figure 4.1 Schematic showing some of the signaling molecules that mediate microglia and monocyte-derived macrophage responses after CNS injury. (1) The earliest response of microglia to injury is mediated by ATP released by astrocytes near the lesion site. (2) Subsequently DAMPs released by damaged cells in this region signal via TLRs on microglia as well as on astrocytes and neurons to release proinflammatory mediators including cytokines, and reactive oxygen species (ROS) via NFκB signaling that can cause damage to neurons and glia. (3) Cytokines together with chemokines induce the recruitment of leukocytes from the peripheral circulation that include neutrophils and monocyte-derived macrophages into the CNS parenchyma. (4) The entry of these leukocytes into the CNS requires the action of MMPs that degrade the ECM around blood vessels, leading to the release of additional DAMPs and a further round of activation of TLRs on CNS glia at the injury site and the expression of cytokines and proinflammatory mediators. Inflammation therefore can proceed for prolonged periods after injury.

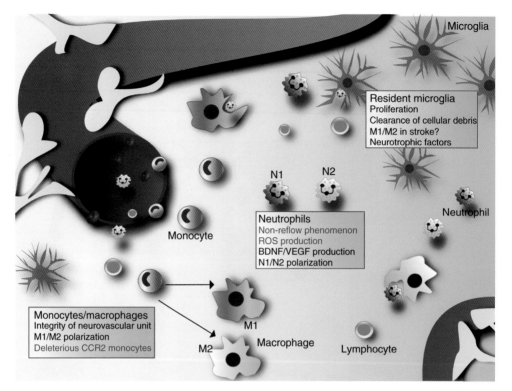

Figure 5.2 Dual role of innate immune system in stroke. The heterogeneity of immune cells population is currently being associated with distinct roles in cerebral brain damage and neurodegeneration. The study of the precise role of different subsets of monocytes, neutrophils, and brain resident macrophages in stroke will help to identify specific therapeutic targets for stroke treatment that can potentiate the benefits of innate immune responses while diminishing their deleterious effects.

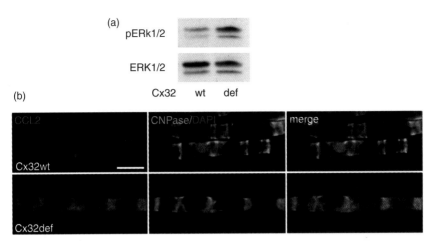

Figure 8.1 Western blot analysis (a) and immunofluorescent labeling of single fiber preparations (b) of femoral quadriceps nerves from age-matched Cx32wt and Cx32def mice. (a) There is increased phosphorylation of ERK in peripheral nerves of Cx32def mice. (b) Mutant myelinating Schwann cells show increased expression of CCL2 (red) in cytoplasmic compartments such as Schmidt–Lanterman incisures which are marked by anti-CNPase reactivity (green). Scale bar: 20 μm.

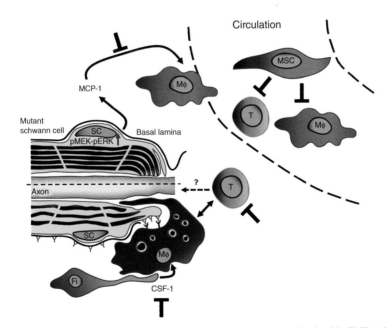

Figure 8.3 Schematic depicting inflammation-related molecular and cellular players involved in CMT pathomechanisms as identified in the mouse models as well as hypothetical targets (**T**) for treatment options. SC, Schwann cell; MΦ, macrophage; Fi, fibroblast; T, T-lymphocyte; Y, antibody; MSC, mesenchymal stem cell. *Source*: Adapted from Martini R, Klein D, Groh J (2013). Similarities between inherited demyelinating neuropathies and Wallerian degeneration: an old repair program may cause myelin and axon perturbation under nonlesion conditions. Am J Pathol 183:655–660.

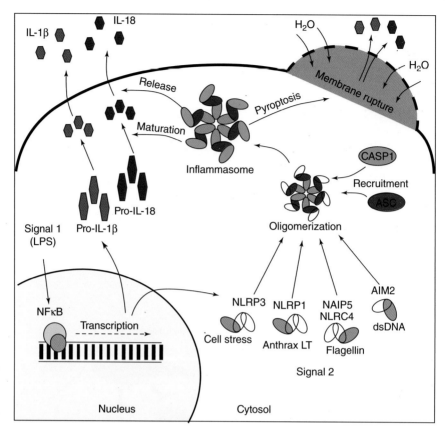

Figure 10.2 Inflammasomes are protein complexes, largely located in macrophage-lineage cells, which act as sensors of infectious or injurious stimuli as well as effectors of innate immune responses, particularly the cleavage and release of IL-1β and IL-18 by caspase-1. Inflammasome activation requires an initial stimulus (Signal 1) to initiate transcription followed by induction of protein assembly by a second stimulus (Signal 2). Multiple inflammasomes are implicated in viral infections including NLRP3 and AIM2.

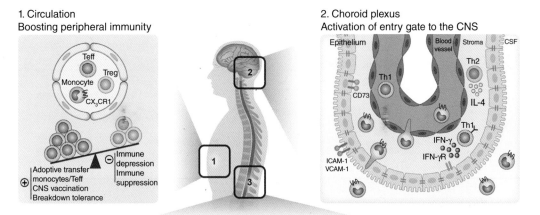

1. Circulation
Boosting peripheral immunity

Teff
Treg
Monocyte
CX_3CR1

Adoptive transfer
monocytes/Teff
CNS vaccination
Breakdown tolerance

⊖ Immune depression
Immune suppression

2. Choroid plexus
Activation of entry gate to the CNS

Epithelium
Blood vessel
Stroma
CSF
Th2
Th1
CD73
IL-4
Th1
IFN-γ
IFN-γR
ICAM-1
VCAM-1

3. Spinal cord lesion site. Infiltration of circulating immune cells

CC
IL-13
TGF-β2

E. Recruitment of Tregs at subacute phase – re-establishment of immunological equilibrium

M2 mo-Mφ
CSPG
Lesion site

A. Removal of debris and apoptotic cells by microglia and mo-Mφ

Cytotoxic mediators demyelination

Microglia
M1 mo-Mφ
IL-1β
TNF-α
ROS

B. Resolution of inflammation by mo-Mφ

Cytotoxic mediators
IL-10

D. Neuronal survival and axonal regeneration

Activin A
BDNF
Oncomodulin
IGF1
Neurotrophic factors

Astrocyte

C. Degradation of glial scar by mo-Mφ

MMP13

Figure 11.1 Protective autoimmunity network following SCI (a model). The immune network works at distinct compartments and phases of the repair process. (1) Immediately following the insult, a balance favoring effector memory CNS-specific T cells (Teff) with decreased immunosuppression is beneficial for recovery and can be achieved using several approaches, including CNS peptide-derived immunization, adoptive transfer of monocytes or Teff, or partial depletion of regulatory T cells (Tregs). (2) The remote choroid plexus is activated by effector Th1 cells, orchestrating the controlled entrance of CX_3CR1^+ healing monocytes. (3) The healing monocytes migrate via the immunoregulatory CP-CSF entry route, reaching the lesion site and maturing into resolving M2 monocyte-derived macrophages (mo-MΦ). (A) The lesion site is markedly proinflammatory, with M1 mo-MΦ and microglia. These cells are needed at the initial repair response for clearance of apoptotic cells and debris. (B) At the acute phase, the M2 mo-MΦ are vital for repair, by resolving the proinflammatory response, and (C) regulate the degradation of the glial scar. (D) The resolving M2 mo-MΦ can also produce numerous neuroprotective molecules, which promote axonal survival and regeneration. (E) During the subacute/chronic phase, the mo-MΦ promote recruitment of regulatory T cells that resolve the effector T cell response, to ensure that its uncontrolled action will not lead to autoimmune disease.

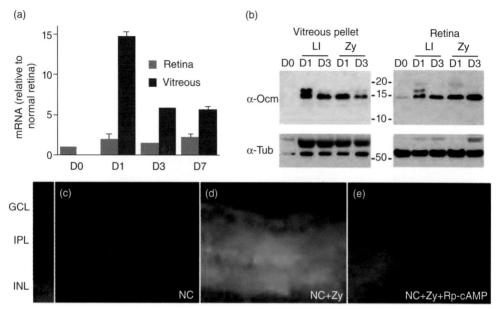

Figure 12.2 Oncomodulin expression in inflammatory cells. (a) Ocm mRNA in cells of the retina (light gray bar) and in cells that infiltrate the posterior chamber of the eye (black bar) following intraocular injection of Zymosan. mRNA levels were determined by quantitative polymerase chain reaction (qPCR) and then normalized by levels of 18S RNA and then to normalized levels in the control retina. While expression in the retina does not change appreciably, infiltrative cells express high levels of Ocm. (b) Western blots show increases in Ocm in infiltrative cells collected from the posterior chamber (left panel) and within the retina (right panel) after either lens injury (LI) or Zymosan injections (Zy). Bottom panels: loading controls, stained for α-Tubulin. (c–e). Immunostaining shows near-absence of Ocm in the untreated retina after optic nerve crush (NC) but high levels 1 day after NC combined with intraocular Zymosan injection (NC, Zy). Levels are diminished by co-injection of the cAMP antagonist Rp-cAMP, which prevents Ocm from binding to its receptor. (f) Most of the cells present in the vitreous 12 h after intraocular Zymosan are neutrophils [Gr-1[high]: compare to 4′,6-diamidino-2-phenylindole (DAPI)] that express high levels of Ocm. However, Ocm levels within Gr-1[high] cells (*arrows* at 72 h) decline over time (*arrowheads* at 72 h). Note increasing appearance of Gr-1[low] cells over time that also express Ocm. (g) Macrophages (F4/80[high]) cells (*arrows*) represent a relatively small percentage of the cells in the vitreous at 12 and 24 h (compare F4/80 staining with DAPI) and express high levels of Ocm (*arrowheads*). Relative frequency of these cells increases at 72 h. Unlike neutrophils, Ocm levels remain high in macrophages, perhaps due to continuous expression or recruitment of new cells. Scale bar: 10 μm. (h) The morphology of cells extracted from the vitreous at 24 h shows the typical lobulated nuclei of Gr-1[high] neutrophils, whereas F4/80[high] macrophages show large, round nuclei. (i) Ocm mRNA expression (normalized by 18S RNA) in FACS-sorted Gr-1[high]/F4/80[low] cells (neutrophils, N) and F4/80[high] cells (macrophages, M) 24 h after Zymosan injection is many times that of the retina. $*p < 0.05$, $***p < 0.001$ relative to the retina (Ret). (j) While almost all Gr-1[high] cells express detectable levels of Ocm 6 h, levels diminish at 24 h; at the same time, the number of Gr-1[low] cells, presumably macrophages, increases and these express Ocm. *Source*: From Kurimoto *et al.* (2013).

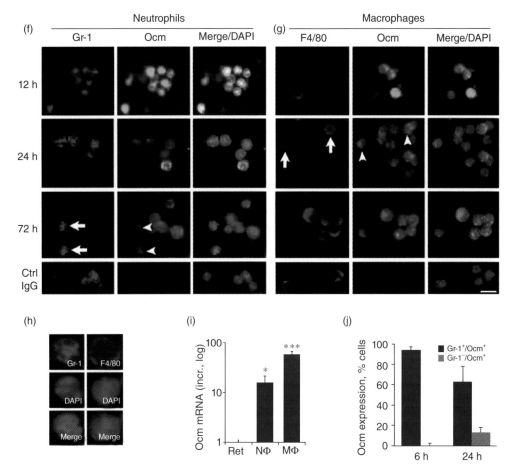

Figure 12.2 (*Continued*)

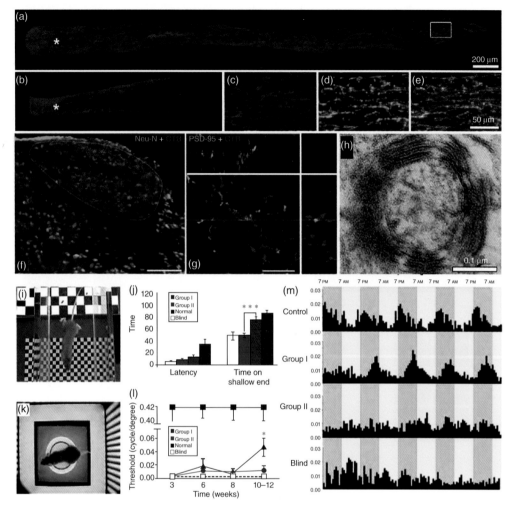

Figure 12.3 Long-distance regeneration, target reinnervation, and partial recovery of vision. (a, b) Regenerating axons 10–12 weeks after optic nerve injury visualized using the anterograde tracer cholera toxin B-fragment (CTB, red). Axons extend the full length of the optic nerve in mice treated with Zymosan, CPT-cAMP, and *pten* gene deletion (Group I) but only part-way in mice receiving similar treatment but without *pten* deletion (Group II). (c–e) Region in the white rectangle of panel(a) double-labeled for CTB and GAP-43. (f) Reinnervation of the lateral geniculate nucleus (DLGN). CTB+ fibers (red) in the DLGN contralateral to the regenerating optic nerve in a Group I mouse. Counterstaining for the neuronal protein NeuN shows CTB+ fibers to be confined to the neuropil of the DLG (dotted line). (g) Preliminary evidence for synapse formation: apposition of CTB+ terminals and PSD-95 positive structures. Side panels show z-stacks of images in the orthogonal planes. Scale bars in (f) and (g), 100 μm. (h) Electron micrographic image showing remyelination of a regenerating axon. (i–m). Partial recovery of visually guided behaviors. (i) Top-down view of visual cliff apparatus. (j) Average latency to step off shallow end (left) and total time spent on shallow end (right). **$P < 0.01$; n.s., not significant. (k) Top-down view of apparatus used to evaluate optomotor response (OMR). (l) Average OMR (response threshold, cycles/degree) as a function of time. Mice in Group I show partial recovery; y-axis in h and i are discontinuous. (m) Circadian photoentrainment: percent of overall activity in 1-h bins (group averages). Mice were maintained on a continuous cycle of lights on at 7 AM and off at 7 PM before testing and for the first 2.5 days in the activity monitor. The light cycle was set back 6 h on day 3. Note entrainment of circadian activity to ambient day–night cycle in Group I, though with a phase shift of approximately 8 h compared to normal mice. Activity in Group II (incomplete regeneration) is asynchronous and resembles blind mice. Error bars: S.E.M. *Source*: From de Lima *et al.* (2012).

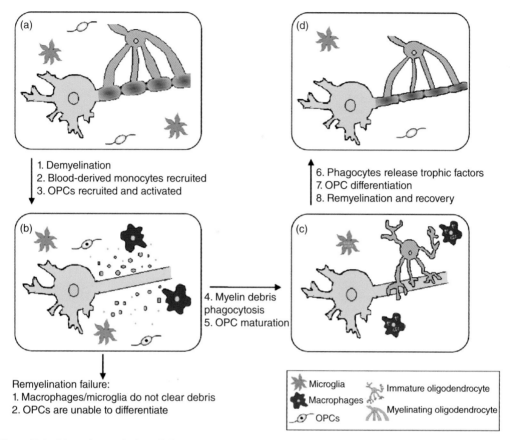

Figure 13.1 Macrophage and microglia involvement in the stages of demyelination to remyelination. (a) Myelinating oligodendrocytes, microglia, and OPCs populate healthy CNS white matter. (b) After demyelination, myelin debris is formed around denuded axons and blood-derived monocytes are recruited to the lesion site. OPCs are recruited and activated as well in response to demyelination. However, if macrophages are not properly recruited and activated, myelin debris is not cleared and OPCs are unable to differentiate causing remyelination to fail. (c) Myelin debris is phagocytosed by macrophages and microglia, clearing the way for OPC differentiation. Phagocytes also release various cytokines and growth factors that promote differentiation and remyelination of the CNS. (d) After proper removal of myelin debris and activation of differentiation cues in OPCs, macrophages, and microglia largely exit the lesion area and return to a resting state. Mature oligodendrocytes effectively remyelinate the exposed axons with a thinner myelin sheath and proper conductance is restored.

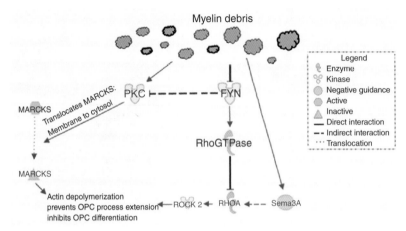

Figure 13.2 Myelin debris prevents OPC differentiation via Sema3A, RhoA, and PKC pathways. The inhibitory effects of degraded myelin on remyelination regulate several pathways in OPCs. Fyn-1 is a positive regulator of OPC differentiation and prevents RhoA phosphorylation by activating Rho-GTPases (O'Meara *et al.*, 2011). When Fyn-1 is dysregulated in the presence of myelin debris, RhoA-GTP activates ROCK2, resulting in actin depolymerization and inhibited remyelination. PKC is also activated when Fyn-1 is dysregulated, and it prevents OPC differentiation by translocating the MARCKS protein from the plasma membrane, where it is active during OPC differentiation, to the cytosol, where it is inactive during OPC quiescence. PKC has also been shown to play a role in RhoA activation. Finally, the negative guidance cue Sema3A has been shown to impair OPC differentiation and remyelination, possibly through activating the RhoA pathway. Myelin debris activates and releases these negative regulators of OPC differentiation to prevent remyelination. Light gray text, activates OPC differentiation; dark gray text, inhibits OPC differentiation.

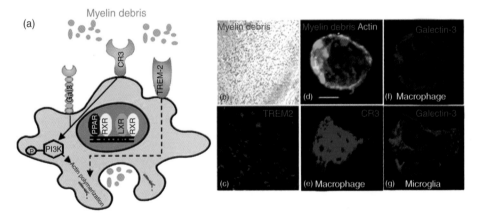

Figure 13.3 (a) Macrophages express unique receptors and compounds that promote myelin debris phagocytosis. Monocytes, macrophages, and microglia are primarily responsible for the removal of inhibitory myelin debris to enhance remyelination. Through signals such as MCP-1 and gelsolin, these myeloid-derived cells are recruited to the CNS and express membrane receptors, nuclear receptors, and complement components to enhance phagocytosis mechanisms. Activation of CR3 and MAC-2 leads to PI3K phosphorylation and phagocytosis. LXR, PPAR, and RXR are activated by lipid-derived ligands and act as transcription factors to enhance phagocytosis and immunoregulation. TREM-2 pathways activate cytoskeletal rearrangement and response to apoptotic cells which results in effective myelin debris clearance. (b) Oil Red O stained myelin debris in a demyelinated lesion; (c) TREM-2 staining of region (b) showing phagocytic TREM-2+ macrophages; (d) actin rearrangement during myelin debris phagocytosis by macrophages; (e) CR3 activation; (f) galectin-3 activation in (c); (g) galectin-3 activation in myelin-phagocytosing microglia. *Source*: Immunostaining adapted from Piccio *et al.* (2008), Hadas *et al.* (2010), and Gitik *et al.* (2011).

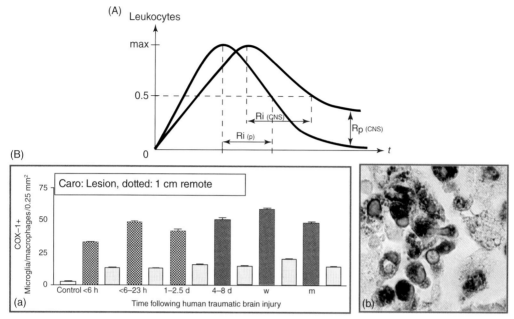

Figure 17.2 Modeling neuroinflammatory resolution phenotypes *in vivo*: Objective measures. (A) Based on cell trafficking into and away from inflammatory lesions, integrative indices were established to quantitatively determine the main events of resolution. These include the Resolution index (Ri) as the time between the maximum and the point when cells numbers are reduced by 50%. In case of a nonresolving CNS acute inflammation, a model of a resolution deficit with respect to the resolution plateau (Rp) can be determined. The black line illustrates the course of an self-limiting inflammatory response (e.g., peritonitis). The blue line illustrates the inflammatory response in CNS lesions as being delayed, sustained and non-self-limiting. (B) Impaired resolution of inflammation is also evident in CNS lesions of noninflammatory origin such as stroke or traumatic brain injury. Following traumatic brain injury, COX-1+ microglia/macrophage numbers remain signficantly elevated at the lesion site (orange colored caro bars) for up to months (m) compared to neuropathological unaltered controls (white bar) and remote areas (dotted bars) (Schwab *et al.*, 2002) (a). The nonresolving CNS lesion milieu is dominated by CD68+ lipid-laden microglia/macrophages (>80%) (brown) coexpressing proinflammatory enzymes such as COX-1 (blue) in areas of ongoing neuronal degeneration (Schwab *et al.*, 2000a) (b).

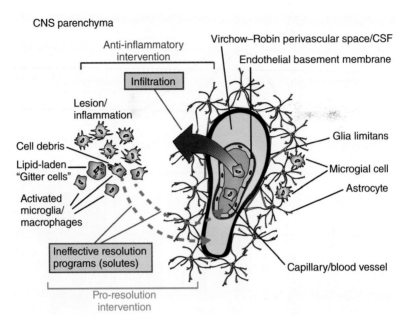

CNS parenchyma

Anti-inflammatory intervention

Virchow–Robin perivascular space/CSF

Endothelial basement membrane

Infiltration

Lesion/inflammation

Cell debris

Lipid-laden "Gitter cells"

Activated microglia/macrophages

Ineffective resolution programs (solutes)

Glia limitans

Microgial cell

Astrocyte

Capillary/blood vessel

Pro-resolution intervention

Figure 17.3 Infiltration and exit routes of inflammatory traffic in the immune-privileged CNS: Targets for anti-inflammatory versus pro-resolution intervention. Traditional anti-inflammatory treatments focussing mostly on leukocyte infiltration (left upper part) are likely to be insufficient if impaired resolution of inflammation is part of the underlying CNS pathophysiology (left lower part). This is supported by the lack of efficacy of classical anti-inflammatory approaches in chronic inflammatory CNS disease such as progressive MS. Published experimental and human neuropathological and neuroimmunological evidence suggests a CNS lesion environment, which blocks effective resolution of inflammation. Given that the acute inflammatory response in CNS lesions is delayed or non-self-limiting, SPMs qualify as good candidates with robust bioactivity to shape a maladaptive immune response. Reducing the exposure time of vulnerable neurons, oligodendrocytes and other neuropil to the hostile milieu of chronic inflammation by treatment with SPMs can be expected to attenuate inflammation-mediated pain and neurodegeneration.

PART III
Beneficial Aspects of Inflammation

11 The Interplay between the Peripheral and Local Immune Response in Recovery from Acute Central Nervous System Injuries

Catarina Raposo and Michal Schwartz

Department of Neurobiology, Weizmann Institute of Science, Rehovot, Israel

Paradigm of Protective Autoimmunity

Inflammation is a natural response of the immune system to stressful events such as tissue damage and is a necessary process aimed at tissue repair. Nevertheless, inflammation has gained a mostly negative reputation in the central nervous system (CNS), in part due to the limited regenerative capacity of the CNS and the inadequate capacity to replenish lost neurons. In addition, the immune-privileged nature of the CNS led to the misconception that immune cell entry into the CNS occurs as a result of pathological inflammation due to disruption of the blood–brain barrier (BBB).

Accumulating evidence over the years contributed to the appreciation that distinct immune cells are pivotal players in the healing process from CNS injuries (Rapalino *et al.*, 1998; Moalem *et al.*, 1999; Leon *et al.*, 2000). Moreover, we now understand that more than obsolete blockades, the system of barriers protecting the brain grants the CNS its immune singularity, and parenchymal infiltration following insult is a result of an active mechanism of recruitment, needed for repair, which occurs at specialized compartments (Shechter *et al.*, 2013a). Similarly to the wound healing response in tissues outside the CNS, a cascade of immune events takes place following CNS injury, with early recruitment of neutrophils, followed by activation of resident microglia and infiltration of monocyte-derived macrophages (mo-MΦ), and late infiltration of T cells (Fleming *et al.*, 2006; Raposo *et al.*, 2014). Early evidence suggested the importance of macrophages for axonal regeneration and motor function recovery (David *et al.*, 1990; Rapalino *et al.*, 1998; Leon *et al.*, 2000). CNS-specific (myelin-specific) T cells were found to promote repair and neuronal survival when transferred to axonally injured mice (Moalem *et al.*, 1999). T-cell-deficient mice showed increased neuronal loss following injury, while higher neuronal survival following injury was observed in transgenic mice overexpressing a T cell receptor to

Neuroinflammation: New Insights into Beneficial and Detrimental Functions, First Edition. Edited by Samuel David.
© 2015 John Wiley & Sons, Inc. Published 2015 by John Wiley & Sons, Inc.

myelin basic protein (MBP) (Yoles *et al.*, 2001; Schori *et al.*, 2002). Furthermore, the outcome of CNS axonal injury (in this case to the optic nerve) was improved when preceded by a primary lesion at a distinct CNS site (Yoles *et al.*, 2001). These and other studies were stepping stones contributing to the development of our theory of "protective autoimmunity," viewing immune response to CNS antigens as a pivotal immune network that is needed to cope with the consequences of injury; only when such a response goes awry, it becomes detrimental leading to pathological rather than physiological autoimmunity (Schwartz and Kipnis, 2001; Raposo *et al.*, 2014).

In this chapter, we discuss the beneficial effects of immune cells following CNS injuries, referring mainly to the model of spinal cord injury (SCI). The detailed understanding of the events occurring after CNS injury will enable the development of novel immune-based interventions, modulating specific inflammatory components in a timely manner.

Dichotomy between Microglia and Infiltrating Monocyte-Derived Macrophages

For decades, microglia and infiltrating mo-MΦ were thought to be a functionally homogenous population; these two populations display similar morphology and phenotypic markers and therefore could not be distinguished using standard techniques. This lack of discrimination contributed to the erroneous belief that all inflammatory responses at the CNS are detrimental and should be inhibited (Popovich *et al.*, 1999, 2002; Gris *et al.*, 2004). Over the years, accumulating data demonstrated that these two myeloid cell populations are functionally distinct and nonredundant (Shechter *et al.*, 2009, 2011) and also differ in their ontogeny (Ginhoux *et al.*, 2010). Infiltrating macrophages derive from the classical hematopoietic stem cells, which persist throughout life in specific stem cell niches, such as the bone marrow, or immune reservoirs such as the spleen (Swirski *et al.*, 2009), and reach their targets via the bloodstream only following insult. In contrast, recent fate-mapping studies demonstrated that the microglial precursors reach the CNS early in embryonic development (Ginhoux *et al.*, 2010; Schulz *et al.*, 2012). Adult microglia derive from primitive erythromyeloid progenitors that arise before embryonic day 8, and these cells gradually assume definitive microglial properties at their CNS destination (Kierdorf *et al.*, 2013). They are a unique tissue-specific macrophage population, consisting of self-renewing cells and with a genetic profile distinct from other populations in the mononuclear phagocyte system (Kierdorf *et al.*, 2013). The evolution of microglia within the brain microenvironment may endow the microglia with specialized functions supporting the homeostasis of the CNS. They are active surveyors of the CNS parenchyma, needed to maintain tissue homeostasis, neuronal integrity, and network functioning in the brain. Given their expression of an abundance of receptors, including sensors of innate immunity, receptors of neurotransmitters, and for a variety of trophic factors, they can interact with neurons, thereby affecting neuronal activity and survival (Kettenmann *et al.*, 2013). Other important functions of microglia that contribute to neuronal plasticity in the developing and adult brain include synaptic stripping (Schafer *et al.*, 2012), mobilization and induction of neurogenic progenitor cells in their niches (Sierra *et al.*, 2010), and production of neurotrophic factors (NFs) (Parkhurst *et al.*, 2013).

In response to pathology, such as injury, the microglial activity is often not optimal, and eventually these cells turn from a friend into a foe and contribute to pathological inflammation and disease progression (Ekdahl *et al.*, 2003; Stirling *et al.*, 2004; Hanisch and Kettenmann, 2007; Heneka *et al.*, 2014). As microglial cells fail to acquire the full spectrum of activities under severe pathological conditions, reprogramming their phenotypes to an adequate activation state or recruiting cells that will bridge the functional gap might be necessary to support recovery.

Overall, an important conclusion drawn from the seminal studies performed in the 1990s is that for successful recovery following mechanical injury to the CNS, the resident microglial response is not sufficient, and subsets of alternatively activated blood macrophages are needed as well (Rapalino *et al.*, 1998). One of the populations of mo-MΦ spontaneously recruited following the insult has vital roles in recovery following SCI, in particular by their regulation of the inflammatory microglial response (Shechter *et al.*, 2009). Yet, their spontaneous recruitment is limited. As such, boosting mo-MΦ recruitment was found to improve recovery following SCI (Shechter *et al.*, 2009). It is important to note that their therapeutic benefit is dependent on the time window between the injury and their administration, highlighting the importance of synchrony in the series of immunological events needed for the post-injury repair (Shechter and Schwartz, 2013).

Infiltrating Macrophages Promote Inflammation Resolution and Axonal Regeneration

Unlike the resident microglia, mo-MΦ can shift their functional state in response to changes in tissue physiology or environmental challenges, highlighting their hallmark, plasticity (Sica and Mantovani, 2012). Following SCI, distinct subsets of mo-MΦ were found at the injured parenchyma. The monocytes that give rise at the lesion site to proinflammatory M1 mo-MΦ infiltrate the injured spinal cord through the adjacent spinal cord leptomeninges, in a CCL2-dependent manner (Shechter *et al.*, 2013b). These $Ly6c^{hi}CX_3CR1^{low}$ mo-MΦ are detected as early as day 1 after injury and produce high levels of tumor necrosis factor alpha (TNF-α) and interleukin (IL)-1β (Shechter *et al.*, 2013b). *In vitro* evidence suggests that proinflammatory macrophages are neurotoxic (Kigerl *et al.*, 2009) and can cause retraction of dystrophic axons of adult dorsal root ganglion neurons (Horn *et al.*, 2008). Nevertheless, caution must be taken when interpreting these results without considering the temporal needs of the tissue. The M1 microglia/mo-MΦ are involved in the clearing of dead cells and damaged tissue, phagocytosis of myelin, and of apoptotic cells at the early stages following injury (Shechter and Schwartz, 2013; Greenhalgh and David, 2014). Furthermore, TNF-α and IL-1β have been implicated in the recruitment and activation of peripheral immune cells and the activation of CNS cells (astrocytes and microglia) (Yang *et al.*, 2004; Pineau and Lacroix, 2007; Kunis *et al.*, 2013). In addition, the subpopulations of macrophages have distinct roles in modulation of the glial scar. Thus, for example, M1-polarized macrophages were found to express high levels of chondroitin sulfate proteoglycan (CSPG) compared to M2-polarized cells (Martinez *et al.*, 2006), which can express matrix-degrading enzymes (Shechter *et al.*, 2011). While CSPG is a major component of the glial scar accounting for regenerative failure (McKeon *et al.*, 1991; Bradbury *et al.*, 2002), the scar tissue plays key beneficial roles at the early stages following injury, in stabilizing the injured parenchyma and preventing the spread of injury-induced toxic molecules to spared neurons (Rolls *et al.*, 2008). Moreover, the scar facilitates the correct spatial location of macrophages and is endowed with immunomodulatory functions (Faulkner *et al.*, 2004; Okada *et al.*, 2006; Rolls *et al.*, 2008; Shechter *et al.*, 2011; Raposo and Schwartz, 2014).

Importantly, however, successful recovery and regeneration are critically affected by the timely accumulation within the lesion area of the inflammation-resolving M2 mo-MΦ. Results from our group suggest that the monocytes that give rise to the M2 mo-MΦ infiltrate the injured CNS through the remote cerebrospinal fluid (CSF) barrier, a process orchestrated by the epithelial brain choroid plexus (CP) (Shechter *et al.*, 2013b). These Ly6C^{low}CX$_3$CR1^{high} mo-MΦ are detected at the injured parenchyma at highest numbers on day 7 after injury and are endowed with an inflammation-resolving activity (Shechter *et al.*, 2013b). They display a myriad of functions vital for tissue repair and remodeling. Thus, for example, their expression of the anti-inflammatory cytokine IL-10 is pivotal for the resolution of the local inflammatory response, in particular the inflammatory microglia, and recovery of the injured CNS (Shechter *et al.*, 2009; London *et al.*, 2011). Importantly, the interaction of mo-MΦ with CSPG is an important process for the final maturation of the mo-MΦ, in particular the expression of IL-10 by mo-MΦ (Shechter *et al.*, 2011). In addition, they express matrix-metalloproteinase-13 (MMP-13) and thus can promote glial scar resolution (Shechter *et al.*, 2011). They display additional immunomodulatory properties by orchestrating recruitment of regulatory T cells (Tregs), key players in maintenance of self-tolerance and immune homeostasis: Tregs are needed at the late stage of tissue remodeling and can control the adaptive inflammatory response (Raposo *et al.*, 2014). Macrophages can further facilitate tissue remodeling by their production of molecules that support neuronal survival, neuroprotection, axonal regeneration, and sprouting, such as oncomodulin (Yin *et al.*, 2006), activin-A (Miron *et al.*, 2013), and an array of NFs (Dougherty *et al.*, 2000; Barrette *et al.*, 2008). NFs stimulate neuronal plasticity, axonal growth, contribute to the establishment of synaptic contacts during development, and support neuronal survival and augment neuronal function in the injured CNS. Finally, macrophages can also support progenitor cell renewal in the injured retina and spinal cord (London *et al.*, 2011; Martino *et al.*, 2011; Cusimano *et al.*, 2012; Kokaia *et al.*, 2012). Importantly, immunization with CNS-derived peptide combined with transplantation of adult neural stem/progenitor cells into the CSF had a synergistic effect, improving recovery from SCI beyond the effect of each treatment separately, through changes in the phenotype of microglia/macrophages that could support neurogenesis (Ziv *et al.*, 2006).

The Two Faces of Tregs in CNS Repair

T cells, including autoimmune T cells, were shown to secrete NFs, including brain-derived neurotrophic factor (BDNF), upon antigen stimulation in models of injury and multiple sclerosis (Ehrhard *et al.*, 1993; Kerschensteiner *et al.*, 1999; Hammarberg *et al.*, 2000; Wolf *et al.*, 2002; Ziemssen *et al.*, 2002; Hohlfeld *et al.*, 2006; Linker *et al.*, 2010); one of the mechanisms by which they contribute to neuroprotection. Nevertheless, given potential detrimental roles of autoimmune T cells in the CNS, their beneficial activity is critically dependent on Tregs, key regulators of immune homeostasis, and immunological self-tolerance, with the vital ability to control autoimmune T cells and prevent autoimmune disease development (Olivares-Villagomez *et al.*, 1998). It is critical, however, that Treg levels are compatible with the needs of the tissue. This explains why Treg activity in the context of recovery from acute insult ranges from inhibitory to supportive, according to the time after injury and location (Kipnis *et al.*, 2002b; Raposo *et al.*, 2014). In a model of ischemic stroke, Tregs were found to have an important immunomodulatory role via their expression of IL-10; their depletion exacerbated brain damage and worsened functional outcome (Liesz *et al.*, 2009, 2013). Importantly, Tregs were also reported to contribute to ischemic neurodegeneration by promoting microvascular dysfunction and thrombosis (Klein-schnitz *et al.*, 2013). These conflicting results might be attributed, at least in part, to different depletion paradigms [Foxp3-DTR versus CD25-specific monoclonal antibody (mAb)] and timing of Treg depletion. For example, although Treg depletion was performed before the insult in both studies, CD25-specific mAb (PC-61) can persist in the circulation for several days (Couper *et al.*, 2007), promoting ongoing clearance of $CD25^+$ cells (which will include both Tregs and effector T cells), even after the treatment is stopped.

We have recently shown that $Foxp3^+$ Treg cells play important but opposing roles at distinct stages of SCI repair: these cells are beneficial at the late chronic phase following insult, preventing an uncontrolled effector response at the injured parenchyma, but their time-dependent reduction at the time of the insult, supporting the initial adaptive effector immune response, improves repair (Raposo *et al.*, 2014). Importantly, Treg reduction before the insult was only beneficial if limited in its duration, otherwise leading to an overwhelming effector response that impaired the recovery process. These results reconcile the apparent discrepancy between previous studies. Protocols that led to reduction of Treg numbers or their suppressive activity were found to improve neuronal survival and neuroprotection, as observed in models of optic nerve injury and glutamate intoxication of the eye (Kipnis *et al.*, 2002b, 2004b; Johnson *et al.*, 2007). On the other hand, the neuroprotective effect of CNS-specific autoimmune T cells on retinal ganglion cell survival was lost when T_{MBP} cells (comprised mainly of Th1 cells) were transferred to neonatally thymectomized (Kipnis *et al.*, 2002a); the beneficial effect was restored following transfer of additional $CD4^+$ populations. Of note, vaccination with a CNS-derived peptide, shown to augment recovery by enhancing infiltration of mo-MΦ (Shechter *et al.*, 2009), was also found to boost infiltration of effector T cells and concomitant recruitment of Tregs (Raposo *et al.*, 2014). Altogether, effector and regulatory T cells are an integral part of the immune network needed to cope with CNS deviations from homeostasis, including injury. A unique balance between these subsets, specific to the location and time after injury, must be achieved in order to promote protection of spared tissue, tissue remodeling, and repair, while avoiding pathological autoimmunity, on one hand, or overwhelming immunosuppression, on the other hand. Our results argue in favor of distinct and opposite roles for Tregs in the periphery and the lesion site in the course of the response to the injury. While at the acute phase a timely reduction in Tregs and shift in favor of autoimmunity are needed, at the subacute/chronic phase this balance should favor Tregs.

Protective Autoimmunity Works at the Specialized Choroid Plexus Gate

As was stated previously, one of the key problems that limits recovery following SCI is the insufficient infiltration of resolving mo-MΦ into the injured parenchyma (Shechter *et al.*, 2009). Beyond the general immune depression observed following injury to the CNS, leading to the increased immunosuppression in the periphery (Meisel *et al.*, 2005), the unique anatomy of the CNS is an additional factor that restricts recruitment of immune cells to the damaged CNS. The CNS contains a specialized system of barriers that strictly controls inflammatory reactions in its territory. These consist of the BBB, formed by highly specialized endothelial cells with an elaborate network of tight junctions, and the blood–cerebrospinal fluid barrier (BCSFB), composed of a monolayer of CP epithelial cells vascularized by blood vessels (Ransohoff *et al.*, 2003).

Under normal physiological conditions, the immune cell infiltration is limited, leaving to the resident microglia the critical role of supporting the optimal functioning of the brain and spinal cord parenchyma. In addition, the naïve CP is enriched with CD4$^+$ T cells, specific for CNS antigens, in particular, memory T cells (Baruch *et al.*, 2013) of the Th1 and Th2 phenotype (Kunis *et al.*, 2013).

Data from several studies further emphasized the importance of the remote CP gateway for recruitment of immune cells upon disturbances to homeostasis, such as injury and neurodegenerative diseases (reviewed in detail in (Schwartz and Baruch, 2014)). Under pathological conditions in the CNS, upregulation of critical adhesion molecules and chemokines occurs at the CP epithelium (Steffen *et al.*, 1996; Reboldi *et al.*, 2009; Szmydynger-Chodobska *et al.*, 2009, 2012; Kunis *et al.*, 2013; Shechter *et al.*, 2013b), allowing the trafficking of different immune subsets such as neutrophils, monocytes, and T cells across the CP–CSF route. Of particular importance for CNS injury, but also immune surveillance, is the crosstalk between circulating effector Th1 cells and the CP endothelial cells. Mice that lack interferon gamma receptor (IFN-γR) in the CNS, or interferon gamma (IFN-γ) expression by circulating immune cells, as well as IFN-γR knockout or Tbx21 (transcription factor that determines IFN-γ production by Th1 cells) knockout transgenic mice, showed impaired activation of key adhesion molecules and chemokines for leukocyte trafficking, including vascular cell adhesion molecule 1 (VCAM-1), intercellular adhesion molecule 1 (ICAM-1), CX$_3$CL1, and CD73 (Kunis *et al.*, 2013; Raposo *et al.*, 2014). The upregulation of these molecules is critical for the recruitment of the inflammation-resolving mo-MΦ into the CNS, which infiltrate via this gate, rather than by breaching the BBB (Shechter *et al.*, 2013b). This explains why Th1-deficient mice have limited numbers of resolving IL-10 producing mo-MΦ at the site of injury, with consequences for resolution of inflammation and the overall repair response and recovery (Raposo *et al.*, 2014). In agreement with these results, passive transfer of T$_{MBP}$ cells (mainly IFN-γ producers) or Th1 cells was associated with an increase of M2 macrophages at the lesion site and improved recovery (Hu *et al.*, 2012; Ishii *et al.*, 2012). Low dose irradiation, a protocol that leads to decreased incidence of Tregs and proliferation of effector T cells (with high expression of IFN-γ), immediately following the insult (optic nerve axotomy, spinal cord contusion, or glutamate toxicity), increased neuronal survival and improved recovery (Kipnis *et al.*, 2004a). Overall, these findings emphasize that Th1 cells contribute to recovery immediately following acute CNS injury. Temporary breakdown of systemic immune suppression at the time of the insult, for example, by timely decrease of Tregs, aims at promoting a more effective Th1 response that can activate the CP, and allows timely and controlled infiltration of healing monocytes into the injured CNS.

Beyond serving as an infiltration gateway, the BCSFB is an educative gate. The CSF milieu is highly immunosuppressive (Taylor and Streilein, 1996; Gordon *et al.*, 1998), enriched in cytokines such as transforming growth factor beta (TGF-β) and IL-13 (Shechter *et al.*, 2013b). The orchestrated recruitment of these cells via the CP ensures that the highly plastic macrophages, encountering this immunosuppressive environment, will be skewed to an inflammation-resolving phenotype before their arrival to the site of injury (Shechter *et al.*, 2013b). The recruitment of immune cells via this fate establishes an active, tissue-protective immune response.

Inflammation, the Old Villain in Spinal Cord Repair

The data accumulated thus far, including the results summarized previously, highlighted the protective roles of immune cells following CNS injury and neurodegenerative diseases, leading to the overall understanding that "nonspecific" immunomodulatory drugs might actually increase secondary damage to the injured spinal cord, as they also inhibit the protective effect of the immune system following SCI. Nevertheless, in the past, inflammatory or edema-forming processes were believed to be major factors contributing to secondary degeneration (Janssen and Hansebout, 1989). Corticosteroids, particularly methylprednisolone (MP), were studied extensively in animal models of SCI, where they were thought to control edema and limit the inflammatory reaction following injury (Amar and Levy, 1999). Following the National Institutes of Health multicenter, randomized, double-blinded clinical trial (National Adult Social Care Intelligence Service, NASCIS) evaluating the effect of MP in spinal cord repair (Bracken et al., 1990), which concluded that high-dose MP can reduce some of the damage that results from acute SCI, MP became widely instituted as the standard of care for nonpenetrating acute SCI in many countries. These reports have been criticized by their lack of sufficient evidence to support the claims, questioning the validity of the findings (Coleman et al., 2000; Hurlbert and Moulton, 2002; Sayer et al., 2006). It is important to note that clinical evidence supporting glucocorticoid therapy for traumatic SCI (and other CNS pathologies including ischemic stroke and traumatic brain injury) did not demonstrate definitive therapeutic effect (Gomes et al., 2005). In addition, this regimen was associated with significant increase in medical complications (including increased fatalities) (McCutcheon et al., 2004), leaving clinicians treating SCI in a difficult position, often not feeling confident prescribing a drug that lacks scientific consensus, but feeling compelled to do so due to peer pressure or fear of litigation (Coleman et al., 2000; Hurlbert and Moulton, 2002). The reason behind the intrinsic failure of steroid therapy may reside in the effect of steroids on the inflammatory response (Can et al., 2009) and their pro-apoptotic activity in a variety of inflammatory cells, including monocytes (Schmidt et al., 1999).

Comprehensive View of the Protective Autoimmune Network: the Link between Autoimmune T Cells and Inflammation-Resolving Cells

The complex immune process involved in SCI repair is part of the protective autoimmune response that is activated following CNS injury (Fig. 11.1). The optimal function of this network requires a balance between effector and regulatory mechanisms synchronized with the needs of the tissue. Immediately following the insult, peripheral immunosuppression must be alleviated to promote activation of the effector response. This effector T cells can then activate the remote CP gate, the activation of which orchestrates the infiltration of healing macrophages to the injured parenchyma. At the lesion site, the initial proinflammatory response is needed for fighting infections, clearing dead cells and damaged tissue, and initiating the healing response. The expression of proinflammatory cytokines might play a fundamental role related to the recruitment of peripheral immune cells into the injured spinal cord (Yang et al., 2004). As this proinflammatory response might result in secondary tissue damage and consequent permanent functional loss

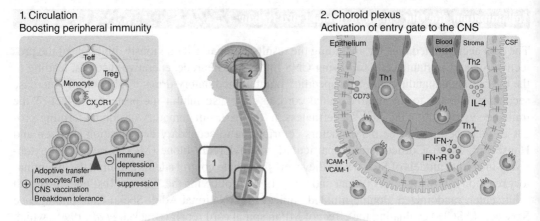

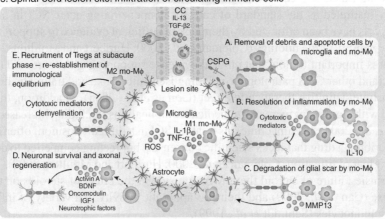

Figure 11.1   Protective autoimmunity network following SCI (a model). The immune network works at distinct compartments and phases of the repair process. (1) Immediately following the insult, a balance favoring effector memory CNS-specific T cells (Teff) with decreased immunosuppression is beneficial for recovery and can be achieved using several approaches, including CNS peptide-derived immunization, adoptive transfer of monocytes or Teff, or partial depletion of regulatory T cells (Tregs). (2) The remote choroid plexus is activated by effector Th1 cells, orchestrating the controlled entrance of CX_3CR1^+ healing monocytes. (3) The healing monocytes migrate via the immunoregulatory CP-CSF entry route, reaching the lesion site and maturing into resolving M2 monocyte-derived macrophages (mo-MΦ). (A) The lesion site is markedly proinflammatory, with M1 mo-MΦ and microglia. These cells are needed at the initial repair response for clearance of apoptotic cells and debris. (B) At the acute phase, the M2 mo-MΦ are vital for repair, by resolving the proinflammatory response, and (C) regulate the degradation of the glial scar. (D) The resolving M2 mo-MΦ can also produce numerous neuroprotective molecules, which promote axonal survival and regeneration. (E) During the subacute/chronic phase, the mo-MΦ promote recruitment of regulatory T cells that resolve the effector T cell response, to ensure that its uncontrolled action will not lead to autoimmune disease. (*See insert for color representation of this figure.*)

in the injured CNS, a switch towards the anti-inflammatory component is necessary at the acute phase, to ensure resolution of the initial inflammatory response. The infiltrating resolving mo-MΦ acquire the healing phenotype as they migrate through the immunosuppressive CSF, and furthermore, on reaching the lesion site, they encounter the educative CNS scar, which further biases their phenotype toward IL-10 production. Besides regulating the inflammatory microglia, resolving mo-MΦ recruit Tregs, which arrive at the subacute/chronic phase, regulating the adaptive inflammatory response, and supporting the return to homeostasis.

Rather than suppressing immune activity, the limited recovery from CNS injury can be enhanced by boosting the immune system, including transfer of activated autoimmune cells, active immunization with CNS-derived peptides, increasing the circulating monocyte pool, or breaking immunosupression at the time of the insult by Treg depletion.

The increase in our basic understanding of the effects of distinct immune populations in CNS repair already resulted in the identification of new therapeutic targets and enabled clinical trials of drugs modulating specific elements of the inflammatory response (David *et al.*, 2012). Enhanced therapeutic approaches should aim at specific populations and time windows, to promote the beneficial effects of the immune response, while minimizing the detrimental bystander effects of the ensuing inflammation.

Acknowledgments

This research was supported by a European Research Council Grant Award (ERC, given to M.S.) and by the Seventh Framework Programme (FP7) HEALTH-2011 Grant (to M.S.). M.S. holds the Maurice and Ilse Katz Professorial Chair in Neuroimmunology. We thank Dr. Shelley Schwarzbaum for editing the manuscript.

References

Amar, A.P. & Levy, M.L. (1999) Pathogenesis and pharmacological strategies for mitigating secondary damage in acute spinal cord injury. *Neurosurgery*, **44**, 1027–1039; discussion 1039–1040.

Barrette, B., Hebert, M.A., Filali, M. *et al.* (2008) Requirement of myeloid cells for axon regeneration. *Journal of Neuroscience*, **28**, 9363–9376.

Baruch, K., Ron-Harel, N., Gal, H. *et al.* (2013) CNS-specific immunity at the choroid plexus shifts toward destructive Th2 inflammation in brain aging. *Proceedings of the National Academy of Sciences of the United States of America*, **110**, 2264–2269.

Bracken, M.B., Shepard, M.J., Collins, W.F. *et al.* (1990) A randomized, controlled trial of methylprednisolone or naloxone in the treatment of acute spinal-cord injury. Results of the Second National Acute Spinal Cord Injury Study. *New England Journal of Medicine*, **322**, 1405–1411.

Bradbury, E.J., Moon, L.D., Popat, R.J. *et al.* (2002) Chondroitinase ABC promotes functional recovery after spinal cord injury. *Nature*, **416**, 636–640.

Can, M., Gul, S., Bektas, S., Hanci, V. & Acikgoz, S. (2009) Effects of dexmedetomidine or methylprednisolone on inflammatory responses in spinal cord injury. *Acta Anaesthesiologica Scandinavica*, **53**, 1068–1072.

Coleman, W.P., Benzel, D., Cahill, D.W. *et al.* (2000) A critical appraisal of the reporting of the National Acute Spinal Cord Injury Studies (II and III) of methylprednisolone in acute spinal cord injury. *Journal of Spinal Disorders*, **13**, 185–199.

Couper, K.N., Blount, D.G., de Souza, J.B., Suffia, I., Belkaid, Y. & Riley, E.M. (2007) Incomplete depletion and rapid regeneration of Foxp3+ regulatory T cells following anti-CD25 treatment in malaria-infected mice. *Journal of Immunology*, **178**, 4136–4146.

Cusimano, M., Biziato, D., Brambilla, E. *et al.* (2012) Transplanted neural stem/precursor cells instruct phagocytes and reduce secondary tissue damage in the injured spinal cord. *Brain*, **135**, 447–460.

David, S., Lopez-Vales, R. & Wee Yong, V. (2012) Harmful and beneficial effects of inflammation after spinal cord injury: Potential therapeutic implications. *Handbook of Clinical Neurology*, **109**, 485–502.

David, S., Bouchard, C., Tsatas, O. & Giftochristos, N. (1990) Macrophages can modify the nonpermissive nature of the adult mammalian central nervous system. *Neuron*, **5**, 463–469.

Dougherty, K.D., Dreyfus, C.F. & Black, I.B. (2000) Brain-derived neurotrophic factor in astrocytes, oligodendrocytes, and microglia/macrophages after spinal cord injury. *Neuromuscular Disorders*, **7**, 574–585.

Ehrhard, P.B., Erb, P., Graumann, U. & Otten, U. (1993) Expression of nerve growth factor and nerve growth factor receptor tyrosine kinase Trk in activated CD4-positive T-cell clones. *Proceedings of the National Academy of Sciences of the United States of America*, **90**, 10984–10988.

Ekdahl, C.T., Claasen, J.H., Bonde, S., Kokaia, Z. & Lindvall, O. (2003) Inflammation is detrimental for neurogenesis in adult brain. *Proceedings of the National Academy of Sciences of the United States of America*, **100**, 13632–13637.

Faulkner, J.R., Herrmann, J.E., Woo, M.J., Tansey, K.E., Doan, N.B. & Sofroniew, M.V. (2004) Reactive astrocytes protect tissue and preserve function after spinal cord injury. *Journal of Neuroscience*, **24**, 2143–2155.

Fleming, J.C., Norenberg, M.D., Ramsay, D.A. *et al.* (2006) The cellular inflammatory response in human spinal cords after injury. *Brain*, **129**, 3249–3269.

Ginhoux, F., Greter, M., Leboeuf, M. *et al.* (2010) Fate mapping analysis reveals that adult microglia derive from primitive macrophages. *Science*, **330**, 841–845.

Gomes, J.A., Stevens, R.D., Lewin, J.J. 3rd, Mirski, M.A. & Bhardwaj, A. (2005) Glucocorticoid therapy in neurologic critical care. *Critical Care Medicine*, **33**, 1214–1224.

Gordon, L.B., Nolan, S.C., Ksander, B.R., Knopf, P.M. & Harling-Berg, C.J. (1998) Normal cerebrospinal fluid suppresses the in vitro development of cytotoxic T cells: Role of the brain microenvironment in CNS immune regulation. *Journal of Neuroimmunology*, **88**, 77–84.

Greenhalgh, A.D. & David, S. (2014) Differences in the phagocytic response of microglia and peripheral macrophages after spinal cord injury and its effects on cell death. *Journal of Neuroscience*, **34**, 6316–6322.

Gris, D., Marsh, D.R., Oatway, M.A. *et al.* (2004) Transient blockade of the CD11d/CD18 integrin reduces secondary damage after spinal cord injury, improving sensory, autonomic, and motor function. *Journal of Neuroscience*, **24**, 4043–4051.

Hammarberg, H., Lidman, O., Lundberg, C. *et al.* (2000) Neuroprotection by encephalomyelitis: Rescue of mechanically injured neurons and neurotrophin production by CNS-infiltrating T and natural killer cells. *Journal of Neuroscience*, **20**, 5283–5291.

Hanisch, U.K. & Kettenmann, H. (2007) Microglia: Active sensor and versatile effector cells in the normal and pathologic brain. *Nature Neuroscience*, **10**, 1387–1394.

Heneka, M.T., Kummer, M.P. & Latz, E. (2014) Innate immune activation in neurodegenerative disease. *Nature Reviews Immunology*, **14**, 463–477.

Hohlfeld, R., Kerschensteiner, M., Stadelmann, C., Lassmann, H. & Wekerle, H. (2006) The neuroprotective effect of inflammation: Implications for the therapy of multiple sclerosis. *Neurological Sciences*, **27** (Suppl 1), S1–S7.

Horn, K.P., Busch, S.A., Hawthorne, A.L., van Rooijen, N. & Silver, J. (2008) Another barrier to regeneration in the CNS: Activated macrophages induce extensive retraction of dystrophic axons through direct physical interactions. *Journal of Neuroscience*, **28**, 9330–9341.

Hu, J.G., Shen, L., Wang, R. *et al.* (2012) Effects of Olig2-overexpressing neural stem cells and myelin basic protein-activated T cells on recovery from spinal cord injury. *Neurotherapeutics*, **9**, 422–445.

Hurlbert, R.J. & Moulton, R. (2002) Why do you prescribe methylprednisolone for acute spinal cord injury? A Canadian perspective and a position statement. *Canadian Journal of Neurological Sciences (Le journal canadien des sciences neurologiques)*, **29**, 236–239.

Ishii, H., Jin, X., Ueno, M. *et al.* (2012) Adoptive transfer of Th1-conditioned lymphocytes promotes axonal remodeling and functional recovery after spinal cord injury. *Cell Death & Disease*, **3**, e363.

Janssen, L. & Hansebout, R.R. (1989) Pathogenesis of spinal cord injury and newer treatments. A review. *Spine*, **14**, 23–32.

Johnson, T.V., Camras, C.B. & Kipnis, J. (2007) Bacterial DNA confers neuroprotection after optic nerve injury by suppressing CD4+CD25+ regulatory T-cell activity. *Investigative Ophthalmology & Visual Science*, **48**, 3441–3449.

Kerschensteiner, M., Gallmeier, E., Behrens, L. *et al.* (1999) Activated human T cells, B cells, and monocytes produce brain-derived neurotrophic factor in vitro and in inflammatory brain lesions: A neuroprotective role of inflammation? *Journal of Experimental Medicine*, **189**, 865–870.

Kettenmann, H., Kirchhoff, F. & Verkhratsky, A. (2013) Microglia: New roles for the synaptic stripper. *Neuron*, **77**, 10–18.

Kierdorf, K. *et al.* (2013) Microglia emerge from erythromyeloid precursors via Pu.1- and Irf8-dependent pathways. *Nature Neuroscience*, **16**, 273–280.

Kigerl, K.A., Gensel, J.C., Ankeny, D.P., Alexander, J.K., Donnelly, D.J. & Popovich, P.G. (2009) Identification of two distinct macrophage subsets with divergent effects causing either neurotoxicity or regeneration in the injured mouse spinal cord. *Journal of Neuroscience*, **29**, 13435–13444.

Kipnis, J., Mizrahi, T., Yoles, E., Ben-Nun, A. & Schwartz, M. (2002a) Myelin specific Th1 cells are necessary for post-traumatic protective autoimmunity. *Journal of Neuroimmunology*, **130**, 78–85.

Kipnis, J., Mizrahi, T., Hauben, E., Shaked, I., Shevach, E. & Schwartz, M. (2002b) Neuroprotective autoimmunity: Naturally occurring CD4+CD25+ regulatory T cells suppress the ability to withstand injury to the central nervous system. *Proceedings of the National Academy of Sciences of the United States of America*, **99**, 15620–15625.

Kipnis, J., Avidan, H., Markovich, Y. *et al.* (2004a) Low-dose gamma-irradiation promotes survival of injured neurons in the central nervous system via homeostasis-driven proliferation of T cells. *European Journal of Neuroscience*, **19**, 1191–1198.

Kipnis, J., Cardon, M., Avidan, H. *et al.* (2004b) Dopamine, through the extracellular signal-regulated kinase pathway, downregulates CD4+CD25+ regulatory T-cell activity: Implications for neurodegeneration. *Journal of Neuroscience*, **24**, 6133–6143.

Kleinschnitz, C. *et al.* (2013) Regulatory T cells are strong promoters of acute ischemic stroke in mice by inducing dysfunction of the cerebral microvasculature. *Blood*, **121**, 679–691.

Kokaia, Z., Martino, G., Schwartz, M. & Lindvall, O. (2012) Cross-talk between neural stem cells and immune cells: The key to better brain repair? *Nature Neuroscience*, **15**, 1078–1087.

Kunis, G., Baruch, K., Rosenzweig, N. *et al.* (2013) IFN-gamma-dependent activation of the brain's choroid plexus for CNS immune surveillance and repair. *Brain*, **136**, 3427–3440.

Leon, S., Yin, Y., Nguyen, J., Irwin, N. & Benowitz, L.I. (2000) Lens injury stimulates axon regeneration in the mature rat optic nerve. *Journal of Neuroscience*, **20**, 4615–4626.

Liesz, A., Suri-Payer, E., Veltkamp, C. *et al.* (2009) Regulatory T cells are key cerebroprotective immunomodulators in acute experimental stroke. *Nature Medicine*, **15**, 192–199.

Liesz, A., Zhou, W., Na, S.Y. *et al.* (2013) Boosting regulatory T cells limits neuroinflammation in permanent cortical stroke. *Journal of Neuroscience*, **33**, 17350–17362.

Linker, R.A., Lee, D.H., Demir, S. *et al.* (2010) Functional role of brain-derived neurotrophic factor in neuroprotective autoimmunity: Therapeutic implications in a model of multiple sclerosis. *Brain*, **133**, 2248–2263.

London, A., Itskovich, E., Benhar, I. *et al.* (2011) Neuroprotection and progenitor cell renewal in the injured adult murine retina requires healing monocyte-derived macrophages. *Journal of Experimental Medicine*, **208**, 23–39.

Martinez, F.O., Gordon, S., Locati, M. & Mantovani, A. (2006) Transcriptional profiling of the human monocyte-to-macrophage differentiation and polarization: New molecules and patterns of gene expression. *Journal of Immunology*, **177**, 7303–7311.

Martino, G., Pluchino, S., Bonfanti, L. & Schwartz, M. (2011) Brain regeneration in physiology and pathology: The immune signature driving therapeutic plasticity of neural stem cells. *Physiological Reviews*, **91**, 1281–1304.

McCutcheon, E.P., Selassie, A.W., Gu, J.K. & Pickelsimer, E.E. (2004) Acute traumatic spinal cord injury, 1993-2000A population-based assessment of methylprednisolone administration and hospitalization. *Journal of Trauma*, **56**, 1076–1083.

McKeon, R.J., Schreiber, R.C., Rudge, J.S. & Silver, J. (1991) Reduction of neurite outgrowth in a model of glial scarring following CNS injury is correlated with the expression of inhibitory molecules on reactive astrocytes. *Journal of Neuroscience*, **11**, 3398–3411.

Meisel, C., Schwab, J.M., Prass, K., Meisel, A. & Dirnagl, U. (2005) Central nervous system injury-induced immune deficiency syndrome. *Nature Reviews Neuroscience*, **6**, 775–786.

Miron, V.E., Boyd, A., Zhao, J.W. *et al.* (2013) M2 microglia and macrophages drive oligodendrocyte differentiation during CNS remyelination. *Nature Neuroscience*, **16**, 1211–1218.

Moalem, G., Leibowitz-Amit, R., Yoles, E., Mor, F., Cohen, I.R. & Schwartz, M. (1999) Autoimmune T cells protect neurons from secondary degeneration after central nervous system axotomy. *Nature Medicine*, **5**, 49–55.

Okada, S., Nakamura, M., Katoh, H. *et al.* (2006) Conditional ablation of Stat3 or Socs3 discloses a dual role for reactive astrocytes after spinal cord injury. *Nature Medicine*, **12**, 829–834.

Olivares-Villagomez, D., Wang, Y. & Lafaille, J.J. (1998) Regulatory CD4(+) T cells expressing endogenous T cell receptor chains protect myelin basic protein-specific transgenic mice from spontaneous autoimmune encephalomyelitis. *Journal of Experimental Medicine*, **188**, 1883–1894.

Parkhurst, C.N., Yang, G., Ninan, I. *et al.* (2013) Microglia promote learning-dependent synapse formation through brain-derived neurotrophic factor. *Cell*, **155**, 1596–1609.

Pineau, I. & Lacroix, S. (2007) Proinflammatory cytokine synthesis in the injured mouse spinal cord: Multiphasic expression pattern and identification of the cell types involved. *Journal of Comparative Neurology*, **500**, 267–285.

Popovich, P.G., Guan, Z., Wei, P., Huitinga, I., van Rooijen, N. & Stokes, B.T. (1999) Depletion of hematogenous macrophages promotes partial hindlimb recovery and neuroanatomical repair after experimental spinal cord injury. *Experimental Neurology*, **158**, 351–365.

Popovich, P.G., Guan, Z., McGaughy, V., Fisher, L., Hickey, W.F. & Basso, D.M. (2002) The neuropathological and behavioral consequences of intraspinal microglial/macrophage activation. *Journal of Neuropathology and Experimental Neurology*, **61**, 623–633.

Ransohoff, R.M., Kivisakk, P. & Kidd, G. (2003) Three or more routes for leukocyte migration into the central nervous system. *Nature Reviews Immunology*, **3**, 569–581.

Rapalino, O., Lazarov-Spiegler, O., Agranov, E. *et al.* (1998) Implantation of stimulated homologous macrophages results in partial recovery of paraplegic rats. *Nature Medicine*, **4**, 814–821.

Raposo, C. & Schwartz, M. (2014) Glial scar and immune cell involvement in tissue remodeling and repair following acute CNS injuries. *Glia*, **62**, 1895–1904.

Raposo, C., Graubardt, N., Cohen, M. *et al.* (2014) CNS repair requires both effector and regulatory T cells with distinct temporal and spatial profiles. *Journal of Neuroscience*, **34**, 10141–10155.

Reboldi, A., Coisne, C., Baumjohann, D. *et al.* (2009) C-C chemokine receptor 6-regulated entry of TH-17 cells into the CNS through the choroid plexus is required for the initiation of EAE. *Nature Immunology*, **10**, 514–523.

Rolls, A., Shechter, R., London, A. *et al.* (2008) Two faces of chondroitin sulfate proteoglycan in spinal cord repair: A role in microglia/macrophage activation. *PLoS Medicine*, **5**, e171.

Sayer, F.T., Kronvall, E. & Nilsson, O.G. (2006) Methylprednisolone treatment in acute spinal cord injury: The myth challenged through a structured analysis of published literature. *Spine Journal*, **6**, 335–343.

Schafer, D.P., Lehrman, E.K., Kautzman, A.G. *et al.* (2012) Microglia sculpt postnatal neural circuits in an activity and complement-dependent manner. *Neuron*, **74**, 691–705.

Schmidt, M., Pauels, H.G., Lugering, N., Lugering, A., Domschke, W. & Kucharzik, T. (1999) Glucocorticoids induce apoptosis in human monocytes: Potential role of IL-1 beta. *Journal of Immunology*, **163**, 3484–3490.

Schori, H., Lantner, F., Shachar, I. & Schwartz, M. (2002) Severe immunodeficiency has opposite effects on neuronal survival in glutamate-susceptible and -resistant mice: Adverse effect of B cells. *Journal of Immunology*, **169**, 2861–2865.

Schulz, C., Gomez Perdiguero, E., Chorro, L. *et al.* (2012) A lineage of myeloid cells independent of Myb and hematopoietic stem cells. *Science*, **336**, 86–90.

Schwartz, M. & Kipnis, J. (2001) Protective autoimmunity: Regulation and prospects for vaccination after brain and spinal cord injuries. *Trends in Molecular Medicine*, **7**, 252–258.

Schwartz, M. & Baruch, K. (2014) The resolution of neuroinflammation in neurodegeneration: Leukocyte recruitment via the choroid plexus. *EMBO Journal*, **33**, 7–22.

Shechter, R. & Schwartz, M. (2013) CNS sterile injury: Just another wound healing? *Trends in Molecular Medicine*, **19**, 135–143.

Shechter, R., London, A. & Schwartz, M. (2013a) Orchestrated leukocyte recruitment to immune-privileged sites: Absolute barriers versus educational gates. *Nature Reviews Immunology*, **13**, 206–218.

Shechter, R., Raposo, C., London, A., Sagi, I. & Schwartz, M. (2011) The glial scar-monocyte interplay: A pivotal resolution phase in spinal cord repair. *PLoS One*, **6**, e27969.

Shechter, R., London, A., Varol, C. *et al.* (2009) Infiltrating blood-derived macrophages are vital cells playing an anti-inflammatory role in recovery from spinal cord injury in mice. *PLoS Medicine*, **6**, e1000113.

Shechter, R., Miller, O., Yovel, G. *et al.* (2013b) Recruitment of beneficial M2 macrophages to injured spinal cord is orchestrated by remote brain choroid plexus. *Immunity*, **38**, 555–569.

Sica, A. & Mantovani, A. (2012) Macrophage plasticity and polarization: In vivo veritas. *Journal of Clinical Investigation*, **122**, 787–795.

Sierra, A., Encinas, J.M., Deudero, J.J. *et al.* (2010) Microglia shape adult hippocampal neurogenesis through apoptosis-coupled phagocytosis. *Cell stem cell*, **7**, 483–495.

Steffen, B.J., Breier, G., Butcher, E.C., Schulz, M. & Engelhardt, B. (1996) ICAM-1, VCAM-1, and MAdCAM-1 are expressed on choroid plexus epithelium but not endothelium and mediate binding of lymphocytes in vitro. *American Journal of Pathology*, **148**, 1819–1838.

Stirling, D.P., Khodarahmi, K., Liu, J. *et al.* (2004) Minocycline treatment reduces delayed oligodendrocyte death, attenuates axonal dieback, and improves functional outcome after spinal cord injury. *Journal of Neuroscience*, **24**, 2182–2190.

Swirski, F.K., Nahrendorf, M., Etzrodt, M. *et al.* (2009) Identification of splenic reservoir monocytes and their deployment to inflammatory sites. *Science*, **325**, 612–616.

Szmydynger-Chodobska, J., Strazielle, N., Zink, B.J., Ghersi-Egea, J.F. & Chodobski, A. (2009) The role of the choroid plexus in neutrophil invasion after traumatic brain injury. *Journal of Cerebral Blood Flow and Metabolism*, **29**, 1503–1516.

Szmydynger-Chodobska, J., Strazielle, N., Gandy, J.R. *et al.* (2012) Posttraumatic invasion of monocytes across the blood-cerebrospinal fluid barrier. *Journal of Cerebral Blood Flow and Metabolism*, **32**, 93–104.

Taylor, A.W. & Streilein, J.W. (1996) Inhibition of antigen-stimulated effector T cells by human cerebrospinal fluid. *Neuroimmunomodulation*, **3**, 112–118.

Wolf, S.A., Fisher, J., Bechmann, I., Steiner, B., Kwidzinski, E. & Nitsch, R. (2002) Neuroprotection by T-cells depends on their subtype and activation state. *Journal of Neuroimmunology*, **133**, 72–80.

Yang, L., Blumbergs, P.C., Jones, N.R., Manavis, J., Sarvestani, G.T. & Ghabriel, M.N. (2004) Early expression and cellular localization of proinflammatory cytokines interleukin-1beta, interleukin-6, and tumor necrosis factor-alpha in human traumatic spinal cord injury. *Spine*, **29**, 966–971.

Yin, Y., Henzl, M.T., Lorber, B. *et al.* (2006) Oncomodulin is a macrophage-derived signal for axon regeneration in retinal ganglion cells. *Nature Neuroscience*, **9**, 843–852.

Yoles, E., Hauben, E., Palgi, O. *et al.* (2001) Protective autoimmunity is a physiological response to CNS trauma. *Journal of Neuroscience*, **21**, 3740–3748.

Ziemssen, T., Kumpfel, T., Klinkert, W.E., Neuhaus, O. & Hohlfeld, R. (2002) Glatiramer acetate-specific T-helper 1- and 2-type cell lines produce BDNF: Implications for multiple sclerosis therapy. Brain-derived neurotrophic factor. *Brain*, **125**, 2381–2391.

Ziv, Y., Avidan, H., Pluchino, S., Martino, G. & Schwartz, M. (2006) Synergy between immune cells and adult neural stem/progenitor cells promotes functional recovery from spinal cord injury. *Proceedings of the National Academy of Sciences of the United States of America*, **103**, 13174–13179.

12   Inflammation and Optic Nerve Regeneration

Lukas Andereggen,[1,2] Ephraim F. Trakhtenberg,[1,2] Yuqin Yin,[1,2] and Larry I. Benowitz[1,2,3,4]

[1]*Laboratories for Neuroscience Research in Neurosurgery, F.M. Kirby Neurobiology Center, Boston Children's Hospital, Boston, MA, USA*
[2]*Department of Neurosurgery, Harvard Medical School, Boston, MA, USA*
[3]*Department of Ophthalmology, Harvard Medical School, Boston, MA, USA*
[4]*Program in Neuroscience, Harvard Medical School, Boston, MA, USA*

Introduction

The optic nerve is a well-established model for investigating factors that prevent or promote axon regeneration in the central nervous system (CNS) (Benowitz and Yin, 2008). This pathway is easily accessible and can be experimentally injured to disrupt the long-projecting axons that convey information from the eye to the brain. In mature mammals, retinal ganglion cells (RGCs), similarly to other CNS neurons, cannot regenerate injured axons over long distances and begin to die within several days after injury, precluding any possibility of visual recovery (Berkelaar *et al.*, 1994). Immature RGCs can regenerate their axons but lose this ability in the early postnatal period (Goldberg *et al.*, 2002). Regenerative failure in the mature CNS has been attributed to the low intrinsic growth potential of mature CNS neurons, the development of an inhibitory extracellular environment, the absence of appropriate trophic support, and the limited presence of guidance cues in the extracellular environment (Harel and Strittmatter, 2006; Yiu and He, 2006; Sun and He, 2010). Several factors that are developmentally regulated in RGCs have been identified as important intrinsic regulators of axon growth, including transcription factors of the Kruppel-like factor (KLF) family (Veldman *et al.*, 2007; Moore *et al.*, 2009), suppressors of key cell-signaling pathways, particularly phosphatase and tensin homolog (PTEN) and suppressor of cytokine signaling 3 (SOCS3) (Sun *et al.*, 2012), and histone acetyl transferases (Gaub *et al.*, 2011). Amacrine cells form synapses onto RGCs shortly after birth and appear to provide an important signal for the decline in RGCs' capacity for robust axon growth (Goldberg *et al.*, 2002). In addition, glial cells contribute to the development of an inhibitory environment for axon regeneration (Yiu and He, 2006). Multiple inhibitory molecules are associated with CNS myelin, including Nogo-A and Nogo-B (Chen *et al.*, 2000), oligodendrocyte-myelin glycoprotein (OMgp) (Wang *et al.*,

Neuroinflammation: New Insights into Beneficial and Detrimental Functions, First Edition. Edited by Samuel David.
© 2015 John Wiley & Sons, Inc. Published 2015 by John Wiley & Sons, Inc.

2002), myelin-associated glycoprotein (MAG) (Arregui *et al.*, 1994), and repulsive guidance molecules (Hsieh *et al.*, 2006) of the semaphorin (Moreau-Fauvarque *et al.*, 2003) and netrin families (Low *et al.*, 2008). Reactive astrocytes at the injury site also express chondroitin sulfate proteoglycans (CSPG) that contribute to the inhibitory effects of the glial scar (Silver and Miller, 2004). Receptors for many of these molecules have been identified, including variant forms of the nogo-66 receptor (NgR) (Fournier *et al.*, 2001; Dickendesher *et al.*, 2012) and receptor tyrosine phosphatases (Shen *et al.*, 2009; Fisher *et al.*, 2011). This review focuses on another aspect of CNS repair, specifically the role of inflammation in promoting axon regeneration in the optic nerve.

Background

Tello, a student of Ramon y Cajal, was the first to discover that mature RGCs retain a capacity to regenerate injured axons. After attaching a sciatic nerve graft to the cut end of the optic nerve, Tello observed that some RGCs were able to extend axons into the graft, leading Cajal to suggest that regenerative failure in the CNS is due to a neuroglial environment that suppresses growth, unlike that of the peripheral nervous system (PNS) (Ramon y Cajal, 1991). In much more systematic studies carried out several decades later, Aguayo *et al.* (1991) showed that mature RGCs not only have the ability to regrow their axons into a peripheral nerve graft, but can also form synapses if the other end of the graft is targeted to the superior colliculus. As a result of these studies, research in the field of neural repair became directed to studying the role of growth-inhibitory molecules associated with oligodendrocyte myelin in suppressing axon regeneration in the CNS (Bandtlow *et al.*, 1990). However, in 1996, Berry *et al.* (1996) reported that simply implanting a fragment of peripheral nerve into the posterior chamber of the eye was sufficient to stimulate extensive axon regeneration through the inhibitory environment of the optic nerve itself. This finding suggested that the main effects of a peripheral nerve graft could be due to Schwann-cell-derived neurotrophic factors. However, the grafts also contained numerous infiltrative cells that could have played a role, which was confirmed in our laboratory a few years later. At the time, we were investigating the molecules that "prime" injured RGCs of lower vertebrates to switch into an active growth state (Schwalb *et al.*, 1995) and tested whether a candidate factor from those studies might account for the proregenerative effects of intravitreal peripheral nerve grafts. Inadvertently, we found that any manipulation that caused intraocular inflammation stimulated appreciable regeneration, whether it was injury to the lens, implanting a peripheral nerve graft, or injecting the yeast cell-wall preparation Zymosan (Fig. 12.1a and 12.1b) (Leon *et al.*, 2000). Intraocular inflammation caused RGCs to undergo dramatic changes in the expression of growth-associated protein-43 (GAP-43), small proline-rich protein 1 (SPRR1), activating transcription factor 3 (ATF-3), and other genes related to axon growth, in a pattern strongly resembling that seen in dorsal root ganglia neurons undergoing axon regeneration after peripheral nerve injury (Fischer *et al.*, 2004b).

We found that the proregenerative effects of intraocular inflammation could not be mimicked by any well-established trophic factor and identified the primary mediator of this phenomenon as oncomodulin (Ocm), a small calcium-binding protein (Yin *et al.*, 2006). Macrophages have long been known to play a major role in regeneration after injury (Lotan and Schwartz, 1994).

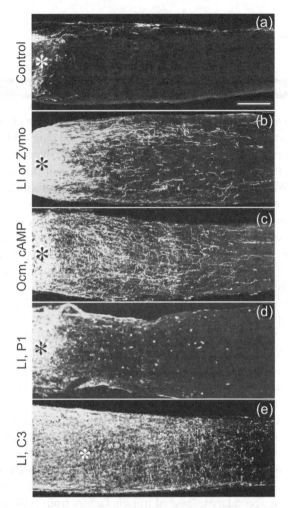

Figure 12.1 Inflammation and oncomodulin (Ocm) induce axon regeneration in the optic nerve. Longitudinal sections are stained with an antibody to the growth-associated protein GAP-43 to visualize axons regenerating beyond the injury site (asterisk) 2 weeks after nerve injury. (a) Absence of regenerating axons in negative controls receiving no further treatments. (b) Induction of inflammation by either lens injury (LI) or Zymosan (Zym) promotes extensive regeneration. (c) Slow release of Ocm and a cAMP analog from polymeric beads fully mimics the effects of Zymosan. (d, e) Regeneration induced by LI is nearly eliminated by intraocular injections of P1, a peptide antagonist based on the N-terminal of Ocm (d) but not by a control peptide (C3). Scale bar in all figs: 250 μm.

David *et al.* (1990) showed that macrophages can act on the inhibitory CNS white matter to enhance axon growth, and Schwartz and colleagues reported that transplantation of macrophages preincubated *ex vivo* with segments of a sciatic nerve could promote axon regeneration in the injured rat optic nerve (Lazarov-Spiegler *et al.*, 1996). Others have subsequently reported on the roles of immune cell toll-like pattern recognition receptors (TLR) and their effectors, as well as various cytokines and downstream molecules, in regulating the effects of inflammation in promoting regeneration after optic nerve injury (Zheng *et al.*, 2012; Wu *et al.*, 2013). Possible cross-talk in downstream pathways and synergistic effects of manipulating Ocm, TLRs, and specific cytokine pathways may be fruitful areas for future research.

Effects of Inflammation on RGC Survival and Optic Nerve Regeneration

The interactions between the immune system and the nervous system after injury are extensive and involve positive and negative effects on CNS protection and repair (Donnelly and Popovich, 2008; Benowitz and Popovich, 2011). Under some circumstances, the immune response can clear cellular debris and limit neuronal degeneration (Montgomery and Bowers, 2012), protect from infections (Greenlee-Wacker et al., 2014), and contribute to neuroprotection and CNS repair (David et al., 1990; Schwartz, 2001; Kerschensteiner et al., 2009). However, the immune response can also result in neurotoxicity, in part by secreting proinflammatory cytokines (Dirnagl et al., 1999; Lucas et al., 2006; Ransohoff, 2009). These varying effects reflect the cellular and molecular complexity of the immune response after CNS injury, which involves the recruitment of resident innate immune cells to the injury site, infiltration of immune cells from the blood, and the activation of adaptive immune response.

The immune response after a lens injury or an intravitreal injection of Zymosan similarly involves both beneficial and deleterious effects. Proinflammatory molecules such as endothelins, tumor necrosis factor alpha (TNF-α), and nitric oxide are secreted by macrophages and reactive astrocytes and are toxic to RGC, whereas attenuation of neuroinflammation, for example, by blocking endothelin-B receptors, can rescue RGCs (Tonari et al., 2012). On the other hand, the net effect of inducing an inflammatory response in the eye is to enhance RGC survival and axon regeneration following optic nerve injury (Leon et al., 2000). However, inflammation within the optic nerve per se can be neuroprotective without promoting axon regeneration (Ahmed et al., 2010). The dissociation between the effects of intraocular and optic nerve inflammation suggests that different immune-derived molecules may mediate the effects of inflammation on RGC survival and axon regeneration, or that different molecules are expressed by inflammatory cells in the environment of the optic nerve versus posterior chamber of the eye, or that intraocular inflammation triggers the secondary release of trophic factors from cells in the retina.

Toll-like pattern recognition receptors (TLRs) are expressed on microglia and macrophages and play a role in the activation of the innate immune system in the CNS. The TLR2 agonist Pam3Cys promotes axon regeneration after optic nerve injury (Hauk et al., 2009), presumably by enhancing inflammation. Regeneration can also be increased somewhat by genetic deletion of a downstream intracellular effector of TLR3 that is expressed in microglia, TIR-domain-containing adapter-inducing interferon-β (TRIF) (Lin et al., 2012). Genetic deletion of TLR4 and TLR2 delays the recruitment of macrophages and clearance of myelin debris, which impairs regeneration after peripheral nerve injury (Wu et al., 2013). TLR4 is also one of the mediators of inflammation after optic nerve injury in mice, although its role in optic nerve regeneration per se remains to be investigated (Zheng et al., 2012).

Cells of the innate immune system also participate in synaptic pruning and in glaucoma. A key mediator of the complement cascade, C1q, marks inappropriate or inactive synapses in the dorsal lateral geniculate nucleus for pruning by microglia during retinal development (Stevens et al., 2007; Schafer et al., 2012). In a mouse model of glaucoma, C1qa is upregulated in the inner plexiform layer of the retina and may contribute to the loss of RGCs, perhaps by the removal of synaptic inputs that are important for maintaining cell viability (Stevens *et al.*, 2007). In addition, microglia infiltrate the optic nerve head at an early stage of the disease, and genetic deletion of C1qa decreases glaucomatous damage to the optic nerve and retina (Howell *et al.*, 2011), as does deleting components of the complement receptor (Nakazawa *et al.*, 2006). The chemokine TNF-α plays a central role in this phenomenon, and deleting the gene for TNF-α or blocking its activity (with a neutralizing antibody or with Etanercept) suppresses microglial activity and attenuates RGC death despite a persistently elevated intraocular pressure (Nakazawa *et al.*, 2006; Roh *et al.*, 2012). The role of complement and microglia in the CNS after injury is an area of active investigation, and its role in traumatic and ischemic optic neuropathies remains to be investigated.

Macrophages infiltrate the site of optic nerve injury and contribute to growth cone dynamics by virtue of EphB3, which is expressed on their cell surface (Liu *et al.*, 2006). Injured RGC terminals express the cognate ligand EphrinB3, which interacts with macrophage EphB3 and stimulates local axonal sprouting (Liu *et al.*, 2006). However, EphrinB3 is also expressed by oligodendrocytes, which inhibit axonal sprouting (Benson *et al.*, 2005), and contributes to the inhibitory effects of myelin (Duffy *et al.*, 2012). Thus, infiltrating macrophages can both promote and inhibit axonal sprouting through EphB3, depending on whether they act on EphrinB3 in axonal terminals or on oligodendrocytes, respectively. Application of the macrophage-recruiting cytokine GM-CSF (granulocyte-macrophage colony-stimulating factor) directly to the ischemically injured optic nerve was not neuroprotective and did not promote axon regeneration, despite increased macrophage activation and recruitment. This study suggests that macrophages may not be the key cell type that mediates the beneficial effects of inflammation, or that macrophages' neuroprotective effects are manifested primarily when they are activated within the environment of the posterior chamber, or that traumatic and ischemic injuries respond differently to macrophage activation (Slater *et al.*, 2013).

Oncomodulin as a Key Mediator of Inflammation-Induced Regeneration

Intraocular inflammation leads to a massive influx of neutrophils and macrophages into the eye, suggesting that one or both of these cell types may be the source of the trophic factor(s) that stimulates axon regeneration after optic nerve injury. Earlier work from our laboratory had shown that mannose, which is abundant in the normal vitreous, stimulates a modest amount of axon outgrowth in dissociated RGCs in culture provided cyclic adenosine monophosphate (cAMP) levels are elevated (Li *et al.*, 2003). The addition of secreted proteins from a macrophage cell line (macrophage-conditioned media, MCM) augmented this outgrowth to a greater extent than any of the classic trophic factors previously reported to act on RGCs [e.g., ciliary neurotrophic factor (CNTF), brain-derived neurotrophic factor (BDNF), basic fibroblast growth factor (bFGF), glial-cell-line-derived neurotrophic factor (GDNF)] (Yin *et al.*, 2003). Chromatographic separation of MCM yielded many high-molecular weight fractions that were toxic to RGCs and a low-molecular weight fraction with high axon-promoting activity. This latter fraction contained a protein that was identified by mass spectrometry as Ocm. Ocm is a small calcium-binding protein that is related to α-parvalbumin, though not to other well-established trophic factors (Yin *et al.*, 2003). Binding assays revealed that Ocm binds to a high-affinity receptor on RGCs in a cAMP-dependent manner ($k_D = 28$ nM) and stimulates lengthy outgrowth at 1/10 this concentration. The requirement for cAMP appears to be due to the translocation of an as-yet unidentified Ocm receptor to the cell surface; the requirement for mannose is not yet understood. In the presence of mannose and forskolin (to elevate intracellular cAMP), recombinant Ocm was as effective as complete MCM in enhancing axon outgrowth from RGCs, while conversely, immunodepletion of Ocm eliminated the activity of MCM (Yin et al., 2006, 2009). In vivo studies also point to Ocm as the principle axon-promoting factor associated with intraocular inflammation. Within 24 h of either injuring the lens or injecting Zymosan into the eye, levels of Ocm mRNA and protein increase dramatically due to the entry of neutrophils and macrophages into the vitreous (Yin et al., 2006, 2009); at the same time, levels of the protein increase many fold in the ganglion cell layer and inner plexiform layer of the retina, containing the somata and dendrites of RGCs, respectively (Fig. 12.2) (Yin et al., 2006, 2009). In gain-of-function studies, slow release of Ocm plus a cAMP analog from polymeric beads induced nearly as much axon regeneration in the rat optic nerve as intraocular inflammation (Fig. 12.1c), whereas either a peptide antagonist of Ocm (P1) or a neutralizing antibody strongly suppressed inflammation-induced regeneration (Fig. 12.1d and 12.1e) (Yin et al., 2006, 2009).

Our initial use of a macrophage cell line to isolate Ocm, combined with the vesicular localization of Ocm in macrophages in vivo (Yin et al., 2006), initially led us to believe that macrophages represent the principal source of the protein. However, levels of Ocm mRNA peak within a day of injecting Zymosan into the eye and then decline (Yin et al., 2009), a time-course that is discrepant with the slow accumulation of macrophages that occurs over the first week. This discordance suggested that Ocm could be associated with neutrophils, the first responders of the innate immune system. This idea was confirmed by immunocytochemistry, reverse transcription polymerase chain reaction (RT-PCR), and flow cytometry. Numerous cells enter the posterior chamber of the eye within 12 h of injecting Zymosan and express high levels of Gr-1, which is characteristic of neutrophils, whereas only a few cells express the macrophage marker F4/80 (Fig. 12.2a and 12.2b) (Kurimoto et al., 2013). These results were confirmed by flow cytometry. Neutrophils express high levels of Ocm mRNA and protein at 12 h. Intracellular Ocm staining decreases by 24 h and is barely detectable at 72 h (Fig. 12.2a and 12.2b), consistent with the protein being secreted and accumulating in the retina, where it binds to a cell-surface receptor on RGCs in a cAMP-dependent manner (Yin et al., 2006, 2009; Kurimoto et al., 2010). Immune depletion of neutrophils, such as use of a peptide antagonist of Ocm, diminished most of the proregenerative effect of Zymosan (Kurimoto et al., 2013). Depletion of neutrophils did not interfere with the delayed entry of macrophages, which also express Ocm mRNA and protein. This finding suggests that although neutrophils and macrophages both express Ocm, neutrophils represent the more biologically important source for regeneration, presumably because of their rapid entry in large numbers. Although the residual macrophage response seen after depleting neutrophils may not be sufficient for extensive regeneration, it may still contribute to maintaining modest levels of Ocm and the continued stimulation of RGCs within the first few days after inducing an inflammatory response.

One group has argued that neither inflammation nor Ocm plays a role in mediating the effects of lens injury on regeneration (Hauk et al., 2008), but their study was highly problematic. The authors of that study reported that a commercial anti-Ocm antibody did not suppress the effect of lens injury on optic nerve regeneration, but they did not test whether the antibody was capable of neutralizing the protein; as noted previously, our experiments nearly eliminated regeneration using a validated neutralizing anti-Ocm antibody (Yin *et al.*, 2009). Their study reported that clodronate liposomes injected systemically or intraocularly did not eliminate the effects of lens injury on axon regeneration, but the liposome injections only had a partial effect on macrophage depletion and unknown effects on intraocular Ocm levels or neutrophils, the primary mediators of inflammation-induced regeneration.

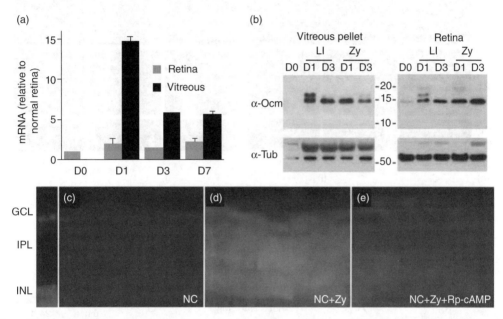

Figure 12.2   Oncomodulin expression in inflammatory cells. (a) Ocm mRNA in cells of the retina (light gray bar) and in cells that infiltrate the posterior chamber of the eye (black bar) following intraocular injection of Zymosan. mRNA levels were determined by quantitative polymerase chain reaction (qPCR) and then normalized by levels of 18S RNA and then to normalized levels in the control retina. While expression in the retina does not change appreciably, infiltrative cells express high levels of Ocm. (b) Western blots show increases in Ocm in infiltrative cells collected from the posterior chamber (left panel) and within the retina (right panel) after either lens injury (LI) or Zymosan injections (Zy). Bottom panels: loading controls, stained for α-Tubulin. (c–e). Immunostaining shows near-absence of Ocm in the untreated retina after optic nerve crush (NC) but high levels 1 day after NC combined with intraocular Zymosan injection (NC, Zy). Levels are diminished by co-injection of the cAMP antagonist Rp-cAMP, which prevents Ocm from binding to its receptor. (f) Most of the cells present in the vitreous 12 h after intraocular Zymosan are neutrophils [Gr-1^{high}: compare to 4′,6-diamidino-2-phenylindole (DAPI)] that express high levels of Ocm. However, Ocm levels within Gr-1^{high} cells (*arrows* at 72 h) decline over time (*arrowheads* at 72 h). Note increasing appearance of Gr-1^{low} cells over time that also express Ocm. (g) Macrophages (F4/80^{high}) cells (*arrows*) represent a relatively small percentage of the cells in the vitreous at 12 and 24 h (compare F4/80 staining with DAPI) and express high levels of Ocm (*arrowheads*). Relative frequency of these cells increases at 72 h. Unlike neutrophils, Ocm levels remain high in macrophages, perhaps due to continuous expression or recruitment of new cells. Scale bar: 10 μm. (h) The morphology of cells extracted from the vitreous at 24 h shows the typical lobulated nuclei of Gr-1^{high} neutrophils, whereas F4/80^{high} macrophages show large, round nuclei. (i) Ocm mRNA expression (normalized by 18S RNA) in FACS-sorted Gr-1^{high}/F4/80^{low} cells (neutrophils, N) and F4/80^{high} cells (macrophages, M) 24 h after Zymosan injection is many times that of the retina. *$p < 0.05$, ***$p < 0.001$ relative to the retina (Ret). (j) While almost all Gr-1^{high} cells express detectable levels of Ocm 6 h, levels diminish at 24 h; at the same time, the number of Gr-1^{low} cells, presumably macrophages, increases and these express Ocm. *Source*: From Kurimoto *et al.* (2013), with permission from Society for NeuroScience. (*See insert for color representation of this figure.*)

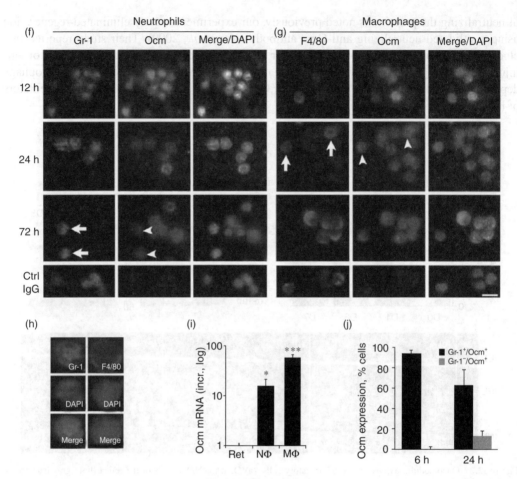

Figure 12.2 *Continued.*

Although neutrophil depletion in our studies decreased Zymosan-induced regeneration substantially, it did not eliminate it altogether (Kurimoto *et al.*, 2010), perhaps because of residual neutrophils or macrophages or other cell types. One group has proposed that factors secreted by retinal glia contribute to the regeneration seen after intraocular inflammation (Lorber *et al.*, 2009), and several lines of evidence suggest that other immune cells can also have an effect. Neonatal thymectomy, which depletes T-cells, enhances RGC survival after optic nerve injury (Luo *et al.*, 2007). On the other hand, systemic injection of T-cells pre-exposed to myelin basic protein was reported to increase T-cell accumulation at the optic nerve injury site and protect RGCs and the optic nerve by reducing secondary damage (Moalem *et al.*, 1999). In normal rats that are resistant to autoimmune disease, pharmacological immunosuppression improved RGC survival and axon regeneration following optic nerve transection and peripheral nerve grafting, whereas this effect was not seen in Lewis rats that are vulnerable to autoimmune disease (Cui *et al.*, 2007).

Neutrophil infiltration has been reported to have a beneficial effect after spinal cord injury, as immune depletion of these cells impairs the healing process and neurological outcome (Stirling *et al.*, 2009). On the other hand, there is evidence that neutrophils exert a detrimental effect in secondary CNS damage, which occurs at a later stage of immune response (Souza-Rodrigues *et al.*, 2008). In the case of peripheral nerve injury, immune depletion of neutrophils does not affect the ability of dorsal root sensory neurons to regenerate their axons (Nadeau *et al.*, 2011), whereas suppressing the macrophage response strongly suppresses regeneration (Barrette *et al.*, 2008; Kwon *et al.*, 2013). In addition to their presence at the site of nerve damage, macrophages infiltrate dorsal root ganglia after a peripheral nerve lesion, and depletion of these cells specifically at this site suppresses the conditioning lesion effect, that is, the ability of dorsal root ganglion (DRG) neurons to regenerate their centrally directed axon branch through the dorsal root after injury to the peripheral branch. Conversely, local induction of an inflammatory response within DRG is a sufficient stimulus to promote axon regeneration through a dorsal root (Lu and Richardson, 1991; Steinmetz *et al.*, 2005). The ability of macrophages to stimulate neurite outgrowth from DRG neurons can also be seen in culture, and immune depletion of Ocm but not other trophic factors eliminates the axon-promoting effects of macrophages (Kwon *et al.*, 2013). This finding accords with earlier studies showing that Ocm has strong neurite-promoting effects on DRG neurons in culture (Yin *et al.*, 2006) and a moderate effect in stimulating dorsal root regeneration when injected into the DRG (Harel *et al.*, 2012). The proregenerative effect of a conditioning lesion and macrophage accumulation are also suppressed by genetic deletion of the receptor for the chemokine CCR2, which is secreted by macrophages (Niemi *et al.*, 2013). Together, these studies point to a major role of the innate immune response in stimulating axon regeneration in the optic nerve and peripheral nerves, although the most important cell types appears to differ in the two systems. In addition, Ocm may play a role in both CNS and PNS repair.

Depletion of either neutrophils or just Ocm alone suppresses the effect of intraocular inflammation on axon regeneration but does not diminish its effects on RGC survival (Kurimoto *et al.*, 2010). One possibility is that other trophic factors associated with inflammation, such as leukemia inhibitory factor (LIF) and/or CNTF could be important in this regard (Leibinger *et al.*, 2009), as well as a yet-to-be identified factor(s) that lead to cAMP elevation within RGCs (Yin *et al.*, 2006). The existence of such a factor can be inferred from the fact that intraocular inflammation results in strong Ocm binding in the retina, which is dependent on cAMP (Fig. 12.2d–12.2f) (Kurimoto *et al.*, 2010). Others have suggested that proinflammatory agents cause CNTF to be secreted from retinal astrocytes and act as the primary mediator of optic nerve regeneration (Muller *et al.*, 2007), but this appears unlikely in view of many studies that demonstrate that intraocularly injected CNTF has only a minor effect on axon regeneration in the mature visual system due to the developmental increase in expression of SOCS3, a suppressor of signaling through the Janus kinase (Jak)– signal transducers and activators of transcription (STAT) pathway (Cohen *et al.*, 1994; Park *et al.*, 2009; Smith *et al.*, 2009; Qin *et al.*, 2013). In one study in which high concentrations of CNTF were found to promote axon regeneration through a peripheral nerve graft, this effect was found to be secondary to the effect of CNTF in recruiting macrophages (Cen *et al.*, 2007), but this issue has not been examined in other studies in which high intravitreal concentrations of CNTF or virally delivered CNTF was found to have some effect (Leaver *et al.*, 2006; Pernet *et al.*, 2013b). Another argument against CNTF or any other trophic factor playing a major role in mediating the effects of inflammation on optic nerve regeneration is the near-complete loss of regeneration seen when the effects of Ocm are blocked (Yin *et al.*, 2009; Kurimoto *et al.*, 2013). However, it remains possible that one or more other factors can bolster the effects of Ocm. The chemokine SDF-1 is also upregulated following intraocular inflammation and augments the effects of zymosan *in vivo* (Y. Yin, Y.Q. Li, L.P. Cen, L. Benowitz, unpublished observations; Heskamp *et al.*, 2013). Unlike Ocm or CNTF, BDNF promotes RGC survival but simultaneously blocks inflammation-induced axon regeneration (Pernet and Di Polo, 2006). Although the basis for this observation remains unknown, it illustrates the dissociation between cell-signaling pathways that lead to cell survival and axon regeneration (Weibel *et al.*, 1995; Malik *et al.*, 2005; Monnier *et al.*, 2011). Blocking the kinase activity of, or deleting the gene for, dual-leucine zipper kinase (DLK) similarly attenuates the death of injured RGCs while blocking regeneration induced by *pten* gene deletion (Watkins *et al.*, 2013). In addition, Bcl-2 overexpression (Chierzi *et al.*, 1999) or inhibition of the unfolded protein response (Hu *et al.*, 2012) promotes RGC survival without affecting regeneration. Thus, the development of therapies to treat optic nerve injury may require separate treatments to target RGC survival and axon regeneration.

Synergistic Effects of Combinatorial Treatments

The effects of Ocm on axon outgrowth involve the activation of several signal transduction pathways. Although pharmacological inhibition of the mitogen-activated protein kinases (MAPK), PI3 kinase, or Jak–STAT signaling pathway alone does not suppress the effects of Ocm on RGC outgrowth, inhibiting all three fully blocks its effects (Yin *et al.*, 2006). Yet, while these results suggest that several pathways need to be active in parallel, they do not tell us whether Ocm actually activates these pathways, nor whether one or more must simply be constitutively active for Ocm to have an effect, nor whether these pathways are only partially activated by Ocm or whether fuller activation would enhance regeneration further. Deleting the gene for *pten* in RGCs de-represses the PI3 kinase–Akt pathway and is sufficient to induce appreciable regeneration (Park *et al.*, 2008). Combining *pten* deletion with Zymosan and a cAMP analog has a strongly synergistic effect (Kurimoto *et al.*, 2010), and by 10–12 weeks, this combination enables some RGCs to regenerate axons the full length of the optic nerve, across the optic chiasm, and on into appropriate central target areas, where they form synapses and partially restore simple visual responses (Fig. 12.3) (de Lima *et al.*, 2012). Many of these axons become myelinated (de Lima *et al.*, 2012). As noted previously, deletion of *socs3* de-represses the Jak–STAT pathway and enables RGCs to respond to CNTF (Smith *et al.*, 2009), and dual deletion of *pten* and *socs3* combined with CNTF also has a strongly synergistic effect (Sun *et al.*, 2012). However, in this case, axons did not cross the chiasm readily. Axonal misguidance or inability to overcome growth-inhibitory signals may partially explain why few axons crossed the chiasm or navigated to their proper destinations in another study that attempted to replicate our work but failed to transect the contralateral intact optic nerve (Luo *et al.*, 2013; Pernet *et al.*, 2013a, 2013b).

Intraocular inflammation also has synergistic effects with treatments that neutralize cell-extrinsic inhibitors of axon growth. The three isoforms of the NgR act as receptors for myelin-associated suppressors of axon growth and/or chondroitin sulfate proteoglycans, and either genetic deletion of these receptors or expression of a dominant-negative form of NgR synergistically enhances the effect of intraocular inflammation, as does expression of a bacterial

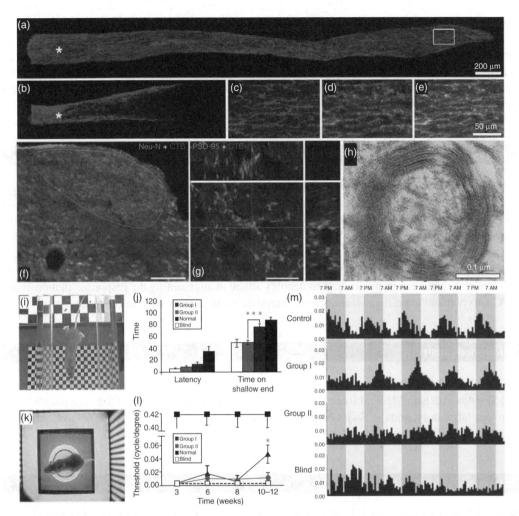

Figure 12.3 Long-distance regeneration, target reinnervation, and partial recovery of vision. (a, b) Regenerating axons 10–12 weeks after optic nerve injury visualized using the anterograde tracer cholera toxin B-fragment (CTB, red). Axons extend the full length of the optic nerve in mice treated with Zymosan, CPT-cAMP, and *pten* gene deletion (Group I) but only part-way in mice receiving similar treatment but without *pten* deletion (Group II). (c–e) Region in the white rectangle of panel(a) double-labeled for CTB and GAP-43. (f) Reinnervation of the lateral geniculate nucleus (DLGN). CTB+ fibers (red) in the DLGN contralateral to the regenerating optic nerve in a Group I mouse. Counterstaining for the neuronal protein NeuN shows CTB+ fibers to be confined to the neuropil of the DLG (dotted line). (g) Preliminary evidence for synapse formation: apposition of CTB+ terminals and PSD-95-positive structures. Side panels show z-stacks of images in the orthogonal planes. Scale bars in (f) and (g), 100 μm. (h) Electron micrographic image showing remyelination of a regenerating axon. (i–m). Partial recovery of visually guided behaviors. (i) Top-down view of visual cliff apparatus. (j) Average latency to step off shallow end (left) and total time spent on shallow end (right). **$P < 0.01$; n.s., not significant. (k) Top-down view of apparatus used to evaluate optomotor response (OMR). (l) Average OMR (response threshold, cycles/degree) as a function of time. Mice in Group I show partial recovery; y-axis in h and i are discontinuous. (m) Circadian photoentrainment: percent of overall activity in 1-h bins (group averages). Mice were maintained on a continuous cycle of lights on at 7 AM and off at 7 PM before testing and for the first 2.5 days in the activity monitor. The light cycle was set back 6 h on day 3. Note entrainment of circadian activity to ambient day–night cycle in Group I, though with a phase shift of approximately 8 h compared to normal mice. Activity in Group II (incomplete regeneration) is asynchronous and resembles blind mice. Error bars: S.E.M. *Source*: From de Lima *et al.* (2012), with permission from PNAS. (*See insert for color representation of this figure.*)

enzyme that inactivates RhoA, a downstream effector of NgR and other cell-extrinsic suppressors of axon growth (Fischer *et al.*, 2004a, 2004b; Dickendesher *et al.*, 2012; Wang *et al.*, 2012). It remains to be determined whether counteracting cell-extrinsic suppressors of axon growth or deleting *socs3* would further augment the regeneration obtained by combining Zymosan with a cAMP analog and *pten* deletion. In addition, it is likely that other major suppressors of axon growth remain to be discovered.

Conclusions

Induction of an inflammatory response following optic nerve injury elicits beneficial and detrimental effects. Some of the components of the inflammatory response have the potential to enhance RGC survival and promote axon regeneration, while other components could lead to secondary damage and RGC death. Future investigations may help identify additional molecules and signaling pathways, enabling us to eventually alter the balance between beneficial and deleterious factors and improve outcome beyond current levels. Ultimately, we expect that this research will lead to selective manipulation of molecules aimed at augmenting the responses that promote RGC survival and axon regeneration while inactivating mediators of cytotoxicity.

Acknowledgments

We are grateful for the support of the National Eye Institute (EY05690 to L.B.), the Dr. Miriam and Sheldon Adelson Medical Research Foundation (to L.B.) for support of the original research from our laboratory, and the Swiss National Science Foundation (PBBEP3-146099 to L.A.). The authors declare that they do not have competing financial interest.

References

Aguayo, A.J., Rasminsky, M., Bray, G.M. *et al.* (1991) Degenerative and regenerative responses of injured neurons in the central nervous system of adult mammals. *Philosophical Transactions of the Royal Society B: Biological Sciences*, **331**, 337–343.

Ahmed, Z., Aslam, M., Lorber, B., Suggate, E.L., Berry, M. & Logan, A. (2010) Optic nerve and vitreal inflammation are both RGC neuroprotective but only the latter is RGC axogenic. *Neurobiology of Disease*, **37**, 441–454.

Arregui, C.O., Carbonetto, S. & McKerracher, L. (1994) Characterization of neural cell adhesion sites: Point contacts are the sites of interaction between integrins and the cytoskeleton in PC12 cells. *Journal of Neuroscience*, **14**, 6967–6977.

Bandtlow, C., Zachleder, T. & Schwab, M.E. (1990) Oligodendrocytes arrest neurite growth by contact inhibition. *Journal of Neuroscience*, **10**, 3837–3848.

Barrette, B., Hebert, M.A., Filali, M. *et al.* (2008) Requirement of myeloid cells for axon regeneration. *Journal of Neuroscience*, **28**, 9363–9376.

Benowitz, L. & Yin, Y. (2008) Rewiring the injured CNS: Lessons from the optic nerve. *Experimental Neurology*, **209**, 389–398.

Benowitz, L.I. & Popovich, P.G. (2011) Inflammation and axon regeneration. *Current Opinion In Neurology*, **24**, 577–583.

Benson, M.D., Romero, M.I., Lush, M.E., Lu, Q.R., Henkemeyer, M. & Parada, L.F. (2005) Ephrin-B3 is a myelin-based inhibitor of neurite outgrowth. *Proceedings of the National Academy of Sciences of the United States of America*, **102**, 10694–10699.

Berkelaar, M., Clarke, D.B., Wang, Y.C., Bray, G.M. & Aguayo, A.J. (1994) Axotomy results in delayed death and apoptosis of retinal ganglion cells in adult rats. *Journal of Neuroscience*, **14**, 4368–4374.

Berry, M., Carlile, J. & Hunter, A. (1996) Peripheral nerve explants grafted into the vitreous body of the eye promote the regeneration of retinal ganglion cell axons severed in the optic nerve. *Journal of Neurocytology*, **25**, 147–170.

Cen, L.P., Luo, J.M., Zhang, C.W. *et al.* (2007) Chemotactic effect of ciliary neurotrophic factor on macrophages in retinal ganglion cell survival and axonal regeneration. *Investigative Ophthalmology & Visual Science*, **48**, 4257–4266.

Chen, M.S., Huber, A.B., van der Haar, M.E. *et al.* (2000) Nogo-A is a myelin-associated neurite outgrowth inhibitor and an antigen for monoclonal antibody IN-1. *Nature*, **403**, 434–439.

Chierzi, S., Strettoi, E., Cenni, M.C. & Maffei, L. (1999) Optic nerve crush: Axonal responses in wild-type and bcl-2 transgenic mice. *Journal of Neuroscience*, **19**, 8367–8376.

Cohen, A., Bray, G.M. & Aguayo, A.J. (1994) Neurotrophin-4/5 (NT-4/5) increases adult rat retinal ganglion cell survival and neurite outgrowth in vitro. *Journal of Neurobiology*, **25**, 953–959.

Cui, Q., Hodgetts, S.I., Hu, Y., Luo, J.M. & Harvey, A.R. (2007) Strain-specific differences in the effects of cyclosporin A and FK506 on the survival and regeneration of axotomized retinal ganglion cells in adult rats. *Neuroscience*, **146**, 986–999.

David, S., Bouchard, C., Tsatas, O. & Giftochristos, N. (1990) Macrophages can modify the nonpermissive nature of the adult mammalian central nervous system. *Neuron*, **5**, 463–469.

de Lima, S., Koriyama, Y., Kurimoto, T. *et al.* (2012) Full-length axon regeneration in the adult mouse optic nerve and partial recovery of simple visual behaviors. *Proceedings of the National Academy of Sciences of the United States of America*, **109**, 9149–9154.

Dickendesher, T.L., Baldwin, K.T., Mironova, Y.A. *et al.* (2012) NgR1 and NgR3 are receptors for chondroitin sulfate proteoglycans. *Nature Neuroscience*, **15**, 703–712.

Dirnagl, U., Iadecola, C. & Moskowitz, M.A. (1999) Pathobiology of ischaemic stroke: An integrated view. *Trends in Neurosciences*, **22**, 391–397.

Donnelly, D.J. & Popovich, P.G. (2008) Inflammation and its role in neuroprotection, axonal regeneration and functional recovery after spinal cord injury. *Experimental Neurology*, **209**, 378–388.

Duffy, P., Wang, X., Siegel, C.S. *et al.* (2012) Myelin-derived ephrinB3 restricts axonal regeneration and recovery after adult CNS injury. *Proceedings of the National Academy of Sciences of the United States of America*, **109**, 5063–5068.

Fischer, D., He, Z. & Benowitz, L.I. (2004a) Counteracting the Nogo receptor enhances optic nerve regeneration if retinal ganglion cells are in an active growth state. *Journal of Neuroscience*, **24**, 1646–1651.

Fischer, D., Petkova, V., Thanos, S. & Benowitz, L.I. (2004b) Switching mature retinal ganglion cells to a robust growth state in vivo: Gene expression and synergy with RhoA inactivation. *Journal of Neuroscience*, **24**, 8726–8740.

Fisher, D., Xing, B., Dill, J. *et al.* (2011) Leukocyte common antigen-related phosphatase is a functional receptor for chondroitin sulfate proteoglycan axon growth inhibitors. *Journal of Neuroscience*, **31**, 14051–14066.

Fournier, A.E., GrandPre, T. & Strittmatter, S.M. (2001) Identification of a receptor mediating Nogo-66 inhibition of axonal regeneration. *Nature*, **409**, 341–346.

Gaub, P., Joshi, Y., Wuttke, A. *et al.* (2011) The histone acetyltransferase p300 promotes intrinsic axonal regeneration. *Brain*, **134**, 2134–2148.

Goldberg, J.L., Klassen, M.P., Hua, Y. & Barres, B.A. (2002) Amacrine-signaled loss of intrinsic axon growth ability by retinal ganglion cells. *Science*, **296**, 1860–1864.

Greenlee-Wacker, M.C., Rigby, K.M., Kobayashi, S.D., Porter, A.R., Deleo, F.R. & Nauseef, W.M. (2014) Phagocytosis of *Staphylococcus aureus* by human neutrophils prevents macrophage efferocytosis and induces programmed necrosis. *Journal of Immunology*, **192**, 4709–4717.

Harel, N.Y. & Strittmatter, S.M. (2006) Can regenerating axons recapitulate developmental guidance during recovery from spinal cord injury? *Nature Reviews Neuroscience*, **7**, 603–616.

Harel, R., Iannotti, C.A., Hoh, D., Clark, M., Silver, J. & Steinmetz, M.P. (2012) Oncomodulin affords limited regeneration to injured sensory axons in vitro and in vivo. *Experimental Neurology*, **233**, 708–716.

Hauk, T.G., Muller, A., Lee, J., Schwendener, R. & Fischer, D. (2008) Neuroprotective and axon growth promoting effects of intraocular inflammation do not depend on oncomodulin or the presence of large numbers of activated macrophages. *Experimental Neurology*, **209**, 469–482.

Hauk, T.G., Leibinger, M., Muller, A., Andreadaki, N., Knippschild, U. & Fischer, D. (2009) Intravitreal application of the Toll-like receptor 2 agonist Pam3Cys stimulates axon regeneration in the mature optic nerve. *Investigative Ophthalmology & Visual Science*, **51**, 459–464.

Heskamp, A., Leibinger, M., Andreadaki, A., Gobrecht, P., Diekmann, H. & Fischer, D. (2013) CXCL12/SDF-1 facilitates optic nerve regeneration. *Neurobiology of Disease*, **55**, 76–86.

Howell, G.R., Macalinao, D.G., Sousa, G.L. *et al.* (2011) Molecular clustering identifies complement and endothelin induction as early events in a mouse model of glaucoma. *Journal of Clinical Investigation*, **121**, 1429–1444.

Hsieh, S.H., Ferraro, G.B. & Fournier, A.E. (2006) Myelin-associated inhibitors regulate cofilin phosphorylation and neuronal inhibition through LIM kinase and Slingshot phosphatase. *Journal of Neuroscience*, **26**, 1006–1015.

Hu, Y., Park, K.K., Yang, L. *et al.* (2012) Differential effects of unfolded protein response pathways on axon injury-induced death of retinal ganglion cells. *Neuron*, **73**, 445–452.

Kerschensteiner, M., Meinl, E. & Hohlfeld, R. (2009) Neuro-immune crosstalk in CNS diseases. *Neuroscience*, **158**, 1122–1132.

Kurimoto, T., Yin, Y., Habboub, G. *et al.* (2013) Neutrophils express oncomodulin and promote optic nerve regeneration. *Journal of Neuroscience*, **33**, 14816–14824.

Kurimoto, T., Yin, Y., Omura, K. *et al.* (2010) Long-distance axon regeneration in the mature optic nerve: Contributions of oncomodulin, cAMP, and pten gene deletion. *Journal of Neuroscience*, **30**, 15654–15663.

Kwon, M.J., Kim, J., Shin, H. *et al.* (2013) Contribution of macrophages to enhanced regenerative capacity of dorsal root ganglia sensory neurons by conditioning injury. *Journal of Neuroscience*, **33**, 15095–15108.

Lazarov-Spiegler, O., Solomon, A.S., Zeev-Brann, A.B., Hirschberg, D.L., Lavie, V. & Schwartz, M. (1996) Transplantation of activated macrophages overcomes central nervous system regrowth failure. *FASEB Journal*, **10**, 1296–1302.

Leaver, S.G., Cui, Q., Bernard, O. & Harvey, A.R. (2006) Cooperative effects of bcl-2 and AAV-mediated expression of CNTF on retinal ganglion cell survival and axonal regeneration in adult transgenic mice. *European Journal of Neuroscience*, **24**, 3323–3332.

Leibinger, M., Muller, A., Andreadaki, A., Hauk, T.G., Kirsch, M. & Fischer, D. (2009) Neuroprotective and axon growth-promoting effects following inflammatory stimulation on mature retinal ganglion cells in mice depend on ciliary neurotrophic factor and leukemia inhibitory factor. *Journal of Neuroscience*, **29**, 14334–14341.

Leon, S., Yin, Y., Nguyen, J., Irwin, N. & Benowitz, L.I. (2000) Lens injury stimulates axon regeneration in the mature rat optic nerve. *Journal of Neuroscience*, **20**, 4615–4626.

Li, Y., Irwin, N., Yin, Y., Lanser, M. & Benowitz, L.I. (2003) Axon regeneration in goldfish and rat retinal ganglion cells: Differential responsiveness to carbohydrates and cAMP. *Journal of Neuroscience*, **23**, 7830–7838.

Lin, S., Liang, Y., Zhang, J. *et al.* (2012) Microglial TIR-domain-containing adapter-inducing interferon-beta (TRIF) deficiency promotes retinal ganglion cell survival and axon regeneration via nuclear factor-kappaB. *Journal of Neuroinflammation*, **9**, 39.

Liu, X., Hawkes, E., Ishimaru, T., Tran, T. & Sretavan, D.W. (2006) EphB3: An endogenous mediator of adult axonal plasticity and regrowth after CNS injury. *Journal of Neuroscience*, **26**, 3087–3101.

Lorber, B., Berry, M., Douglas, M.R., Nakazawa, T. & Logan, A. (2009) Activated retinal glia promote neurite outgrowth of retinal ganglion cells via apolipoprotein E. *Journal of Neuroscience Research*, **87**, 2645–2652.

Lotan, M. & Schwartz, M. (1994) Cross talk between the immune system and the nervous system in response to injury: Implications for regeneration. *FASEB Journal*, **8**, 1026–1033.

Low, K., Culbertson, M., Bradke, F., Tessier-Lavigne, M. & Tuszynski, M.H. (2008) Netrin-1 is a novel myelin-associated inhibitor to axon growth. *Journal of Neuroscience*, **28**, 1099–1108.

Lu, X. & Richardson, P.M. (1991) Inflammation near the nerve cell body enhances axonal regeneration. *Journal of Neuroscience*, **11**, 972–978.

Lucas, S.M., Rothwell, N.J. & Gibson, R.M. (2006) The role of inflammation in CNS injury and disease. *British Journal of Pharmacology*, **147** (Suppl 1), S232–S240.

Luo, J.M., Zhi, Y., Chen, Q. *et al.* (2007) Influence of macrophages and lymphocytes on the survival and axon regeneration of injured retinal ganglion cells in rats from different autoimmune backgrounds. *European Journal of Neuroscience*, **26**, 3475–3485.

Luo, X., Salgueiro, Y., Beckerman, S.R., Lemmon, V.P., Tsoulfas, P. & Park, K.K. (2013) Three-dimensional evaluation of retinal ganglion cell axon regeneration and pathfinding in whole mouse tissue after injury. *Experimental Neurology*, **247**, 653–662.

Malik, J.M., Shevtsova, Z., Bahr, M. & Kugler, S. (2005) Long-term in vivo inhibition of CNS neurodegeneration by Bcl-XL gene transfer. *Molecular Therapy*, **11**, 373–381.

Moalem, G., Leibowitz-Amit, R., Yoles, E., Mor, F., Cohen, I.R. & Schwartz, M. (1999) Autoimmune T cells protect neurons from secondary degeneration after central nervous system axotomy. *Nature Medicine*, **5**, 49–55.

Monnier, P.P., D'Onofrio, P.M., Magharious, M. *et al.* (2011) Involvement of caspase-6 and caspase-8 in neuronal apoptosis and the regenerative failure of injured retinal ganglion cells. *Journal of Neuroscience*, **31**, 10494–10505.

Montgomery, S.L. & Bowers, W.J. (2012) Tumor necrosis factor-alpha and the roles it plays in homeostatic and degenerative processes within the central nervous system. *Journal of Neuroimmune Pharmacology*, **7**, 42–59.

Moore, D.L., Blackmore, M.G., Hu, Y. *et al.* (2009) KLF family members regulate intrinsic axon regeneration ability. *Science*, **326**, 298–301.

Moreau-Fauvarque, C., Kumanogoh, A., Camand, E. *et al.* (2003) The transmembrane semaphorin Sema4D/CD100, an inhibitor of axonal growth, is expressed on oligodendrocytes and upregulated after CNS lesion. *Journal of Neuroscience*, **23**, 9229–9239.

Muller, A., Hauk, T.G. & Fischer, D. (2007) Astrocyte-derived CNTF switches mature RGCs to a regenerative state following inflammatory stimulation. *Brain*, **130**, 3308–3320.

Nadeau, S., Filali, M., Zhang, J. *et al.* (2011) Functional recovery after peripheral nerve injury is dependent on the pro-inflammatory cytokines IL-1beta and TNF: Implications for neuropathic pain. *Journal of Neuroscience*, **31**, 12533–12542.

Nakazawa, T., Nakazawa, C., Matsubara, A. *et al.* (2006) Tumor necrosis factor-alpha mediates oligodendrocyte death and delayed retinal ganglion cell loss in a mouse model of glaucoma. *Journal of Neuroscience*, **26**, 12633–12641.

Niemi, J.P., DeFrancesco-Lisowitz, A., Roldan-Hernandez, L., Lindborg, J.A., Mandell, D. & Zigmond, R.E. (2013) A critical role for macrophages near axotomized neuronal cell bodies in stimulating nerve regeneration. *Journal of Neuroscience*, **33**, 16236–16248.

Park, K.K., Hu, Y., Muhling, J. *et al.* (2009) Cytokine-induced SOCS expression is inhibited by cAMP analogue: Impact on regeneration in injured retina. *Molecular and Cellular Neuroscience*, **41**, 313–324.

Park, K.K., Liu, K., Hu, Y. *et al.* (2008) Promoting axon regeneration in the adult CNS by modulation of the PTEN/mTOR pathway. *Science*, **322**, 963–966.

Pernet, V. & Di Polo, A. (2006) Synergistic action of brain-derived neurotrophic factor and lens injury promotes retinal ganglion cell survival, but leads to optic nerve dystrophy in vivo. *Brain*, **129**, 1014–1026.

Pernet, V., Joly, S., Jordi, N. *et al.* (2013a) Misguidance and modulation of axonal regeneration by Stat3 and Rho/ROCK signaling in the transparent optic nerve. *Cell Death & Disease*, **4**, e734.

Pernet, V., Joly, S., Dalkara, D. *et al.* (2013b) Long-distance axonal regeneration induced by CNTF gene transfer is impaired by axonal misguidance in the injured adult optic nerve. *Neurobiology of Disease*, **51**, 202–213.

Qin, S., Zou, Y. & Zhang, C.L. (2013) Cross-talk between KLF4 and STAT3 regulates axon regeneration. *Nature Communications*, **4**, 2633.

Ramon y Cajal, S. (1991) *Degeneration and Regeneration of the Nervous System*. Oxford University Press, New York.

Ransohoff, R.M. (2009) Chemokines and chemokine receptors: Standing at the crossroads of immunobiology and neurobiology. *Immunity*, **31**, 711–721.

Roh, M., Yang, J., Murakami, Y. *et al.* (2012) Etanercept, a widely used inhibitor of tumor necrosis factor-α (TNF-a), prevents retinal ganglion cell loss in a rat model of glaucoma. *PLoS One*, **3**, e40065.

Schafer, D.P., Lehrman, E.K., Kautzman, A.G. *et al.* (2012) Microglia sculpt postnatal neural circuits in an activity and complement-dependent manner. *Neuron*, **74**, 691–705.

Schwalb, J.M., Boulis, N.M., Gu, M.F. *et al.* (1995) Two factors secreted by the goldfish optic nerve induce retinal ganglion cells to regenerate axons in culture. *Journal of Neuroscience*, **15**, 5514–5525.

Schwartz, M. (2001) Harnessing the immune system for neuroprotection: Therapeutic vaccines for acute and chronic neurodegenerative disorders. *Cellular and Molecular Neurobiology*, **21**, 617–627.

Shen, Y., Tenney, A.P., Busch, S.A. *et al.* (2009) PTPsigma is a receptor for chondroitin sulfate proteoglycan, an inhibitor of neural regeneration. *Science*, **326**, 592–596.

Silver, J. & Miller, J.H. (2004) Regeneration beyond the glial scar. *Nature Reviews Neuroscience*, **5**, 146–156.

Slater, B.J., Vilson, F.L., Guo, Y., Weinreich, D., Hwang, S. & Bernstein, S.L. (2013) Optic nerve inflammation and demyelination in a rodent model of nonarteritic anterior ischemic optic neuropathy. *Investigative Ophthalmology & Visual Science*, **54**, 7952–7961.

Smith, P.D., Sun, F., Park, K.K. *et al.* (2009) SOCS3 deletion promotes optic nerve regeneration in vivo. *Neuron*, **64**, 617–623.

Souza-Rodrigues, R.D., Costa, A.M., Lima, R.R., Dos Santos, C.D., Picanco-Diniz, C.W. & Gomes-Leal, W. (2008) Inflammatory response and white matter damage after microinjections of endothelin-1 into the rat striatum. *Brain Research*, **1200**, 78–88.

Steinmetz, M.P., Horn, K.P., Tom, V.J. *et al.* (2005) Chronic enhancement of the intrinsic growth capacity of sensory neurons combined with the degradation of inhibitory proteoglycans allows functional regeneration of sensory axons through the dorsal root entry zone in the mammalian spinal cord. *Journal of Neuroscience*, **25**, 8066–8076.

Stevens, B., Allen, N.J., Vazquez, L.E. *et al.* (2007) The classical complement cascade mediates CNS synapse elimination. *Cell*, **131**, 1164–1178.

Stirling, D.P., Liu, S., Kubes, P. & Yong, V.W. (2009) Depletion of Ly6G/Gr-1 leukocytes after spinal cord injury in mice alters wound healing and worsens neurological outcome. *Journal of Neuroscience*, **29**, 753–764.

Sun, F. & He, Z. (2010) Neuronal intrinsic barriers for axon regeneration in the adult CNS. *Current Opinion in Neurobiology*, **20**, 510–518.

Sun, F., Park, K.K., Belin, S. *et al.* (2012) Sustained axon regeneration induced by co-deletion of PTEN and SOCS3. *Nature,* **480**, 372–375.

Tonari, M., Kurimoto, T., Horie, T., Sugiyama, T., Ikeda, T. & Oku, H. (2012) Blocking endothelin-B receptors rescues retinal ganglion cells from optic nerve injury through suppression of neuroinflammation. *Investigative Ophthalmology & Visual Science,* **53**, 3490–3500.

Veldman, M.B., Bemben, M.A., Thompson, R.C. & Goldman, D. (2007) Gene expression analysis of zebrafish retinal ganglion cells during optic nerve regeneration identifies KLF6a and KLF7a as important regulators of axon regeneration. *Developmental Biology,* **312**, 596–612.

Wang, K.C., Koprivica, V., Kim, J.A. *et al.* (2002) Oligodendrocyte-myelin glycoprotein is a Nogo receptor ligand that inhibits neurite outgrowth. *Nature,* **417**, 941–944.

Wang, X., Hasan, O., Arzeno, A., Benowitz, L.I., Cafferty, W.B. & Strittmatter, S.M. (2012) Axonal regeneration induced by blockade of glial inhibitors coupled with activation of intrinsic neuronal growth pathways. *Experimental Neurology,* **237**, 55–69.

Watkins, T.A., Wang, B., Huntwork-Rodriguez, S. *et al.* (2013) DLK initiates a transcriptional program that couples apoptotic and regenerative responses to axonal injury. *Proceedings of the National Academy of Sciences of the United States of America,* **110**, 4039–4044.

Weibel, D., Kreutzberg, G.W. & Schwab, M.E. (1995) Brain-derived neurotrophic factor (BDNF) prevents lesion-induced axonal die-back in young rat optic nerve. *Brain Research,* **679**, 249–254.

Wu, S.C., Rau, C.S., Lu, T.H. *et al.* (2013) Knockout of TLR4 and TLR2 impair the nerve regeneration by delayed demyelination but not remyelination. *Journal of Biomedical Science,* **20**, 62.

Yin, Y., Cui, Q., Li, Y. *et al.* (2003) Macrophage-derived factors stimulate optic nerve regeneration. *Journal of Neuroscience,* **23**, 2284–2293.

Yin, Y., Henzl, M.T., Lorber, B. *et al.* (2006) Oncomodulin is a macrophage-derived signal for axon regeneration in retinal ganglion cells. *Nature Neuroscience,* **9**, 843–852.

Yin, Y., Cui, Q., Gilbert, H.Y. *et al.* (2009) Oncomodulin links inflammation to optic nerve regeneration. *Proceedings of the National Academy of Sciences of the United States of America,* **106**, 19587–19592.

Yiu, G. & He, Z. (2006) Glial inhibition of CNS axon regeneration. *Nature Reviews Neuroscience,* **7**, 617–627.

Zheng, Z., Yuan, R., Song, M. *et al.* (2012) The toll-like receptor 4-mediated signaling pathway is activated following optic nerve injury in mice. *Brain Research,* **1489**, 90–97.

13 Effects of Macrophages and Monocytes in Remyelination of the CNS

Muktha Natrajan,[1] Bibiana Bielekova,[2] and Robin J.M. Franklin[1]

[1]*Department of Clinical Neurosciences, Wellcome Trust-MRC Cambridge Stem Cell Institute, University of Cambridge, Cambridge, UK*
[2]*Neuroimmunology Branch, National Institute of Neurological Disorders and Stroke, National Institutes of Health, Bethesda, MD, USA*

Introduction

Neuroinflammation is considered one of the major underlying causes of demyelinating diseases of the central nervous system (CNS). In these diseases, such as multiple sclerosis (MS), symptoms occur due to the loss of myelin mediated by an autoimmune response (Griffiths *et al.*, 1998). Although immune cells such as monocytes and microglia are involved in demyelinating events, these cells can also play a prominent role in robust regeneration of new myelin sheaths, a process known as remyelination (Kotter *et al.*, 2005; Ruckh *et al.*, 2012; Miron *et al.*, 2013). Remyelination allows for recovery from demyelinating disorders by preventing axonal loss, protecting vulnerable axons, and organizing the neural environment for optimal signal conduction. Although this process generally results in thinner myelin sheaths, the exception being the smallest diameter myelinated axons (Stidworthy *et al.*, 2003), remyelination can completely restore saltatory conduction across axons (Franklin and Ffrench-Constant, 2008).

Myelin is formed by oligodendrocytes in the CNS to ensheath axons and serves two main functions. Firstly, myelin allows for rapid saltatory conduction by providing insulation to axons in the electrically charged environment. It is primarily composed of lipids, which make up almost 80% of its dry weight, in order to increase the speed of impulses up to 100-fold (Edgar *et al.*, 2009). In addition, myelin also preserves the long-term integrity of the axon (Griffiths *et al.*, 1998). In the developing nervous system, myelinating oligodendrocytes form from the response of oligodendrocyte progenitor cells (OPCs) to differentiation cues. OPCs are also prevalent in the adult CNS and remain a quiescent stem cell population until inductive cues cause them to differentiate (Warrington *et al.*, 1993; Zhang *et al.*, 1999). In diseases such as MS, demyelination occurs and oligodendrocytes and their processes are degraded, but remyelination and functional recovery can take place when OPCs are recruited and differentiated in the lesion sites. In the

Neuroinflammation: New Insights into Beneficial and Detrimental Functions, First Edition. Edited by Samuel David.
© 2015 John Wiley & Sons, Inc. Published 2015 by John Wiley & Sons, Inc.

recruitment stage, OPCs migrate to the demyelinated area of the axon. Then, these cells respond to both intrinsic and extrinsic factors to differentiate into oligodendrocytes and remyelinate axons (Groves *et al.*, 1993; Franklin and Ffrench-Constant, 2008).When remyelination fails in clinical disorders, OPC recruitment is often not greatly affected; it is generally due to a failure in the maturation and differentiation of OPCs (Kuhlmann *et al.*, 2008; Dyall *et al.*, 2010; Fancy *et al.*, 2010).

There are multiple extrinsic factors involved in the failure of OPC differentiation, including the accumulation of inhibitory myelin debris and the lack of growth factor signaling in the demyelinated area (Robinson and Miller, 1999; Hinks and Franklin, 2000; Kotter *et al.*, 2006). During demyelination, myelin debris is formed and accumulates around the denuded axon. In order to prevent axonal degradation, these fragments must be cleared away so OPCs are allowed to activate and differentiate (Kotter *et al.*, 2006; Clarner *et al.*, 2012; Ruckh *et al.*, 2012; Plemel *et al.*, 2013). This clearance is mainly through an innate immune response performed by monocyte-derived macrophages and microglia. Macrophages and microglia have many roles in the CNS, including monitoring the tissue environment for pathogens, maintaining homeostasis, and phagocytosing dead cells (Giulian *et al.*, 1989; Diemel *et al.*, 1998; Rawji and Yong, 2013). Although macrophages and microglia are both myeloid cells, they are derived from different origins and maintain unique markers within the CNS. Microglia are derived from the yolk sac during early development and reside in the CNS through adulthood, whereas blood-derived monocytes are differentiated from bone marrow cells and are usually recruited to the CNS in response to an insult (Neumann *et al.*, 2009; Ginhoux *et al.*, 2010; Ousman and Kubes, 2012). These cells are difficult to distinguish once they are activated, but studies have suggested that monocyte-derived macrophages have been shown to play the pivotal role in myelin debris clearance and CNS remyelination (Kotter *et al.*, 2005; Ruckh *et al.*, 2012), although both cell types are able to phagocytose debris (Neumann *et al.*, 2009; Olah *et al.*, 2012).

In demyelinating disorders, phagocytes respond to the destruction of myelin and remove myelin debris. It has been hypothesized that these macrophages then act to encourage remyelination by clearing the way for OPCs to differentiate. Once these cells are recruited to the demyelinated area, they release cytokines and phagocytose myelin debris in the early stages of remyelination, which then allows for differentiation of OPCs and restoration of proper conductance (Kotter *et al.*, 2001; Syed *et al.*, 2008; Pohl *et al.*, 2011). After myelin phagocytosis, macrophages can alter their own function and change their cytokine profiles. Myelin-phagocytosing macrophages may then exert beneficial effects by releasing protective cytokines that have immunoregulatory functions, orchestrate phagocytosis, and promote tissue repair and remodeling (Boven *et al.*, 2006; Mikita *et al.*, 2011). Phagocytes can release multiple growth factors, including insulin-like growth factor 1 (IGF-1) and transforming growth factor β (TGFβ), which encourage differentiation by acting through receptors and downstream pathways in OPCs (Hinks and Franklin, 1999; Franklin *et al.*, 2001).

Ultimately, microglia and macrophages can provide valuable functions that result in remyelination (Fig. 13.1). The role of macrophages in neuroimmunological disorders is a complex topic, and determining the best method to harness the benefits of phagocytes in remyelination is an important step in identifying the therapeutic capability of these cells. This chapter highlights the ability of macrophages to remove environmental barriers and provide extrinsic stimuli to promote oligodendrocyte differentiation and remyelination.

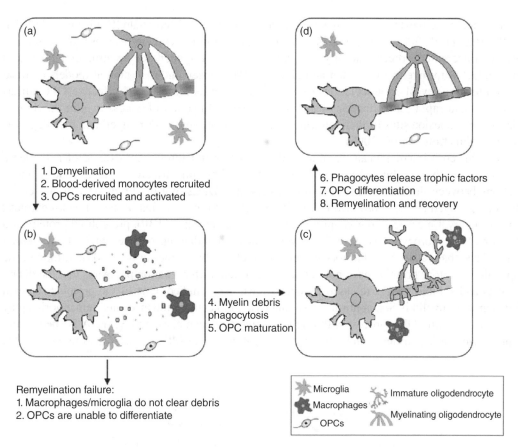

Figure 13.1 Macrophage and microglia involvement in the stages of demyelination to remyelination. (a) Myelinating oligo-dendrocytes, microglia, and OPCs populate healthy CNS white matter. (b) After demyelination, myelin debris is formed around denuded axons and blood-derived monocytes are recruited to the lesion site. OPCs are recruited and activated as well in response to demyelination. However, if macrophages are not properly recruited and activated, myelin debris is not cleared and OPCs are unable to differentiate causing remyelination to fail. (c) Myelin debris is phagocytosed by macrophages and microglia, clearing the way for OPC differentiation. Phagocytes also release various cytokines and growth factors that promote differ-entiation and remyelination of the CNS. (d) After proper removal of myelin debris and activation of differentiation cues in OPCs, macrophages, and microglia largely exit the lesion area and return to a resting state. Mature oligodendrocytes effec-tively remyelinate the exposed axons with a thinner myelin sheath and proper conductance is restored. (*See insert for color representation of this figure.*)

Myelin Debris Inhibits OPC Differentiation and Remyelination

Primary demyelination produces large amounts of debris as myelin sheaths degrade. On demyeli-nation of the CNS, degenerating oligodendrocytes form debris around denuded axons. This debris can create a dense matrix that may present a physical barrier to the demyelinated axon (although this has not been formally demonstrated). Previous studies have shown that myelin debris does not affect the number of OPCs recruited to the lesion site; however, differentiation of OPCs into myelinating oligodendrocytes is impaired by the extracellular accumulation of debris (Franklin and Kotter, 2008; Kuhlmann *et al.*, 2008). Cultured OPCs plated onto CNS myelin substrates and myelin protein extracts *in vitro* were unable to effectively differentiate (Robinson and Miller, 1999; Baer *et al.*, 2009). Increased intracellular calcium in the OPC in response to myelin also leads to decreased process motility and collapse of the oligodendrocyte structural formation on contact with myelin (Moorman and Hume, 1994). Observations in animal models of focal demyelination reveal an association between myelin debris removal and effective OPC differentiation and rapid remyelination (Fancy *et al.*, 2010). Injection of excess myelin debris into demyelinated lesion sites further confirmed impairment of rapid CNS remyelination by degenerated myelin (Kotter *et al.*, 2006).

Myelin debris is a major cause of impaired OPC maturation through the expression and release of molecules that inhibit differentiation (Fig. 13.2). This impairment is mainly due to interactions between the protein extracts from myelin and OPCs, not the lipids or salts present in the debris (Syed *et al.*, 2008). More than 100 proteins were identified in these myelin extracts, including myelin-associated glycoprotein, myelin basic protein (MBP), proteolipid protein, and myelin oligodendrocyte glycoprotein; however, the current datasets only reveal a list of potential candidates that cause the inhibitory effects of myelin debris (Baer *et al.*, 2009). Although the specific inhibitory proteins have not yet been identified, differentiation pathways that the debris targets and soluble factors released by debris have been studied. One of the proteins secreted by degraded myelin is Semaphorin-3A (Sema3A), a molecular guidance cue. Semaphorins play a role in diverting OPC processes through negative guidance cues, and Sema3A is specifically upregulated in active demyelinating lesions of patients with MS. Sema3A also prevents OPC

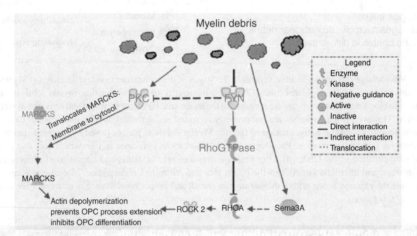

Figure 13.2 Myelin debris prevents OPC differentiation via Sema3A, RhoA, and PKC pathways. The inhibitory effects of degraded myelin on remyelination regulate several pathways in OPCs. Fyn-1 is a positive regulator of OPC differentiation and prevents RhoA phosphorylation by activating Rho-GTPases (O'Meara *et al.*, 2011). When Fyn-1 is dysregulated in the presence of myelin debris, RhoA-GTP activates ROCK2, resulting in actin depolymerization and inhibited remyelination. PKC is also activated when Fyn-1 is dysregulated, and it prevents OPC differentiation by translocating the MARCKS protein from the plasma membrane, where it is active during OPC differentiation, to the cytosol, where it is inactive during OPC quiescence. PKC has also been shown to play a role in RhoA activation. Finally, the negative guidance cue Sema3A has been shown to impair OPC differentiation and remyelination, possibly through activating the RhoA pathway. Myelin debris activates and releases these negative regulators of OPC differentiation to prevent remyelination. Light gray text, activates OPC differentiation; dark gray text, inhibits OPC differentiation. (*See insert for color representation of this figure.*)

differentiation *in vitro* in OPC cultures and *in vivo* in animal models of demyelination. Artificially increasing Sema3A in demyelinated lesions leads to more demyelination and further induces failure of remyelination (Syed *et al.*, 2011). Several signaling processes activated by myelin debris proteins also result in a similar failure of remyelination. Protein kinase C (PKC) signaling is involved in translocation of myristoylated alanine-rich C-kinase substrate (MARCKS) from the OPC membrane to the cytosol, which is known to regulate differentiation. In differentiating OPCs, MARCKS is present in the cell membrane, and in OPC inhibition, it is localized to the cytosol (Baron *et al.*, 1999). Myelin protein extracts activate PKC signaling, thereby promoting MARCKS translocation to the cytosol and impairing OPC differentiation.

Fyn-1 is a Src family tyrosine kinase, and activation of this molecule is one of the earliest events triggered in OPC differentiation. This receptor regulates process extension of OPCs to form myelin sheaths, and myelin debris inhibits phosphorylation and activation of this kinase. Impairment of Fyn-1 allows for activation of RhoA, an important negative regulator of oligo-dendrocyte differentiation. RhoA activates Rho-associated, coiled-coil containing protein kinase 2 (ROCKII), which leads to actin depolymerization and prevents OPC process extensions from expanding and forming new myelin sheaths (Baer *et al.*, 2009). Effective removal of myelin debris to prevent activation of PKC, Sema3A, and RhoA/ROCKII signaling will improve OPC differentiation and enhance effective remyelination.

Monocyte-Derived Macrophages are the Main Actors in Myelin Debris Phagocytosis

Monocyte- and microglia-derived macrophages act as efficient phagocytes in response to demyelination by removing excess myelin debris. Other cell types, such as astrocytes and Schwann cells, may also be involved in debris clearance, but the major actors in the CNS are macrophages. Phagocytically active macrophages containing myelin degradation products are present both in animal models of demyelination and in actively demyelinating MS lesions (Shi *et al.*, 2011; Vogel *et al.*, 2013). When macrophages are artificially depleted before inducing demyelination, a greater number of axons remain demyelinated and remyelination is impaired (Kotter *et al.*, 2001). Persistent myelin debris after spinal cord injury is correlated with a decrease in infiltrating monocytes (Imai *et al.*, 2008). Release of chemotactic factors, such as monocyte chemoattractant protein 1 (MCP-1) and gelsolin, is also impaired in the presence of degenerated myelin. Gelsolin is necessary for macrophage motility and actin polymerization, so it has a role in phagocytosis after monocyte recruitment. Gelsolin knockouts experience both impaired recruitment of monocytes and delayed remyelination of the PNS due to a decreased macrophage response (Goncalves *et al.*, 2010). Myelin debris phagocytosis by myeloid cells is a vital component of remyelination; therefore, macrophages provide an essential role in enhancing OPC differentiation and recovery.

The mechanisms of myelin phagocytosis are dependent on macrophage expression of multiple receptors and soluble compounds, most importantly complement receptor 3 (CR3), galectin-3 (MAC-2), C1q, nuclear receptors, and triggering receptor expressed on myeloid cells (TREM-2) (Fig. 13.3). The presence of complement component 3 (C3) on degenerating myelin encourages phagocytosis via CR3 (Carroll, 2009). CR3 is expressed by myelin-phagocytosing, monocyte-derived macrophages, and microglia in experimental autoimmune encephalomyelitis

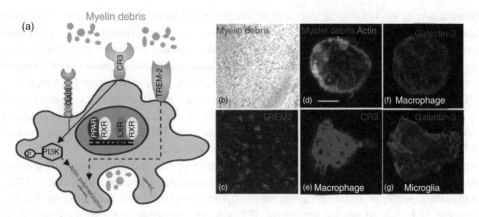

Figure 13.3   (a) Macrophages express unique receptors and compounds that promote myelin debris phagocytosis. Monocytes, macrophages, and microglia are primarily responsible for the removal of inhibitory myelin debris to enhance remyelination. Through signals such as MCP-1 and gelsolin, these myeloid-derived cells are recruited to the CNS and express membrane receptors, nuclear receptors, and complement components to enhance phagocytosis mechanisms. Activation of CR3 and MAC-2 leads to PI3K phosphorylation and phagocytosis. LXR, PPAR, and RXR are activated by lipid-derived ligands and act as transcription factors to enhance phagocytosis and immunoregulation. TREM-2 pathways activate cytoskeletal rearrangement and response to apoptotic cells which results in effective myelin debris clearance. (b) Oil Red O stained myelin debris in a demyelinated lesion; (c) TREM-2 staining of region (b) showing phagocytic TREM-2+ macrophages; (d) actin rearrangement during myelin debris phagocytosis by macrophages; (e) CR3 activation; (f) galectin-3 activation in (c); (g) galectin-3 activation in myelin-phagocytosing microglia. *Source*: Immunostaining adapted from Piccio *et al.* (2008), Hadas *et al.* (2010), and Gitik *et al.* (2011). (*See insert for color representation of this figure.*)

(EAE) models. As an integrin composed of two transmembrane subunits, CD11b and CD18, CR3 mediates many cell functions including adhesion, motility, and phagocytosis. After binding to ligands from myelin debris such as C3, CR3 transmits signals across the cell membrane to engage filamentous actin, resulting in actin rearrangement and phagocytic activity (Reichert *et al.*, 2001). Expression of this receptor has proven to be essential in myelin debris removal via phosphatidylinositol-3-kinase (PI3K)-dependent phagocytosis (Lutz and Correll, 2003). PI3K is also controlled by the galectin-3 (MAC-2) pathway. Galectins are a family of β-galactosidases binding lectins, with MAC-2 perpetually expressed in macrophages and microglia that phagocytose myelin. When conditioned media from MAC-2-expressing microglia is added to OPC cultures, it promotes oligodendrocyte differentiation in culture (Pasquini *et al.*, 2011). MAC-2 regulates scavenger receptor II and Fcγ receptors, which are both involved in myelin phagocytosis, and stabilize Ras GTPases, which phosphorylate PI3K. When PI3K pathways are enhanced, actin polymerization and myelin debris phagocytosis are also enhanced (Rotshenker *et al.*, 2008). Another component of the complement system, complement component 1q (C1q), is importantly linked to phagocytosis mechanisms and is upregulated after myelin phagocytosis. Macrophages release C1q, and it then binds and opsonizes apoptotic cells to signal phagocytosis (Nauta *et al.*, 2003; Bogie *et al.*, 2012).

Macrophages also upregulate many members of the nuclear receptor subfamily in response to myelin phagocytosis. Nuclear receptors contain both a DNA-binding domain and a ligand-binding domain, allowing them to act as transcription factors to directly activate gene expression by binding to low-affinity ligands (Nagy and Schwabe, 2004). Liver X receptors (LXRs), peroxisome-proliferator-activated receptors (PPARs), and retinoid X receptors (RXRs) are members of the nuclear receptor family. All three of these receptors have been implicated in myelin debris phagocytosis. LXRs are activated by oxysterols and lipoproteins such as those in myelin fragments, and their downstream genes have been linked to immunoregulatory functions in monocytes and macrophages. PPARs have been shown to ameliorate symptoms in mouse models of MS, and they also regulate anti-inflammatory gene function in macrophages. RXRs form a heterodimer with both of these receptors to enhance their functions. Upregulated gene expression of these receptors is seen in myelin-phagocytosing macrophages and causes suppressed inflammation and activated lipid metabolism after debris clearance (Bogie et al., 2012, 2013). Modulating expression of TREM-2 also enhances myelin debris clearance. TREM-2 is a receptor belonging to the Ig superfamily and serves to induce cytoskeletal reorganization, augment phagocytosis, and reduce tumor necrosis factor α (TNF-α) and nitric oxide synthase production in monocytes, macrophages, and microglia. Blocking TREM-2 results in exacerbation of demyelination in EAE mice by removing the protective functions of macrophages, such as the control of local inflammation and clearance of debris (Piccio et al., 2007). Enhancing TREM-2 function in EAE limits tissue destruction and allows macrophages to maintain CNS homeostasis after demyelination. These TREM-2-enhanced macrophages also maintain an anti-inflammatory cytokine profile, further proving their regulatory and regenerative capacity (Takahashi et al., 2007; Neumann et al., 2009). These receptors and proteins specifically expressed in myeloid-derived cells respond to myelin debris signals and show the particular role of macrophages and microglia in the phagocytosis of degraded myelin.

Switching from M1 to M2 Macrophages Promotes CNS Remyelination

The phagocytosis of cellular debris is considered to be mainly an anti-inflammatory process. Two extreme types of macrophages have been identified and are classified into distinct categories on the basis of their inflammatory properties such as induction factors, cytokine production, and phagocytosis type. However, macrophages show phenotypic plasticity and may fall anywhere along this continuum (Olah et al., 2012). For simplicity, the hallmarks of the two major polarization states are discussed in this section. M1 macrophages are classically activated macrophages that express proinflammatory cytokines and cell markers, while M2 macrophages are alternatively activated macrophages that express anti-inflammatory and immunomodulatory markers. M1 polarization is induced by interferon γ (IFNγ) and TNF-α from Th1 cells and lipopolysaccharide (LPS) released by bacteria. Activation by these three molecules results in a high production of proinflammatory mediators and destruction of micro-organisms and tumor cells. M1 macrophages express CD80 and CD86 co-stimulatory molecules as well as chemokine receptor 7 (CCR7), resulting in efficient antigen presentation. They also release TNF-α, nitric oxide (NO), interleukin (IL)-6, and IL-1β in response to stimulation. When they produce NO, they create cytotoxic reactive oxygen species (ROS) and also stimulate the secretion if IL-12, another proinflammatory cytokine. These cytokines increase antigen-presenting activity and may assist in perpetuating the autoimmune response (Mikita et al., 2011; Vereyken et al., 2011; Shechter and Schwartz, 2013).

The switch from M1 to M2 macrophages occurs between the recruitment of OPCs and differentiation stages of remyelination and is central to the recovery after demyelination (Miron et al., 2013). M2 macrophages are induced by IL-4, IL-10, IL-13, lipid mediators from Th2-type inflammation, which are inhibitors of the Th1 response. Their primary functions are scavenging cellular debris and apoptotic cells, remodeling tissues, and expressing anti-inflammatory molecules (Vereyken et al., 2011). In remyelination, myelin-containing foamy macrophages are characterized as M2 macrophages conferring immunoregulatory functions. These foam cells in MS lesions express anti-inflammatory molecules and lack proinflammatory cytokines (Boven et al., 2006). Various surface markers such as CD209 (on microglia), CD23, CD163, CD206, and mannose receptors indicate M2 macrophages, which are known to be better at phagocytosing opsonized particles. They also produce growth factors that assist in tissue remodeling and repair (Laskin, 2009).

M2 cytokines are known to reduce inflammation and have higher angiogenic potential. They express high levels of arginase-1 (Arg-1), an enzyme that competes with inducible nitric oxide synthase (iNOS). iNOS converts L-arginine to NO and exacerbates inflammation, while Arg-1 consumes L-arginine by converting it to ornithine and urea, both noninflammatory molecules. Higher levels of Arg-1 in M2 macrophages are associated with phagocytosis of myelin debris in EAE and contribute to modulating neuroinflammation. The increase in iNOS levels at early and peak stages of the disease is followed by a decrease during recovery and high arginase-1 levels, suggesting that M2 macrophages are important for remyelination (Ahn et al., 2012; Durafourt et al., 2012). Arg-1 positive macrophages also express the M2 cytokine activin A, which is a member of the TGFβ family known to be a neuroprotective cytokine expressed in the CNS. Addition of activin A to microglia cultures also reduced NO production and down-regulated IL-6 and IL-18, showing its anti-inflammatory characteristics (Sugama et al., 2007; Wilms et al., 2010). Blocking activin A expression inhibits OPC differentiation in vitro and is associated with inhibited remyelination in vivo, while adding M2-conditioned media containing activin A enhanced OPC differentiation by binding to ACvr2, the activin receptor on OPCs (Miron et al., 2013). Thus, macrophages polarized to the M2 phenotype have reparative properties to help induce remyelination through the phagocytosis of myelin debris, the release of trophic factors, and the production of regenerative cytokines.

Ageing Impairs Macrophage Function, Myelin Debris Clearance, and Remyelination

Similarly to many mammalian tissues, the CNS experiences declining regenerative capacity with increasing age. CNS remyelination occurs more rapidly in young animals partly due to extrinsic factors such as the macrophage response, so it is important to consider the effects of age on these cells (Hinks and Franklin, 2000; Sim et al., 2002). Ageing has a profound impact on the immune system, and several studies have shown significant changes in the gene expression profiles of innate immune cells as they age (Lloberas and Celada, 2002; Stout and Suttles, 2005). Recruited monocytes and macrophages display impaired phagocytic function in respiratory disorders, and wound-healing macrophages show a considerable reduction in phagocytosis of cell debris in response to age. The tissue remodeling and repair function of macrophages declines through decreased release of growth factors and impaired cytoskeletal rearrangement in these models (Ashcroft *et al.*, 1997; Mancuso *et al.*, 2001; Swift *et al.*, 2001). Human monocytes are also altered with age, and these age-related changes include impaired phagocytosis, shortened telomeres, and weakened anti-inflammatory functions (Hearps *et al.*, 2012). Similarly to other systems, the macrophage response to demyelination declines with age (Hinks and Franklin, 2000). Lesions in old animals contain more myelin debris, while lesions in young animals contain less debris and more remyelinated axons (Shields *et al.*, 1999). There was a delay in both the recruitment and proliferation of monocyte-derived macrophages in aged animals; however, there was an increase in expression of various proinflammatory cytokines, including M1-related TNF-α, IL-1β, IL-6, IL-12, and IL-23. These proinflammatory macrophages contribute to the decline in remyelination of aged animals (Shields *et al.*, 1999; Zhao *et al.*, 2006).

Monocytes and blood-derived macrophages appear to be the key regulators in the age-related decline in remyelination. By connecting the circulatory systems of young and aged animals, a model called heterochronic parabiosis, aged mice were exposed to the systemic milieu of young mice. Young mice were GFP+, so Ruckh *et al.* were able to distinguish the young cells recruited to the demyelinated lesions in the aged partner. These cells proved to be blood-derived monocytes; impairing recruitment of young monocytes to demyelinated lesions prevented effective remyelination, and recruitment of young monocytes improved remyelination in this model. In addition, there was significantly more myelin debris in the lesions of old animals compared to that of young animals, indicating that the efficiency of myelin debris clearance is impaired with age. However, when myelin debris clearance in old mice is accelerated with monocytes from young mice, there is a significant decrease in fractionated myelin and a considerable increase in remyelination (Ruckh *et al.*, 2012). This study proved that in CNS biology, signals from the systemic environment, such as those from young macrophages, are able to override age-related deficits in myelin debris phagocytosis and CNS remyelination.

Macrophages Release Growth and Neurotrophic Factors that Promote Remyelination

Monocytes and macrophages can enhance remyelination through the release of protective cytokines and growth factors in response to demyelination. Macrophages have been shown to release growth factors that specifically promote OPC differentiation thereby stimulating recovery (highlighted in Table 13.1). In a study looking for growth factors upregulated during remyelination, IGF-1 and TGFβ were both released by myelin-phagocytosing macrophages and had been shown to enhance OPC differentiation in culture. The release of IGF-1 by M2 microglia *in vitro* exerts beneficial effects on neural progenitor cells and encourages oligodendrogenesis (Butovsky *et al.*, 2006). Both growth factors become more abundant after monocyte-derived macrophage infiltration rather than astrocyte activation, indicating that they are primarily produced by blood-derived phagocytes. IGF-1 and TGFβ exhibit increased expression in a similar temporal pattern as new myelin sheaths are formed, so they appear to share a similar function in OPC maturation (Hinks and Franklin, 1999). These growth factors also show lowered peak expression in aged animals and are associated with delayed remyelination, indicating their expression is importation for effective recovery (Hinks and Franklin, 2000).

Leukemia inhibitory factor (LIF) is released by macrophages as a member of the IL6 family and is known to be a neuropoeitic cytokine that encourages OPC differentiation both *in vitro* and

Table 13.1   Factors released by myelin-phagocytosing macrophages and microglia that promote OPC differentiation and remyelination

Released factor	Mechanisms causing OPC differentiation	Reference
IGF-1	Binds IGF1R to enhance both CNP and MBP expression	Mozell and McMorris, 1991; Barres *et al.*, 1993
TGFβ	Downregulates PDGF and FGF, both of which promote OPC proliferation and precursor cell state, thereby promoting maturation	McKinnon *et al.*, 1993a, 1993b
LIF	Limits ROS production; activates gp130 on OPCs	Hendriks *et al.*, 2008
ET-2	Activates endothelin receptor A and B on OPCs, which mediate ERK and CREB phosphorylation and transcription of mature oligodendrocyte genes	Gadea *et al.*, 2009; Yuen *et al.*, 2013
Iron/ferritin	Acts in oxidative metabolism to cause cell cycle arrest in OPCs and promote maturation	Todorich *et al.*, 2008

Abbreviations: CNP, $2'-3'$ cyclic nucleotide $3'$-phosphohydrolase; MBP, myelin basic protein; PDGF, platelet-derived growth factor; FGF, fibroblast growth factor; IGF-1, insulin-like growth factor 1; TGFβ, transforming growth factor β; LIF, leukemia inhibitory factor; ET-2, endothelin 2; ERK, extracellular-signal-regulated kinases; CREB, cAMP response element-binding protein.

in vivo (Deverman and Patterson, 2012). When LIF binds to receptor complexes on macrophages, it activates PI3K pathways known to activate myelin debris phagocytosis and has been shown to stimulate phagocytosis in models of demyelination and remyelination. Release of LIF inhibits production of reactive oxygen species and stimulates proliferation and differentiation of OPCs through the activation of the gp130 receptor (Hendriks *et al.*, 2008). Another secretory peptide released by macrophages is endothelin 2 (ET-2). ET-2 is a cytokine and growth factor that regulates chemotaxis and activation of macrophages and affects their inflammatory capacity. In cerebellar slice cultures, ET-2 was released by macrophages in demyelinated environments and promoted remyelination. The receptor for ET-2, endothelin receptor B, responds to this release and is expressed on oligodendrocytes during remyelination. Blocking ET-2 activity using an antagonist for this receptor inhibited OPC maturation, indicating that ET-2 release is necessary for efficient remyelination (Yuen *et al.*, 2013). The cysteine protease inhibitor cystatin F is activated during acute demyelination and stays active in remyelinating areas. Cystatin F is expressed by macrophages and microglia, and myelin debris phagocytosis induces its release. This induction is specific to the phagocytosis of myelin debris and results in the overexpression of cystatin F specifically in remyelinating areas, indicating that its expression in phagocytes may play a unique role in OPC differentiation (Ma *et al.*, 2011).

In addition to growth factors and cytokines, macrophages can also regulate other molecules that encourage OPC differentiation. Iron is required for the proliferation and maturation of cells due to its role in DNA synthesis and oxidative metabolism. Regulation of iron content is also specifically involved in oligodendrogenesis and is necessary for OPC differentiation and remyelination (Schulz *et al.*, 2012). Ferritin, an effective iron storage component, is present in activated macrophages and allows them to colocalize with areas of cell genesis in a dose-dependent manner.

Ferritin can sequester thousands or iron atoms and functions to oxidize the more toxic Fe^{2+} to the less reactive Fe^{3+}. Because iron is a pro-oxidant and oxidation causes cell cycle arrest, the release of iron from macrophages can help enhance OPC differentiation. M2 myelin-phagocytosing macrophages release iron after myelin debris phagocytosis and are the main source of iron for OPCs. Excess ferritin can also negatively regulate OPC differentiation, but when iron is released by macrophages at the appropriate timepoint after demyelination, it improves OPC maturation and helps replace lost oligodendrocytes (Schonberg *et al.*, 2012; Mehta *et al.*, 2013). By enhancing OPC differentiation, all of these trophic factors can encourage recovery in demyelinating disorders and confirm the beneficial effects of macrophages in remyelination.

Concluding Remarks

Macrophages and microglia comprise the main innate immune cells in the CNS that play a prominent role in the initiation and resolution of neuroinflammation. Findings thus far have shown the importance of these phagocytes in the removal of myelin debris and initiation of remyelination. Although they also have a role in demyelinating events, it cannot be denied that these cells serve many functions to resolve demyelination. Through their ability to remain flexible, these cells can change their cytokine profiles on the basis of extrinsic cues. On phagocytosis of cellular debris, they are able to produce immunoregulatory cytokines that promote tissue repair and OPC differentiation. In addition, they can interact with many receptors on OPCs to stall the cell cycle and promote maturation, resulting in effective remyelination. Although proinflammatory functions in these cells can cause destruction of myelin, proper control of the immunoregulatory functions of macrophages can lead to the formation of new myelin sheaths. Monocytes, microglia and the macrophages they give rise to have many protective aspects and activating these cells to release anti-inflammatory molecules, trophic factors, and phagocytic signals to promote oligodendrocyte differentiation can lead to efficient remyelination of the CNS. The ability to target peripheral cells and modify their function to enhance CNS recovery provides a unique therapeutic tool for demyelinating diseases. Questions remain on how the beneficial functions of monocytes can be harnessed, and future studies can improve our knowledge on modulating monocyte function to override age-related deficiencies in remyelination.

References

Ahn, M., Yang, W., Kim, H., Jin, J.K., Moon, C. & Shin, T. (2012) Immunohistochemical study of arginase-1 in the spinal cords of Lewis rats with experimental autoimmune encephalomyelitis. *Brain Research*, **1453**, 77–86.

Ashcroft, G.S., Horan, M.A. & Ferguson, M.W. (1997) The effects of ageing on wound healing: immunolocalisation of growth factors and their receptors in a murine incisional model. *Journal of Anatomy*, **190** (Pt 3), 351–365.

Baer, A.S., Syed, Y.A., Kang, S.U. *et al.* (2009) Myelin-mediated inhibition of oligodendrocyte precursor differentiation can be overcome by pharmacological modulation of Fyn-RhoA and protein kinase C signalling. *Brain*, **132**, 465–481.

Baron, W., de Vries, E.J., de Vries, H. & Hoekstra, D. (1999) Protein kinase C prevents oligodendrocyte differentiation: modulation of actin cytoskeleton and cognate polarized membrane traffic. *Journal of Neurobiology*, **41**, 385–398.

Barres, B.A., Schmid, R., Sendtner, M. & Raff, M.C. (1993) Multiple extracellular signals are required for long-term oligodendrocyte survival. *Development*, **118**, 283–295.

Bogie, J.F., Jorissen, W., Mailleux, J. *et al.* (2013) Myelin alters the inflammatory phenotype of macrophages by activating PPARs. *Acta Neuropathologica*, **1**, 43.

Bogie, J.F., Timmermans, S., Huynh-Thu, V.A. *et al.* (2012) Myelin-derived lipids modulate macrophage activity by liver X receptor activation. *PLoS One*, **7**, e44998.

Boven, L.A., Van Meurs, M., Van Zwam, M. *et al.* (2006) Myelin-laden macrophages are anti-inflammatory, consistent with foam cells in multiple sclerosis. *Brain*, **129**, 517–526.

Butovsky, O., Ziv, Y., Schwartz, A. *et al.* (2006) Microglia activated by IL-4 or IFN-gamma differentially induce neurogenesis and oligodendrogenesis from adult stem/progenitor cells. *Molecular and Cellular Neurosciences*, **31**, 149–160.

Carroll, S.J. (2009) *Handbook of the Neuroscience of Aging.* Academic Press (Elsevier), London, UK.

Clarner, T., Diederichs, F., Berger, K. *et al.* (2012) Myelin debris regulates inflammatory responses in an experimental demyelination animal model and multiple sclerosis lesions. *Glia*, **60**, 1468–1480.

Deverman, B.E. & Patterson, P.H. (2012) Exogenous leukemia inhibitory factor stimulates oligodendrocyte progenitor cell proliferation and enhances hippocampal remyelination. *Journal of Neuroscience*, **32**, 2100–2109.

Diemel, L.T., Copelman, C.A. & Cuzner, M.L. (1998) Macrophages in CNS remyelination: Friend or foe? *Neurochemical Research*, **23**, 341–347.

Durafourt, B.A., Moore, C.S., Zammit, D.A. *et al.* (2012) Comparison of polarization properties of human adult microglia and blood-derived macrophages. *Glia*, **60**, 717–727.

Dyall, S.C., Michael, G.J. & Michael-Titus, A.T. (2010) Omega-3 fatty acids reverse age-related decreases in nuclear receptors and increase neurogenesis in old rats. *Journal of Neuroscience Research*, **88**, 2091–2102.

Edgar, J.M., McLaughlin, M., Werner, H.B. *et al.* (2009) Early ultrastructural defects of axons and axon-glia junctions in mice lacking expression of Cnp1. *Glia*, **57**, 1815–1824.

Fancy, S.P., Kotter, M.R., Harrington, E.P. *et al.* (2010) Overcoming remyelination failure in multiple sclerosis and other myelin disorders. *Experimental Neurology*, **225**, 18–23.

Franklin, R.J. & Ffrench-Constant, C. (2008) Remyelination in the CNS: from biology to therapy. *Nature Reviews Neuroscience*, **9**, 839–855.

Franklin, R.J., Hinks, G.L., Woodruff, R.H. & O'Leary, M.T. (2001) What roles do growth factors play in CNS remyelination? *Progress in Brain Research*, **132**, 185–193.

Franklin, R.J. & Kotter, M.R. (2008) The biology of CNS remyelination: The key to therapeutic advances. *Journal of Neurology*, **255** (Suppl 1), 19–25.

Gadea, A., Aguirre, A., Haydar, T.F. & Gallo, V. (2009) Endothelin-1 regulates oligodendrocyte development. *The Journal of Neuroscience*, **29**, 10047–10062.

Ginhoux, F., Greter, M., Leboeuf, M. *et al.* (2010) Fate mapping analysis reveals that adult microglia derive from primitive macrophages. *Science*, **330**, 841–845.

Gitik, M., Liraz-Zaltsman, S., Oldenborg, P.A., Reichert, F. & Rotshenker, S. (2011) Myelin down-regulates myelin phagocytosis by microglia and macrophages through interactions between CD47 on myelin and SIRPalpha (signal regulatory protein-alpha) on phagocytes. *Journal of Neuroinflammation*, **8**, 24.

Giulian, D., Chen, J., Ingeman, J.E., George, J.K. & Noponen, M. (1989) The role of mononuclear phagocytes in wound healing after traumatic injury to adult mammalian brain. *Journal of Neuroscience*, **9**, 4416–4429.

Goncalves, A.F., Dias, N.G., Moransard, M. *et al.* (2010) Gelsolin is required for macrophage recruitment during remyelination of the peripheral nervous system. *Glia*, **58**, 706–715.

Griffiths, I., Klugmann, M., Anderson, T. *et al.* (1998) Axonal swellings and degeneration in mice lacking the major proteolipid of myelin. *Science*, **280**, 1610–1613.

Groves, A.K., Barnett, S.C., Franklin, R.J. *et al.* (1993) Repair of demyelinated lesions by transplantation of purified O-2A progenitor cells. *Nature*, **362**, 453–455.

Hadas, S., Reichert, F. & Rotshenker, S. (2010) Dissimilar and similar functional properties of complement receptor-3 in microglia and macrophages in combating yeast pathogens by phagocytosis. *Glia*, **58**, 823–830.

Hearps, A.C., Martin, G.E., Angelovich, T.A. *et al.* (2012) Aging is associated with chronic innate immune activation and dysregulation of monocyte phenotype and function. *Aging Cell*, **11**, 867–875.

Hendriks, J.J., Slaets, H., Carmans, S. *et al.* (2008) Leukemia inhibitory factor modulates production of inflammatory mediators and myelin phagocytosis by macrophages. *Journal of Neuroimmunology*, **204**, 52–57.

Hinks, G.L. & Franklin, R.J. (1999) Distinctive patterns of PDGF-A, FGF-2, IGF-I, and TGF-beta1 gene expression during remyelination of experimentally-induced spinal cord demyelination. *Molecular and Cellular Neurosciences*, **14**, 153–168.

Hinks, G.L. & Franklin, R.J. (2000) Delayed changes in growth factor gene expression during slow remyelination in the CNS of aged rats. *Molecular and Cellular Neurosciences*, **16**, 542–556.

Imai, M., Watanabe, M., Suyama, K. *et al.* (2008) Delayed accumulation of activated macrophages and inhibition of remyelination after spinal cord injury in an adult rodent model. *Journal of Neurosurgery Spine*, **8**, 58–66.

Kotter, M.R., Li, W.W., Zhao, C. & Franklin, R.J. (2006) Myelin impairs CNS remyelination by inhibiting oligodendrocyte precursor cell differentiation. *Journal of Neuroscience*, **26**, 328–332.

Kotter, M.R., Setzu, A., Sim, F.J., Van Rooijen, N. & Franklin, R.J. (2001) Macrophage depletion impairs oligodendrocyte remyelination following lysolecithin-induced demyelination. *Glia*, **35**, 204–212.

Kotter, M.R., Zhao, C., van Rooijen, N. & Franklin, R.J. (2005) Macrophage-depletion induced impairment of experimental CNS remyelination is associated with a reduced oligodendrocyte progenitor cell response and altered growth factor expression. *Neurobiology of Disease*, **18**, 166–175.

Kuhlmann, T., Miron, V., Cui, Q., Wegner, C., Antel, J. & Bruck, W. (2008) Differentiation block of oligodendroglial progenitor cells as a cause for remyelination failure in chronic multiple sclerosis. *Brain*, **131**, 1749–1758.

Laskin, D.L. (2009) Macrophages and inflammatory mediators in chemical toxicity: A battle of forces. *Chemical Research in Toxicology*, **22**, 1376–1385.

Lloberas, J. & Celada, A. (2002) Effect of aging on macrophage function. *Experimental Gerontology*, **37**, 1325–1331.

Lutz, M.A. & Correll, P.H. (2003) Activation of CR3-mediated phagocytosis by MSP requires the RON receptor, tyrosine kinase activity, phosphatidylinositol 3-kinase, and protein kinase C zeta. *Journal of Leukocyte Biology*, **73**, 802–814.

Ma, J., Tanaka, K.F., Shimizu, T. *et al.* (2011) Microglial cystatin F expression is a sensitive indicator for ongoing demyelination with concurrent remyelination. *Journal of Neuroscience Research*, **89**, 639–649.

Mancuso, P., McNish, R.W., Peters-Golden, M. & Brock, T.G. (2001) Evaluation of phagocytosis and arachidonate metabolism by alveolar macrophages and recruited neutrophils from F344xBN rats of different ages. *Mechanisms of Ageing and Development*, **122**, 1899–1913.

McKinnon, R.D., Piras, G., Ida, J.A. Jr. & Dubois-Dalcq, M. (1993a) A role for TGF-beta in oligodendrocyte differentiation. *Journal of Cell Biology*, **121**, 1397–1407.

McKinnon, R.D., Smith, C., Behar, T., Smith, T. & Dubois-Dalcq, M. (1993b) Distinct effects of bFGF and PDGF on oligodendrocyte progenitor cells. *Glia*, **7**, 245–254.

Mehta, V., Pei, W., Yang, G. *et al.* (2013) Iron is a sensitive biomarker for inflammation in multiple sclerosis lesions. *PLoS One*, **8**, e57573.

Mikita, J., Dubourdieu-Cassagno, N., Deloire, M.S. *et al.* (2011) Altered M1/M2 activation patterns of monocytes in severe relapsing experimental rat model of multiple sclerosis. Amelioration of clinical status by M2 activated monocyte administration. *Multiple Sclerosis*, **17**, 2–15.

Miron, V.E., Boyd, A., Zhao, J.W. *et al.* (2013) M2 microglia and macrophages drive oligodendrocyte differentiation during CNS remyelination. *Nature Neuroscience*, **16**, 1211–1218.

Moorman, S.J. & Hume, R.I. (1994) Contact with myelin evokes a release of calcium from internal stores in neonatal rat oligodendrocytes in vitro. *Glia*, **10**, 202–210.

Mozell, R.L. & McMorris, F.A. (1991) Insulin-like growth factor I stimulates oligodendrocyte development and myelination in rat brain aggregate cultures. *Journal of Neuroscience Research*, **30**, 382–390.

Nagy, L. & Schwabe, J.W. (2004) Mechanism of the nuclear receptor molecular switch. *Trends in Biochemical Sciences*, **29**, 317–324.

Nauta, A.J., Raaschou-Jensen, N., Roos, A. *et al.* (2003) Mannose-binding lectin engagement with late apoptotic and necrotic cells. *European Journal of Immunology*, **33**, 2853–2863.

Neumann, H., Kotter, M.R. & Franklin, R.J. (2009) Debris clearance by microglia: an essential link between degeneration and regeneration. *Brain*, **132**, 288–295.

O'Meara, R.W., Michalski, J.P. & Kothary, R. (2011) Integrin signaling in oligodendrocytes and its importance in CNS myelination. *Journal of Signal Transduction*, **2011**, 354091.

Olah, M., Amor, S., Brouwer, N. *et al.* (2012) Identification of a microglia phenotype supportive of remyelination. *Glia*, **60**, 306–321.

Ousman, S.S. & Kubes, P. (2012) Immune surveillance in the central nervous system. *Nature Neuroscience*, **15**, 1096–1101.

Pasquini, L.A., Millet, V., Hoyos, H.C. *et al.* (2011) Galectin-3 drives oligodendrocyte differentiation to control myelin integrity and function. *Cell Death and Differentiation*, **18**, 1746–1756.

Piccio, L., Buonsanti, C., Cella, M. *et al.* (2008) Identification of soluble TREM-2 in the cerebrospinal fluid and its association with multiple sclerosis and CNS inflammation. *Brain*, **131**, 3081–3091.

Piccio, L., Buonsanti, C., Mariani, M. *et al.* (2007) Blockade of TREM-2 exacerbates experimental autoimmune encephalomyelitis. *European Journal of Immunology*, **37**, 1290–1301.

Plemel, J.R., Manesh, S.B., Sparling, J.S. & Tetzlaff, W. (2013) Myelin inhibits oligodendroglial maturation and regulates oligodendrocytic transcription factor expression. *Glia*, **61**, 1471–1487.

Pohl, H.B., Porcheri, C., Mueggler, T. *et al.* (2011) Genetically induced adult oligodendrocyte cell death is associated with poor myelin clearance, reduced remyelination, and axonal damage. *Journal of Neuroscience*, **31**, 1069–1080.

Rawji, K.S. & Yong, V.W. (2013) The benefits and detriments of macrophages/microglia in models of multiple sclerosis. *Clinical & Developmental Immunology*, **2013**, 948976.

Reichert, F., Slobodov, U., Makranz, C. & Rotshenker, S. (2001) Modulation (inhibition and augmentation) of complement receptor-3-mediated myelin phagocytosis. *Neurobiology of Disease*, **8**, 504–512.

Robinson, S. & Miller, R.H. (1999) Contact with central nervous system myelin inhibits oligodendrocyte progenitor maturation. *Developmental Biology*, **216**, 359–368.

Rotshenker, S., Reichert, F., Gitik, M., Haklai, R., Elad-Sfadia, G. & Kloog, Y. (2008) Galectin-3/MAC-2, Ras and PI3K activate complement receptor-3 and scavenger receptor-AI/II mediated myelin phagocytosis in microglia. *Glia*, **56**, 1607–1613.

Ruckh, J.M., Zhao, J.W., Shadrach, J.L. *et al.* (2012) Rejuvenation of regeneration in the aging central nervous system. *Cell Stem Cell*, **10**, 96–103.

Schonberg, D.L., Goldstein, E.Z., Sahinkaya, F.R., Wei, P., Popovich, P.G. & McTigue, D.M. (2012) Ferritin stimulates oligodendrocyte genesis in the adult spinal cord and can be transferred from macrophages to NG2 cells in vivo. *Journal of Neuroscience*, **32**, 5374–5384.

Schulz, K., Kroner, A. & David, S. (2012) Iron efflux from astrocytes plays a role in remyelination. *Journal of Neuroscience*, **32**, 4841–4847.

Shechter, R. & Schwartz, M. (2013) Harnessing monocyte-derived macrophages to control central nervous system pathologies: no longer 'if' but 'how'. *Journal of Pathology*, **229**, 332–346.

Shi, Y., Zhang, D., Huff, T.B. *et al.* (2011) Longitudinal in vivo coherent anti-Stokes Raman scattering imaging of demyelination and remyelination in injured spinal cord. *Journal of Biomedical Optics*, **16**, 106012.

Shields, S.A., Gilson, J.M., Blakemore, W.F. & Franklin, R.J. (1999) Remyelination occurs as extensively but more slowly in old rats compared to young rats following gliotoxin-induced CNS demyelination. *Glia*, **28**, 77–83.

Sim, F.J., Zhao, C., Penderis, J. & Franklin, R.J. (2002) The age-related decrease in CNS remyelination efficiency is attributable to an impairment of both oligodendrocyte progenitor recruitment and differentiation. *Journal of Neuroscience*, **22**, 2451–2459.

Stidworthy, M.F., Genoud, S., Suter, U., Mantei, N. & Franklin, R.J. (2003) Quantifying the early stages of remyelination following cuprizone-induced demyelination. *Brain Pathology*, **13**, 329–339.

Stout, R.D. & Suttles, J. (2005) Immunosenescence and macrophage functional plasticity: Dysregulation of macrophage function by age-associated microenvironmental changes. *Immunological Reviews*, **205**, 60–71.

Sugama, S., Takenouchi, T., Kitani, H., Fujita, M. & Hashimoto, M. (2007) Activin as an anti-inflammatory cytokine produced by microglia. *Journal of Neuroimmunology*, **192**, 31–39.

Swift, M.E., Burns, A.L., Gray, K.L. & DiPietro, L.A. (2001) Age-related alterations in the inflammatory response to dermal injury. *Journal of Investigative Dermatology*, **117**, 1027–1035.

Syed, Y.A., Baer, A.S., Lubec, G., Hoeger, H., Widhalm, G. & Kotter, M.R. (2008) Inhibition of oligodendrocyte precursor cell differentiation by myelin-associated proteins. *Neurosurgical Focus*, **24**, E5.

Syed, Y.A., Hand, E., Mobius, W. *et al.* (2011) Inhibition of CNS remyelination by the presence of semaphorin 3A. *Journal of Neuroscience*, **31**, 3719–3728.

Takahashi, K., Prinz, M., Stagi, M., Chechneva, O. & Neumann, H. (2007) TREM2-transduced myeloid precursors mediate nervous tissue debris clearance and facilitate recovery in an animal model of multiple sclerosis. *PLoS Medicine*, **4**, e124.

Todorich, B., Zhang, X., Slagle-Webb, B., Seaman, W.E. & Connor, J.R. (2008) Tim-2 is the receptor for H-ferritin on oligodendrocytes. *Journal of Neurochemistry*, **107**, 1495–1505.

Vereyken, E.J., Heijnen, P.D., Baron, W., de Vries, E.H., Dijkstra, C.D. & Teunissen, C.E. (2011) Classically and alternatively activated bone marrow derived macrophages differ in cytoskeletal functions and migration towards specific CNS cell types. *Journal of Neuroinflammation*, **8**, 58.

Vogel, D.Y., Vereyken, E.J., Glim, J.E. *et al.* (2013) Macrophages in inflammatory multiple sclerosis lesions have an intermediate activation status. *Journal of Neuroinflammation*, **10**, 35.

Warrington, A.E., Barbarese, E. & Pfeiffer, S.E. (1993) Differential myelinogenic capacity of specific developmental stages of the oligodendrocyte lineage upon transplantation into hypomyelinating hosts. *Journal of Neuroscience Research*, **34**, 1–13.

Wilms, H., Schwark, T., Brandenburg, L.O. *et al.* (2010) Regulation of activin A synthesis in microglial cells: Pathophysiological implications for bacterial meningitis. *Journal of Neuroscience Research*, **88**, 16–23.

Yuen, T.J., Johnson, K.R., Miron, V.E. *et al.* (2013) Identification of endothelin 2 as an inflammatory factor that promotes central nervous system remyelination. *Brain*, **136**, 1035–1047.

Zhang, S.C., Ge, B. & Duncan, I.D. (1999) Adult brain retains the potential to generate oligodendroglial progenitors with extensive myelination capacity. *Proceedings of the National Academy of Sciences of the United States of America*, **96**, 4089–4094.

Zhao, C., Li, W.W. & Franklin, R.J. (2006) Differences in the early inflammatory responses to toxin-induced demyelination are associated with the age-related decline in CNS remyelination. *Neurobiology of Aging*, **27**, 1298–1307.

14   Microglia Involvement in Rett Syndrome

Noël C. Derecki,[1] James C. Cronk,[1,2] and Jonathan Kipnis[1,2]

[1]Center for Brain Immunology and Glia, Department of Neuroscience, School of Medicine, University of Virginia, Charlottesville, VA, USA
[2]Graduate Program in Neuroscience and Medical Scientist Training Program, School of Medicine, University of Virginia, Charlottesville, VA, USA

Introduction to Rett Syndrome and MeCP2

Rett syndrome is named after pediatrician Andreas Rett, who first described the disorder in 1966 (Rett, 1966) after noticing a cluster of symptoms in several young girls he was treating; his initial writings were lost to the scientific community until the 1980s, when Bengt Hagberg connected Rett's original observations to his own work with over 200 girls (Hagberg *et al.*, 1983; Hagberg and Witt-Engerstrom, 1986). Hagberg graciously named the pathology after Rett. The disease is characterized as a neurodevelopmental disorder, with symptoms including seizures, motor dysfunction and stereotypies, respiratory abnormalities (waking apneas/breath holding), gastrointestinal pathology, osteopenia, scoliosis, and general growth deficit (Glaze, 2005; Chahrour and Zoghbi, 2007). Most patients develop no or poor speech skills, making communication difficult. Thus, the ability of caregivers to understand the precise nature of what patients experience is particularly difficult (Chahrour and Zoghbi, 2007). The vast majority of patients are female, because the disease is caused by mutations of an X-linked gene encoding for methyl-CpG-binding protein 2 (MeCP2); an association discovered in the laboratory of Huda Zoghbi in 1999 (Amir *et al.*, 1999). Owing to X-inactivation, female patients (who are heterozygous for MeCP2 mutations) are born with a mix of cells expressing only normal MeCP2 or mutant MeCP2. In contrast, male patients inheriting MeCP2 mutations will express the mutant version of the protein in all cells, as they possess only the single X chromosome from their mothers containing the mutant version of the gene (and are therefore hemizygous for MeCP2 mutation). Consequently, hemizygous male patients inheriting mutant MeCP2 experience significantly more severe pathology than heterozygous female patients, with most male patients dying within the first year of life (Chahrour and Zoghbi, 2007). Heterozygous female patients survive within a wide age range; some patients

Neuroinflammation: New Insights into Beneficial and Detrimental Functions, First Edition. Edited by Samuel David.
© 2015 John Wiley & Sons, Inc. Published 2015 by John Wiley & Sons, Inc.

succumb early, although many live well into adulthood (Chahrour and Zoghbi, 2007). The exact cause(s) of death is not known; however, they are presumed to be combinations of seizure, respiratory failure, and autonomic failure (Glaze, 2005).

MeCP2 functions by binding to methylated CpG sites in DNA and recruits factors that alter nearby gene expression (Adkins and Georgel, 2011). The protein appears to bind ubiquitously across the genome in the cells in which it is expressed (Nan *et al.*, 1997) and was initially believed to be responsible primarily for recruitment of complexes involved in transcriptional repression, with the most prominent binding partner being Sin3a (Nan *et al.*, 1997, 1998; Jones *et al.*, 1998). However, it was later discovered that MeCP2 could also activate genetic transcription via an association with CREB1 (Chahrour *et al.*, 2008). Interestingly, MeCP2 has also been shown to bind PU.1 (Suzuki *et al.*, 2003) and to mediate expression of PU.1-associated genes via recruitment of the mSin3a–histone deacetylase (HDAC) complex. This is notable for the purposes of this discussion, because PU.1 is necessary for the development of not only microglia specifically (Kierdorf *et al.*, 2013), but also the entire myeloid lineage, of which microglia are a part (McKercher *et al.*, 1996; Anderson *et al.*, 1998). This opens the possibility that MeCP2 may in fact be playing an important role in microglia, and potentially myeloid cells as a whole, via interactions with a critical transcription factor in the development and function of myeloid cells, PU.1. In addition to being a key binding partner for PU.1, *Mecp2* was also shown to be involved in regulation of other immune players including nuclear factor κB (NFκB), FoxP3, peroxisome proliferator-activated receptor gamma (PPARγ), interferon γ IFNγ, and T-Bet (Tong *et al.*, 2005; Lal *et al.*, 2009; Mann *et al.*, 2010; Yang *et al.*, 2012; O'Driscoll *et al.*, 2013), thereby suggesting the possibility of pleiotropic effects on immune regulation as a result of loss or changes in expression of *Mecp2*.

Experimental Mouse Models Used in the Study of Rett Syndrome

Animal models of Rett syndrome (Table 14.1) have focused on *Mecp2*-null mice, with the two major genetic strains having been produced in the laboratories of Adrian Bird (Guy *et al.*, 2001) and Rudolph Jaenisch (Chen *et al.*, 2001), both first published in 2001. In these *Mecp2*-null mouse strains, *Mecp2*-null male mice, predictably, are much sicker than heterozygous female mice. *Mecp2*-null male mice typically survive in the range of 6–12 weeks, with initiation of pathology at about 4 weeks of age and progressing until death. Heterozygous female mice exhibit delayed and then slower disease progression, with pathology beginning about 4–6 months of age. Both male and female mice experience seizures, breathing abnormalities, motor dysfunction, and osteopenia, similar to human patients. However, only male mice exhibit significant somatic growth deficits, and the onset of pathology in male mice occurs before adulthood as in the human female condition. Owing to the faster progression of disease in male mice, and lower degree of variability in disease phenotype, they have been used most commonly in experimentation. The degree to which the completely *Mecp2*-null male mice are directly relevant to the heterozygous human female disease is not clear; it is entirely possible that interactions between MeCP2-normal and mutant cells in heterozygous human female individuals (and mice) may create unique situations and pathologies that are not present in *Mecp2*-null male mice. However, it should be noted that *Mecp2*-null male mice allow scientists to ask more direct questions regarding the function and roles for *Mecp2*, because they are not a mixed experimental system as in the case of

Table 14.1 Amelioration of Rett pathology upon cell-specific rescue of MeCP2 expression in *Mecp2*-null mice

Mouse model	Symptoms improved	Survival
Mecp2-null (Chen *et al.*, 2001; Guy *et al.*, 2001)	—	6–12 weeks
Postnatal Mecp2 expression, all cells (Guy *et al.*, 2007)	Neurologic, general health, and body weight	Near wild type
Mecp2 expression, neurons only (Luikenhuis *et al.*, 2004; Giacometti *et al.*, 2007)	Brain weight, body weight, open field movement	Near wild type (Luikenhuis *et al.*, 2004) or up to 9 months (Giacometti *et al.*, 2007)
Postnatal Mecp2 expression, astrocytes (Lioy *et al.*, 2011)	Open field movement, breathing, neuron soma size	Up to 15 months (all animals euthanized by this age)
Wild-type bone marrow transplant into *Mecp2*-null, including CNS engraftment (Derecki *et al.*, 2012)	Open field movement, breathing, body weight, gait, tremors	Average ~6–7 months, oldest mouse aged 11.5 months
Genetic expression of Mecp2 in only oligodendrocytes (Nguyen *et al.*, 2013)	Hindlimb clasping, body weight, coordination	16 weeks (3 week increase over controls)

heterozygous female mice. Ideally, however, research performed in *Mecp2*-null male mice should be further expanded to Mecp2-heterozygous female mice in order to better understand how the mixed *Mecp2*-normal and -null condition may contribute to pathology and experimental results.

The Cellular Players in Central Nervous System Pathology of Rett Syndrome

Early studies indicated that within the brain, neurons were the only major cell type to express MeCP2 (Shahbazian and Zoghbi, 2002). As such, glial cells were largely ignored for nearly a decade as potential contributors to disease pathogenesis. However, in 2009 and 2011 publications from the laboratory of Gail Mandel indicated that astrocytes may be contributing to the disease by failing to support neurons (Ballas *et al.*, 2009; Lioy *et al.*, 2011). Firstly, in a series of *in vitro* experiments using cultured neurons, astrocytes, and astrocyte-conditioned media from wild-type and *Mecp2*-null mouse brains, Mandel's laboratory demonstrated that wild-type astrocytes or conditioned media could support normal dendritic branching of normally stunted *Mecp2*-null neurons (Ballas *et al.*, 2009). Later *in vivo* experiments using a genetic approach showed that reexpression of *Mecp2* solely in astrocytes of otherwise *Mecp2*-null mice attenuated deficits in several neurologic parameters and significantly increased lifespan (Lioy *et al.*, 2011). These works were the first to suggest that glia, and not only neurons, play a significant role in the pathogenesis of disease in *Mecp2*-deficient mouse models. More recently, in 2013, it was shown that oligodendrocytes may also play a role in pathology, with either specific restoration or removal of *Mecp2* from these cells leading to improvement or initiation of pathology (Nguyen *et al.*, 2013).

Microglia [which are non-neural cells, derived from a separate cellular source as compared to neurons, astrocytes, and oligodendrocytes (Ginhoux *et al.*, 2010)] are the resident mononuclear phagocytes of the central nervous system (CNS). In 2010, it was suggested that *Mecp2*-null microglia may actually cause damage to neuronal dendrites and synapses via increased levels of glutamate release (Maezawa and Jin, 2010a). We subsequently demonstrated that transplant of wild-type microglia-like cells into the brains of *Mecp2*-null mice greatly improved survival, breathing, and locomotor deficits (Derecki *et al.*, 2012). This result was further confirmed using a genetic approach targeting myeloid cells, including a large fraction of microglia for expression of wild-type Mecp2 in otherwise *Mecp2*-null mice. In this work, failure of *Mecp2*-null microglia to properly phagocytose apoptotic cells was implicated as a cause of pathology (Derecki *et al.*, 2012).

It had been known since 2004 that expression of Mecp2 in neurons (under the Tau promoter) could rescue much of the disease in otherwise *Mecp2*-null mice (Luikenhuis *et al.*, 2004). Restoration of Mecp2 in all cells of an otherwise *Mecp2*-null mouse was also shown to reverse pathology in symptomatic mice (Guy *et al.*, 2007). On the basis of these results, it was largely assumed that Rett syndrome was a disease of only neurons; however, the recent works discussed in this chapter have shown that Rett syndrome is a far more complex disorder and certainly is not a single-cell-type pathology. This is exemplified by the incomplete rescue by neuron-only reexpression of Mecp2 and varying therapeutic effects of Mecp2 expression in all three major glia subtypes (Lioy *et al.*, 2011; Derecki *et al.*, 2012; Nguyen *et al.*, 2013); when taken together, the aggregate data may indicate that in Rett syndrome, malfunctioning neurons are impaired both intrinsically and extrinsically via failure of the MeCP2-expressing glia that surround and support them. Glia-specific rescues may in part improve disease outcomes by providing support to critically malfunctioning neurons, enhancing and supporting their function.

Future work should be aimed at understanding the exact mechanisms whereby glial–neuronal and even glial–glial interactions may contribute to pathology or therapy in Rett syndrome. However, the role of glia in the brain, and how they interact with their cellular partners in the normal, healthy condition, is still an active area of research; this makes the study of the roles glia may play in pathology a difficult task, as it is not fully understood what these cells should be doing in the healthy brain. This is especially true for microglia, the focus of this chapter, as they have only recently been recognized as important players in both brain development and homeostasis, as will be discussed in the following section.

Microglia: From Footnote to First-Line

The brain has long been chiefly considered from the point-of-view that neurons are the primary players. This basic concept has not changed (and rightfully so) but lately, glial cells have been increasingly recognized as important in supporting roles: oligodendrocytes are indispensable in myelination and facilitators of neuronal transmission; astrocytes are buffers of the extracellular milieu and are therefore important in maintaining the space within which neurons must function. Along these lines, oligodendrocytes and astrocytes are almost universally accepted as "benign" cells (except, perhaps in the case of glioma). Accordingly, they are frequently examined as regulators of homeostasis and are routinely investigated in terms of their ability to support healthy brain function.

Microglia, however, have remained the odd cell out in this recent elucidation of glial support for the larger CNS. Indeed, for a long time after their initial description by Pio del Rio-Hortega – the "father" of microglial biology (Rio-Hortega, 1932) – microglia were more or less ignored completely. At best, microglia were believed to be quiescent cells, simply doing nothing for long stretches of time in the absence of exogenous stimulation. At worst, if they

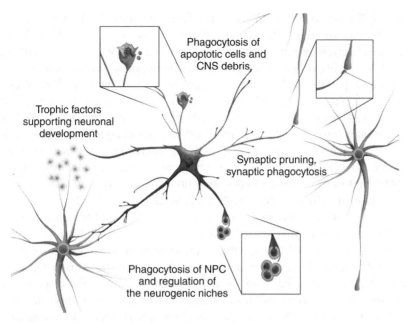

Phagocytosis of
apoptotic cells and
CNS debris

Trophic factors
supporting neuronal
development

Synaptic pruning,
synaptic phagocytosis

Phagocytosis of NPC
and regulation of
the neurogenic niches

Figure 14.1 Supporting functions of microglia in healthy brain. Microglia support neuronal survival by secretion of trophic factors such as insulin-like growth factor (IGF)-1 (Giacometti *et al.*, 2007; Ueno *et al.*, 2013) and brain-derived neurotrophic factor (BDNF; Ferrini and De Koninck, 2013; Parkhurst *et al.*, 2013); microglia are the major phagocytes responsible for clearance of apoptotic corpses and cellular debris (Okazawa *et al.*, 1996); microglia were shown to phagocytose, and possibly even "prune" neuronal synapses (Tremblay *et al.*, 2010; Schafer *et al.*, 2012); microglia are one of the primary phagocytic cells involved in cell clearance and trophic support in the neurogenic niches (Cunningham *et al.*, 2013).

were provoked into activation, microglia were seen as bad actors, even referred to as "the enemy within" because of their ability to cause damage to delicate neurons through their production of proinflammatory factors in response to pathogens or CNS injury (Gehrmann *et al.*, 1995; Zielasek and Hartung, 1996).

It was only with the advent of *in vivo* two-photon microscopy that microglia were finally thrust into the spotlight as likely having a role in day-to-day maintenance of the brain. Time-lapse imaging conclusively revealed that microglia, far from being inactive and quiescent cells, were constantly sampling their environment and responding dynamically to molecular cues (Nimmerjahn *et al.*, 2005). Work since then, using diverse methodologies, has confirmed that microglia perform myriad duties – from shaping neurogenesis and regulating the neuronal progenitor cell niche, to pruning synapses during brain development, to secretion of growth factors in support of behavior and network function (Schafer *et al.*, 2012; Ferrini and De Koninck, 2013; Parkhurst *et al.*, 2013). Therefore, microglia have been revealed to be far more complex and integral to healthy brain function than ever imagined, and a more balanced role for these cells has emerged (Fig. 14.1).

Microglia: the Tissue-Resident Macrophages of the Brain

These recent studies of microglia function have also been complemented by several major works that now elucidate the true origins of these previously enigmatic cells. Microglia have been conclusively shown to belong to the larger family of long-lived phagocytic cells known as tissue-resident macrophages (Schulz *et al.*, 2012; Yona *et al.*, 2013). Tissue-resident macrophages arise during primitive hematopoiesis, with progenitor cells first appearing in the yolk sac; these events occur before definitive hematopoiesis in the bone marrow (Schulz *et al.*, 2012; Yona *et al.*, 2013). Therefore, microglia share provenance with Kupffer cells in the liver, red pulp macrophages in the spleen, and alveolar macrophages in the lungs, rather than bone-marrow-derived monocytes, as was originally posited. Even from this partial list, one can clearly see the tremendous diversity of tissue-resident macrophages depending on final resting tissue. However, their diversity belies their unifying characteristic, which is in homeostatic regulation of the tissues within which they reside and their essential role in development (Ashwell, 1990; Naito *et al.*, 2004; Gordon and Taylor, 2005; Mebius and Kraal, 2005; Gow *et al.*, 2010; Sierra *et al.*, 2010; Erblich *et al.*, 2011; Schafer *et al.*, 2012).

Microglia, as the tissue-resident macrophages of the CNS, would be expected to be involved during brain development as professional phagocytes, and this is indeed the case. Studies of this phenomenon have indicated that apoptotic corpse removal in the brain is similar to that in other tissues, in that recognition is mediated largely by phosphatidylserine exposure by target cells. Interestingly, however, it has also been shown that the microglial response to apoptotic neurons is not strictly stereotyped and involves several nuances. For example, it was shown that microglial cells were able to protect cerebellar granule neurons from excitotoxic death by shifting a high-potassium-depolarizing environment to a low-potassium-hyperpolarizing environment. Strikingly, serial medium transfer experiments indicated that neuronally derived signals were critical to microglial ion-buffering action, suggesting active communication between the two cell types underlying the ability of microglia to preserve neurons in ionically imbalanced environments (Polazzi *et al.*, 2001). Recent works also show that microglial activation phenotype, as indicated by up-regulation of CD11b and DAP12, is necessary for proper brain development; studies using mice with microglia deficient in these key proteins demonstrate concomitant impairment in hippocampal development linked to defective targeting and clearance of superfluous neurons (Wakselman *et al.*, 2008). Similarly, it was demonstrated that microglia promote Purkinje neuron death in cerebellum through contact-dependent mechanisms involving cleaved caspase-3 expression (Marin-Teva *et al.*, 2004).

Although historically Rett syndrome has not been linked to deficits in neuronal corpse removal, our recent data suggest this might be an unrealized phenomenon contributing to neuronal pathology common to both the human Rett syndrome and *Mecp2*-mutant and *Mecp2*-null mouse models of the disease. We demonstrated that directed expression of wild-type Mecp2 in microglia of otherwise *Mecp2*-null mice was sufficient to significantly blunt phenotypic progression of symptoms. However, chronic injection of otherwise genetically rescued mice with annexin V – a factor which binds to exposed phosphatidylserine residues on apoptotic cells and blocks recognition and uptake – completely abrogated rescue and resulted in increased levels of TUNEL-positive debris in brains of injected mice (Derecki *et al.*, 2012). These results indicate that corpse and debris removal may be a key factor by which normally functioning microglia are able to provide amelioration of symptoms in otherwise *Mecp2*-null mouse brain.

Interestingly, neurons in *Mecp2*-null mice have been shown by numerous investigators to exhibit significantly reduced soma size (Chen *et al.*, 2001; Guy *et al.*, 2001; Amit *et al.*, 2009), and visual comparisons of brain slices from wild-type and *Mecp2*-null mice suggest increased packing density of neurons. Accordingly, it has been shown that microglia are a key cell type involved in removal of apoptotic corpses, as well as initiation of the cell death cascade in supernumerary neurons. It may be that malfunctioning microglia, similar to the results shown by Wakselman *et al.*, previously, in DAP-12- and CD11b-impaired mice, could contribute to the abnormal cell morphology seen in *Mecp2*-null mice and patients with Rett syndrome. Similarly, in the absence of proper cell removal, it is possible that neurotransmitters might be insufficiently scavenged from synaptic spaces, and diffusion of soluble factors that support normal neural functioning could be impaired. These specific possibilities have not been examined, however, so remain within the realm of conjecture at this time.

While corpse removal is a key facet of brain development, with estimates of between 20% and 80% of all neurons born being eliminated (Okazawa *et al.*, 1996), it should be noted that whole cells are not the only targets for phagocytosis in the developing brain. Synapses are also remodeled during development. The first reports of microglia functioning in synapse removal were following facial nerve axotomy wherein microglia were visualized removing morphologically intact synaptic terminals (Blinzinger and Kreutzberg, 1968). Synaptic stripping has also been studied following bacterial pathogen injection into cortex. Interestingly, because neuronal pathology was not a feature of the aftermath of the manipulation, the authors hypothesized that microglia might be functioning in a neuroprotective role (Trapp *et al.*, 2007). Most recently, microglia were identified as the key phagocytes involved in the removal of supernumerary synapses during visual system development (Tremblay *et al.*, 2010; Schafer *et al.*, 2012). This finding was notable for several reasons: firstly, it had previously been largely assumed that synaptic removal was limited to a response to traumatic insult or pathogen introduction, following the widely held notion that microglia were essentially inert unless provoked; secondly, it was shown that this synapse removal was activity dependent, which is well documented as driving specification of neuronal inputs during visual system patterning. This is significant because it suggests crosstalk between multiple cell types in service of building a functional circuit, rather than a neuron-intrinsic process simply supported by glial cells. In fact, a subsequent finding revealed that astrocytes, microglia, and neurons were linked by transforming growth factor beta (TGF-β) signaling in support of visual system synaptic removal (Bialas and Stevens, 2013). These data are particularly interesting in the context of Rett syndrome, which, far from being a pathology involving solely neurons, has now been shown to be a result of improper activity by multiple cell types, including astrocytes and microglia (Ballas *et al.*, 2009; Maezawa and Jin, 2010b; Lioy *et al.*, 2011; Derecki *et al.*, 2012). The importance of a single molecule in this tricellular interaction is also notable given recent work implicating TGF-β as indispensable for microglial gene expression profile, phenotype, and population maintenance within the CNS (Butovsky *et al.*, 2014), perhaps underlying the ability of reexpression of *Mecp2* in astrocytes, microglia, or neurons to potently and positively affect disease phenotype in mouse models of Rett syndrome.

It was recently suggested that *Mecp2*-null microglia could be adversely affecting neuronal fate and function by excess glutamate production. While this might conceivably lead to a scenario wherein extensive neuronal death could occur, frank neurodegeneration is not a recognized phenotype seen in Rett syndrome. However, supranormal – but sublethal levels of glutamate might result in downregulation of glutamatergic receptors on neurons as a self-protective response.

Indeed, significantly reduced glutamatergic receptor levels have been indicated by immunofluorescent labeling on neurons in phenotypic *Mecp2*-null mice (Lioy *et al.*, 2011).

Replacement/Augmentation of MICROGLIA as A Potential Therapy in Rett Syndrome

As previously discussed, in 2012, we showed that either engraftment of wild-type microglia via bone marrow transplant or genetic rescue of microglia in otherwise *Mecp2*-null mice significantly abrogates disease and extends lifespan (Derecki *et al.*, 2012). Only 1 year prior, a similar beneficial effect was published using genetic rescue of astrocytes (Lioy *et al.*, 2011), therefore these combined works solidified glia as important, previously unappreciated players in the development of Rett pathology.

In mice, bone marrow transplant is achieved by lethal irradiation, followed by intravenous injection of whole bone marrow single cell suspension. This procedure results in both replacement of the peripheral, bone-marrow-derived immune system, and also engraftment of microglia-like cells in the brain, which develop from $CCR2^+Ly6C^{hi}$ monocytes (Mildner *et al.*, 2007). Engraftment of these microglia-like cells depends critically on irradiation of the brain (Mildner *et al.*, 2007), although the exact reasons for this are still unknown. It is postulated that irradiation may lead to changes in the blood–brain barrier, allowing for entry of peripheral cells; that irradiation may impair microglia from self-renewing, triggering their replacement by peripheral immune cells; or even that irradiation may induce inflammatory or chemokine signals, which call the $CCR2^+Ly6C^{hi}$ progenitors into the brain, leading to their eventual differentiation into resident, long-lasting microglia-like cells. Regardless of the etiology, these microglia-like cells are ramified, resident cells, appearing very similar to microglia with increasing proportion of the total brain tissue-resident mononuclear phagocyte pool as the animal ages. These cells should not, however, be directly equated with true microglia, which as previously discussed are derived from an entirely different cellular source early in embryonic development (Ginhoux *et al.*, 2010). Regardless, these engrafted microglia-like cells have been shown to provide benefit in several disease models, including obsessive–compulsive disorder (Chen *et al.*, 2010), lysosomal and peroxisomal storage diseases (Krivit *et al.*, 1995), and, of course, Rett syndrome (Derecki *et al.*, 2012).

The most surprising finding regarding wild-type microglia-like cell engraftment in *Mecp2*-null mice was the significant increase in lifespan (Derecki *et al.*, 2012). However, the relevance of this finding to disease in heterozygous *MeCP2*-mutant human female individuals is yet to be shown. Although both male humans and mice with either *MeCP2* mutation or complete loss of *Mecp2*, respectively, almost universally experience early mortality, this is not a consistent phenotype in the human female Rett syndrome (Chahrour and Zoghbi, 2007). However, it was also shown that several health, behavioral, and neurologic parameters were improved in Mecp2 heterozygous female mice, including weight, coordination (rotarod), open field movement, and number of apneas (Derecki *et al.*, 2012), suggesting that transplant of normal, healthy microglia into the brains of heterozygous female mice can facilitate improvements in health and neurologic function.

Exactly how microglia mediate benefit in *Mecp2*-deficient mice is still an open question. Although it was shown that *Mecp2*-null microglia are impaired in phagocytosis (Derecki *et al.*, 2012), this is likely not the sole explanation for pathology related to microglia. For instance, it was also demonstrated that *Mecp2*-null microglia may be actively damaging neurons via glutamate release (Maezawa and Jin, 2010a). Failure of microglial phagocytosis could lead to defects of both nervous system development and homeostasis. Augmentation or replacement of *Mecp2*-null microglia with wild-type microglia-like cells could provide benefit by providing necessary homeostatic function, which is absent or insufficient in *Mecp2*-null microglia, or even by mitigating damage that would have otherwise been actively caused by *Mecp2*-null microglia.

Despite the potential for improvement in Rett syndrome pathology, there is great risk involved in the procedure due to the fact that engraftment of new microglia-like cells into the brain necessitates the use of irradiation in young children. Irradiation in children has been associated with craniofacial abnormalities (Dahllof, 1998), endocrine dysfunction (Duffner, 2004), and later development of malignancy (Tucker *et al.*, 1987; Socie *et al.*, 2000). For this reason, further studies should be performed both to confirm the potential for benefit in human Rett syndrome patients and also to reduce the risks posed by, or even eliminate the need for, irradiation altogether. In addition to the risks posed by irradiation, heterologous bone marrow transplant from human leukocyte antigen (HLA)-matched donors is not without inherent risk of rejection, sometimes a lethal consequence. For this reason, scenarios in which autologous bone marrow transplant might be used, either with ablation of the mutant fraction of cells from the patient before reinjection, or with *ex vivo* genetic manipulation of bone marrow in order to "fix" mutant progenitor cells before reimplantation should be explored.

Gene Therapy

There has been a prevailing concept in the scientific community that gene therapy may represent the best way to treat Rett syndrome. While in theory, this makes sense – replacement of normal MeCP2 expression in mutant cells would potentially cure the disease – it may be much more complicated in practice. In mice, it has been shown that virally delivered *Mecp2* can improve disease outcomes in heterozygous female mice (Garg *et al.*, 2013), giving hope to the idea that gene therapy may work for Rett syndrome. However, there are significant concerns regarding gene dosage. In addition to Rett syndrome, there is another disorder caused by aberrant MeCP2 activity – MeCP2-duplication syndrome (Van Esch *et al.*, 2005; Ramocki *et al.*, 2010). In this genetic disorder, instead of mutations in MeCP2, patients have undergone a duplication of the Xq28 chromosomal region, which includes the gene encoding MeCP2 (Ramocki *et al.*, 2010). It has been shown using genetic mouse models that overexpression of Mecp2 directly results in many of the disease phenotypes seen in human patients (Collins *et al.*, 2004). Unlike Rett syndrome, MeCP2-duplication syndrome largely affects male patients, because female patients inheriting the duplication have X chromosome skewing that heavily favors the normal chromosome (Ramocki *et al.*, 2010). Male patients with MeCP2-duplication syndrome experience similar symptoms to female patients with Rett syndrome, including seizures, motor dysfunction, and motor abnormalities, in addition to cognitive impairment (Ramocki *et al.*, 2010). Because of the severe disease caused by MeCP2 overexpression, any endeavors to use gene therapy in Rett syndrome must be particularly concerned with the potential to introduce more than one copy, or induce excessive expression, of *MeCP2*. These potential dangers make microglia-like cell transplant an attractive alternative approach to treating Rett syndrome, although this potential therapy comes with its own set of hurdles to be overcome, as has been discussed.

Conclusions

Scientific and clinical understanding of Rett syndrome has undergone significant advances since 1999 when mutations in *MeCP2* were first identified as the major causative factor in this devastating neurodevelopmental disorder (Amir *et al.*, 1999). While first thought to be absent from glia (Shahbazian and Zoghbi, 2002), MeCP2 has been shown to not only be present in glia, but that glia also contribute to pathology associated with *Mecp2*-deficiency (Ballas *et al.*, 2009; Maezawa and Jin, 2010a; Lioy *et al.*, 2011; Derecki *et al.*, 2012; Nguyen *et al.*, 2013). Microglia, however, represent a unique potential for therapy as compared to other types of glia or neurons. Unlike other major cell types of the CNS, only microglia (or more accurately, microglia-like cells) have been effectively transplanted into the CNS using techniques that can be used in human patients, meaning that real tools exist to augment, or potentially even replace, microglia in the brains of patients with Rett syndrome. Unfortunately, transplantation of microglia-like cells into the brains of patients with Rett syndrome would currently necessitate the use of irradiation in young children, which may lead to serious downstream complications (Tucker *et al.*, 1987; Dahllof, 1998; Socie *et al.*, 2000; Duffner, 2004). In addition, the exact functions that are altered or impaired by *Mecp2* deficiency in microglia are still unclear, and future work should focus on elucidating how *Mecp2* influences microglial behavior and interactions. A better understanding of the function of *Mecp2* in microglia, and how its loss causes pathology, may lead to alternative approaches and therapies in addition to direct transplantation of healthy microglia-like cells into the CNS. Transplantation, however, might become a more attractive therapeutic option if methods for achieving engraftment of microglia-like cells into the brain that obviate the need for irradiation were developed. It is certain, however, that microglia represent a promising therapeutic target for Rett syndrome.

References

Adkins, N.L. & Georgel, P.T. (2011) MeCP2: Structure and function. *Biochemistry and Cell Biology (Biochimie et biologie cellulaire)*, **89**, 1–11.

Amir, R.E., Van den Veyver, I.B., Wan, M., Tran, C.Q., Francke, U. & Zoghbi, H.Y. (1999) Rett syndrome is caused by mutations in X-linked MECP2, encoding methyl-CpG-binding protein 2. *Nature Genetics*, **23**, 185–188.

Amit, I. *et al.* (2009) Unbiased reconstruction of a mammalian transcriptional network mediating pathogen responses. *Science*, **326**, 257–263.

Anderson, K.L., Smith, K.A., Conners, K., McKercher, S.R., Maki, R.A. & Torbett, B.E. (1998) Myeloid development is selectively disrupted in PU.1 null mice. *Blood*, **91**, 3702–3710.

Ashwell, K. (1990) Microglia and cell death in the developing mouse cerebellum. *Brain Research. Developmental Brain Research*, **55**, 219–230.

Ballas, N., Lioy, D.T., Grunseich, C. & Mandel, G. (2009) Non-cell autonomous influence of MeCP2-deficient glia on neuronal dendritic morphology. *Nature Neuroscience*, **12**, 311–317.

Bialas, A.R. & Stevens, B. (2013) TGF-beta signaling regulates neuronal C1q expression and developmental synaptic refinement. *Nature Neuroscience*, **16**, 1773–1782.

Blinzinger, K. & Kreutzberg, G. (1968) Displacement of synaptic terminals from regenerating motoneurons by microglial cells. *Zeitschrift für Zellforschung und mikroskopische Anatomie*, **85**, 145–157.

Butovsky, O., Jedrychowski, M.P., Moore, C.S. *et al.* (2014) Identification of a unique TGF-beta-dependent molecular and functional signature in microglia. *Nature Neuroscience*, **17**, 131–143.

Chahrour, M. & Zoghbi, H.Y. (2007) The story of Rett syndrome: From clinic to neurobiology. *Neuron*, **56**, 422–437.

Chahrour, M., Jung, S.Y., Shaw, C. *et al.* (2008) MeCP2, a key contributor to neurological disease, activates and represses transcription. *Science*, **320**, 1224–1229.

Chen, R.Z., Akbarian, S., Tudor, M. & Jaenisch, R. (2001) Deficiency of methyl-CpG binding protein-2 in CNS neurons results in a Rett-like phenotype in mice. *Nature Genetics*, **27**, 327–331.

Chen, S.K., Tvrdik, P., Peden, E. *et al.* (2010) Hematopoietic origin of pathological grooming in Hoxb8 mutant mice. *Cell*, **141**, 775–785.

Collins, A.L., Levenson, J.M., Vilaythong, A.P. *et al.* (2004) Mild overexpression of MeCP2 causes a progressive neurological disorder in mice. *Human Molecular Genetics*, **13**, 2679–2689.

Cunningham, C.L., Martinez-Cerdeno, V. & Noctor, S.C. (2013) Microglia regulate the number of neural precursor cells in the developing cerebral cortex. *Journal of Neuroscience*, **33**, 4216–4233.

Dahllof, G. (1998) Craniofacial growth in children treated for malignant diseases. *Acta Odontologica Scandinavica*, **56**, 378–382.

Del Rio-Hortega, P. (1932) *Cytology and Cellular Pathology of the Nervous System*. P. B. Hoebaer, New York, NY.

Derecki, N.C., Cronk, J.C., Lu, Z. *et al.* (2012) Wild-type microglia arrest pathology in a mouse model of Rett syndrome. *Nature*, **484**, 105–109.

Duffner, P.K. (2004) Long-term effects of radiation therapy on cognitive and endocrine function in children with leukemia and brain tumors. *Neurologist*, **10**, 293–310.

Erblich, B., Zhu, L., Etgen, A.M., Dobrenis, K. & Pollard, J.W. (2011) Absence of colony stimulation factor-1 receptor results in loss of microglia, disrupted brain development and olfactory deficits. *PLoS One*, **6**, e26317.

Ferrini, F. & De Koninck, Y. (2013) Microglia control neuronal network excitability via BDNF signalling. *Neural Plasticity*, **2013**, 429815.

Garg, S.K., Lioy, D.T., Cheval, H. *et al.* (2013) Systemic delivery of MeCP2 rescues behavioral and cellular deficits in female mouse models of Rett syndrome. *Journal of Neuroscience*, **33**, 13612–13620.

Gehrmann, J., Matsumoto, Y. & Kreutzberg, G.W. (1995) Microglia: Intrinsic immuneffector cell of the brain. *Brain Research Reviews*, **20**, 269–287.

Giacometti, E., Luikenhuis, S., Beard, C. & Jaenisch, R. (2007) Partial rescue of MeCP2 deficiency by postnatal activation of MeCP2. *Proceedings of the National Academy of Sciences of the United States of America*, **104**, 1931–1936.

Ginhoux, F., Greter, M., Leboeuf, M. *et al.* (2010) Fate mapping analysis reveals that adult microglia derive from primitive macrophages. *Science*, **330**, 841–845.

Glaze, D.G. (2005) Neurophysiology of Rett syndrome. *Journal of Child Neurology*, **20**, 740–746.

Gordon, S. & Taylor, P.R. (2005) Monocyte and macrophage heterogeneity. *Nature Reviews Immunology*, **5**, 953–964.

Gow, D.J., Sester, D.P. & Hume, D.A. (2010) CSF-1, IGF-1, and the control of postnatal growth and development. *Journal of Leukocyte Biology*, **88**, 475–481.

Guy, J., Hendrich, B., Holmes, M., Martin, J.E. & Bird, A. (2001) A mouse Mecp2-null mutation causes neurological symptoms that mimic Rett syndrome. *Nature Genetics*, **27**, 322–326.

Guy, J., Gan, J., Selfridge, J., Cobb, S. & Bird, A. (2007) Reversal of neurological defects in a mouse model of Rett syndrome. *Science*, **315**, 1143–1147.

Hagberg, B. & Witt-Engerstrom, I. (1986) Rett syndrome: A suggested staging system for describing impairment profile with increasing age towards adolescence. *American Journal of Medical Genetics. Supplement*, **1**, 47–59.

Hagberg, B., Aicardi, J., Dias, K. & Ramos, O. (1983) A progressive syndrome of autism, dementia, ataxia, and loss of purposeful hand use in girls: Rett's syndrome: Report of 35 cases. *Annals of Neurology*, **14**, 471–479.

Jones, P.L., Veenstra, G.J., Wade, P.A. *et al.* (1998) Methylated DNA and MeCP2 recruit histone deacetylase to repress transcription. *Nature Genetics*, **19**, 187–191.

Kierdorf, K. *et al.* (2013) Microglia emerge from erythromyeloid precursors via Pu.1- and Irf8-dependent pathways. *Nature Neuroscience*, **16**, 273–280.

Krivit, W., Sung, J.H., Shapiro, E.G. & Lockman, L.A. (1995) Microglia: The effector cell for reconstitution of the central nervous system following bone marrow transplantation for lysosomal and peroxisomal storage diseases. *Cell Transplantation*, **4**, 385–392.

Lal, G., Zhang, N., van der Touw, W. *et al.* (2009) Epigenetic regulation of Foxp3 expression in regulatory T cells by DNA methylation. *Journal of Immunology*, **182**, 259–273.

Lioy, D.T., Garg, S.K., Monaghan, C.E. *et al.* (2011) A role for glia in the progression of Rett's syndrome. *Nature*, **475**, 497–500.

Luikenhuis, S., Giacometti, E., Beard, C.F. & Jaenisch, R. (2004) Expression of MeCP2 in postmitotic neurons rescues Rett syndrome in mice. *Proceedings of the National Academy of Sciences of the United States of America*, **101**, 6033–6038.

Maezawa, I. & Jin, L.W. (2010a) Rett syndrome microglia damage dendrites and synapses by the elevated release of glutamate. *Journal of Neuroscience*, **30**, 5346–5356.

Maezawa, I. & Jin, L.W. (2010b) Rett syndrome microglia damage dendrites and synapses by the elevated release of glutamate. *Journal of Neuroscience*, **30**, 5346–5356.

Mann, J., Chu, D.C., Maxwell, A. *et al.* (2010) MeCP2 controls an epigenetic pathway that promotes myofibroblast transdifferentiation and fibrosis. *Gastroenterology*, **138**, 705–714, 714.e1–4.

Marin-Teva, J.L., Dusart, I., Colin, C., Gervais, A., van Rooijen, N. & Mallat, M. (2004) Microglia promote the death of developing Purkinje cells. *Neuron*, **41**, 535–547.

McKercher, S.R., Torbett, B.E., Anderson, K.L. *et al.* (1996) Targeted disruption of the PU.1 gene results in multiple hematopoietic abnormalities. *EMBO Journal*, **15**, 5647–5658.

Mebius, R.E. & Kraal, G. (2005) Structure and function of the spleen. *Nature Reviews Immunology*, **5**, 606–616.

Mildner, A., Schmidt, H., Nitsche, M. *et al.* (2007) Microglia in the adult brain arise from Ly-6ChiCCR2+ monocytes only under defined host conditions. *Nature Neuroscience*, **10**, 1544–1553.

Naito, M., Hasegawa, G., Ebe, Y. & Yamamoto, T. (2004) Differentiation and function of Kupffer cells. *Medical Electron Microscopy*, **37**, 16–28.

Nan, X., Campoy, F.J. & Bird, A. (1997) MeCP2 is a transcriptional repressor with abundant binding sites in genomic chromatin. *Cell*, **88**, 471–481.

Nan, X., Ng, H.H., Johnson, C.A. *et al.* (1998) Transcriptional repression by the methyl-CpG-binding protein MeCP2 involves a histone deacetylase complex. *Nature*, **393**, 386–389.

Nguyen, M.V., Felice, C.A., Du, F. *et al.* (2013) Oligodendrocyte lineage cells contribute unique features to Rett syndrome neuropathology. *Journal of Neuroscience*, **33**, 18764–18774.

Nimmerjahn, A., Kirchhoff, F. & Helmchen, F. (2005) Resting microglial cells are highly dynamic surveillants of brain parenchyma in vivo. *Science*, **308**, 1314–1318.

O'Driscoll, C., Kaufmann, W.E. & Bressler, J. (2013) Relationship between Mecp2 and NFkappab signaling during neural differentiation of P19 cells. *Brain Research*, **1490**, 35–42.

Okazawa, H., Shimizu, J., Kamei, M., Imafuku, I., Hamada, H. & Kanazawa, I. (1996) Bcl-2 inhibits retinoic acid-induced apoptosis during the neural differentiation of embryonal stem cells. *Journal of Cell Biology*, **132**, 955–968.

Parkhurst, C.N., Yang, G., Ninan, I. *et al.* (2013) Microglia promote learning-dependent synapse formation through brain-derived neurotrophic factor. *Cell*, **155**, 1596–1609.

Polazzi, E., Gianni, T. & Contestabile, A. (2001) Microglial cells protect cerebellar granule neurons from apoptosis: Evidence for reciprocal signaling. *Glia*, **36**, 271–280.

Ramocki, M.B., Tavyev, Y.J. & Peters, S.U. (2010) The MECP2 duplication syndrome. *American Journal of Medical Genetics Part A*, **152A**, 1079–1088.

Rett, A. (1966) On a unusual brain atrophy syndrome in hyperammonemia in childhood. *Wiener medizinische Wochenschrift*, **116**, 723–726.

Schafer, D.P., Lehrman, E.K., Kautzman, A.G. *et al.* (2012) Microglia sculpt postnatal neural circuits in an activity and complement-dependent manner. *Neuron*, **74**, 691–705.

Schulz, C., Gomez Perdiguero, E., Chorro, L. *et al.* (2012) A lineage of myeloid cells independent of Myb and hematopoietic stem cells. *Science*, **336**, 86–90.

Shahbazian, M.D. & Zoghbi, H.Y. (2002) Rett syndrome and MeCP2: Linking epigenetics and neuronal function. *American Journal of Human Genetics*, **71**, 1259–1272.

Sierra, A., Encinas, J.M., Deudero, J.J. *et al.* (2010) Microglia shape adult hippocampal neurogenesis through apoptosis-coupled phagocytosis. *Cell Stem Cell*, **7**, 483–495.

Socie, G., Curtis, R.E., Deeg, H.J. *et al.* (2000) New malignant diseases after allogeneic marrow transplantation for childhood acute leukemia. *Journal of Clinical Oncology*, **18**, 348–357.

Suzuki, M., Yamada, T., Kihara-Negishi, F., Sakurai, T. & Oikawa, T. (2003) Direct association between PU.1 and MeCP2 that recruits mSin3A-HDAC complex for PU.1-mediated transcriptional repression. *Oncogene*, **22**, 8688–8698.

Tong, Y., Aune, T. & Boothby, M. (2005) T bet antagonizes mSin3a recruitment and transactivates a fully methylated IFN-gamma promoter via a conserved T-box half-site. *Proceedings of the National Academy of Sciences of the United States of America*, **102**, 2034–2039.

Trapp, B.D., Wujek, J.R., Criste, G.A. *et al.* (2007) Evidence for synaptic stripping by cortical microglia. *Glia*, **55**, 360–368.

Tremblay, M.E., Lowery, R.L. & Majewska, A.K. (2010) Microglial interactions with synapses are modulated by visual experience. *PLoS Biology*, **8**, e1000527.

Tucker, M.A., D'Angio, G.J., Boice, J.D. Jr. *et al.* (1987) Bone sarcomas linked to radiotherapy and chemotherapy in children. *New England Journal of Medicine*, **317**, 588–593.

Ueno, M., Fujita, Y., Tanaka, T. *et al.* (2013) Layer V cortical neurons require microglial support for survival during postnatal development. *Nature Neuroscience*, **16**, 543–551.

Van Esch, H., Bauters, M., Ignatius, J. *et al.* (2005) Duplication of the MECP2 region is a frequent cause of severe mental retardation and progressive neurological symptoms in males. *American Journal of Human Genetics*, **77**, 442–453.

Wakselman, S., Bechade, C., Roumier, A., Bernard, D., Triller, A. & Bessis, A. (2008) Developmental neuronal death in hippocampus requires the microglial CD11b integrin and DAP12 immunoreceptor. *Journal of Neuroscience*, **28**, 8138–8143.

Yang, T., Ramocki, M.B., Neul, J.L. *et al.* (2012) Overexpression of methyl-CpG binding protein 2 impairs T(H)1 responses. *Science Translational Medicine*, **4**, 163ra158.

Yona, S., Kim, K.W., Wolf, Y. *et al.* (2013) Fate mapping reveals origins and dynamics of monocytes and tissue macrophages under homeostasis. *Immunity*, **38**, 79–91.

Zielasek, J. & Hartung, H.P. (1996) Molecular mechanisms of microglial activation. *Advances in Neuroimmunology*, **6**, 191–122.

15 The Role of Regulatory T Cells and Microglia in Amyotrophic Lateral Sclerosis

David R. Beers,[1] Weihua Zhao,[1] Kristopher G. Hooten,[2] and Stanley H. Appel[1]

[1] Department of Neurology, Houston Methodist Neurological Institute, Houston Methodist Hospital Research Institute, Houston Methodist Hospital, Weill Cornell Medical College, Houston, TX, USA
[2] Department of Neurological Surgery, University of Florida, Gainesville, FL, USA

Overview of Amyotrophic Lateral Sclerosis

Amyotrophic lateral sclerosis (ALS), first described by Charcot in the nineteenth century, is a member of a group of adult-onset anterior horn disorders that cause a rapidly progressive and irreversible neurodegenerative disease resulting in the selective degeneration of both upper and lower motoneurons in the cerebral cortex, brainstem, and spinal cord (Rowland, 2001). Colloquially known as Lou Gehrig's disease after the famous New York Yankees first baseman who died of the disease less than 2 years after diagnosis, ALS is one of the most common neurodegenerative disorders and is the most common adult-onset motoneuron disease. ALS is a heterogeneic disease that initiates focally and then spreads to neighboring structures resulting in muscle weakness and atrophy, hyperreflexia with spasticity, dysphagia, dysarthria, progressive paralysis, and ultimately death due to respiratory failure typically within 4–6 years after the first clinical signs. Before motoneuron cell body loss in the spinal cord, denervation at the neuromuscular junction is observed, followed by a "dying back" of distal branches (Fischer *et al.*, 2004). At autopsy, motoneuron loss in the central nervous system (CNS) is evident, while the remaining neurons contain numerous inclusions composed of misfolded proteins, swelling of the perikaryon and proximal axon, mitochondria swellings, vacuoles, and neurofilament accumulations. In general, this accumulation of intracellular or extracellular misfolded proteins in the CNS is a common feature of neurodegenerative disorders. In addition to the well-described motoneuron pathologies, the surrounding glia are also affected; microglia are highly activated containing numerous inclusions.

Neuroinflammation: New Insights into Beneficial and Detrimental Functions, First Edition. Edited by Samuel David.
© 2015 John Wiley & Sons, Inc. Published 2015 by John Wiley & Sons, Inc.

The worldwide incidence of ALS is approximately two per 100,000 individuals and is fairly uniform except for a few high-incidence regions such as the Kii peninsula and Guam (Worms, 2001; Cronin *et al.*, 2007). The mean age of onset is between 55 and 60 years and commonly affects more men than women until after the age of 70 when the ratio approaches 1 : 1. ALS was traditionally considered to be a pure motoneuron disorder; however, a subset of patients have involvement of their frontal and temporal lobes and, to a lesser extent, sensory and spinocerebellar pathways, as well as the substantia nigra and hippocampal dentate gyrus. Thus, ALS is now regarded as a multisystem disorder in which motoneurons are affected the earliest and most severely.

The pathogenic processes underlying ALS are multifactorial and, at present, not fully understood. Most forms of ALS are idiopathic having no obvious genetic basis for the disease and are known as nonhereditary ALS or more commonly referred to as sporadic amyotrophic lateral sclerosis (sALS) (Andersen and Al-Chalabi, 2011). Approximately 10% of patients have heritable forms, referred to as familial amyotrophic lateral sclerosis (fALS) (Traub *et al.*, 2011). ALS, a phenotypically variable syndrome, is a genetically heterogeneous disease with multiple genes initiating motoneuron degeneration through separate but convergent biological pathways leading to one clinical phenotype; the converse is also correct, that is, multiple clinical ALS phenotypes may be caused by one gene.

Within fALS, there are more than 20 Mendelian gene mutations encoding proteins in disparate pathways that appear to be minimally interconnected; however, the genetic penetrance of these genes is not 100%. Most of the genes associated with fALS code for proteins involved in axonal transport or vesicle trafficking (spatacsin, vesicle-associated membrane protein (VAMP)), abrogating or reducing cellular oxidative stress (superoxide dismutase), RNA transcription, processing, and function (angiogenin, TAR DNA binding (TDP-43), fused in sarcoma (FUS)), endosomal trafficking (alsin, FIG4 homolog), and protein degradation pathways (valosin-containing protein, ubiquilin-2). Interestingly, these genes often code for proteins whose mutation or malfunction results in macromolecular cellular aggregates. Several other less common mutations have been described in that include Ataxin-2, and the Unc-13 vesicular protein.

The first identified gene accounting for 20% of fALS was a mutation in the gene encoding the Cu^{2+}/Zn^{2+} superoxide dismutase 1 (SOD1) enzyme (Rosen *et al.*, 1993). SOD1 is a ubiquitously expressed cytosolic enzyme that converts highly reactive and toxic superoxide radicals ($O_2^{\cdot-}$) to hydrogen peroxide (H_2O_2), which is subsequently converted to water and oxygen by a catalase. To date, over 165 mutations have been identified in SOD1 that induce disease by a toxic gain-of-function and not by a loss of enzymatic activity.

In 6–10% of sALS cases, and 30–50% of fALS cases, there is the presence of hexanucleotide repeats in chromosome 9, open reading frame 72 (C9ORF72) that is highly conserved across species that encodes an uncharacterized protein with no known function (DeJesus-Hernandez *et al.*, 2011; Renton *et al.*, 2011). The hexanucleotide repeat expansion prevents expression of the C9ORF72 transcript variant 1 from the mutant allele; however, the defect may also impair RNA processing in general. While little is known about the C9ORF72-encoded protein, it appears to be expressed in the regions of affected neurons in cytoplasmic and synaptic localizations. The mechanism of disease mediated by the GGGGCC repeat is still unresolved but has been attributed to haploinsufficiency, a toxic gain-of-function, or to the synthesis of toxic dipeptide repeat proteins.

The third most common cause of fALS involve mutations in the related genes TARDBP and FUS encoding the DNA/RNA-binding proteins TAR DNA binding protein (TDP-43) and FUS/translocated in liposarcoma (TLS), respectively (Neumann *et al.*, 2006). TDP-43 is a multifunctional DNA/RNA-binding protein involved RNA processing, stabilization, and transport. Since their initial discovery, many other mutations in TARDBP and FUS have been found and comprise approximately 4–5% of fALS cases. Proteomic studies have revealed TDP-43 to be the major aggregating disease protein in ALS. Over 90% of all ALS cases exhibit pathological lesions containing detergent insoluble deposits of phosphorylated, truncated, and ubiquitinated TDP-43 protein.

The definitive diagnosis of ALS relies on a combination of primary clinical findings, systematic inclusion/exclusion of potential genetic factors, and environmental explanations. Unfortunately, the present therapies are mainly supportive and fail to halt disease progression. Riluzole, the first and only US Food and Drug Administration (FDA)-approved medication for ALS, only modestly prolongs survival. The absence of an effective treatment can be explained in part by the complex and heterogeneous genetic, biochemical, and clinical features of ALS.

Different mechanisms of motoneuron injury in ALS have been proposed. These include misfolded protein toxicity – particularly misfolded SOD1 or TDP-43 toxicity, glutamate/calcium-mediated excitotoxicity, mitochondrial dysfunction, neurofilament/cytoskeletal alterations affecting axonal transport, RNA processing and handling defects, endoplasmic reticulum (ER) and golgi dysfunction resulting in ER stress and protein degradation malfunction. Neuroinflammation has also been proposed as a mechanism of motoneuron injury; this chapter discusses these mechanisms in the context of both injury and protection that accompany the inflammatory responses.

Neuroinflammation, including microglial activation and T cell infiltration, is a neuropathological hallmark of ALS. This inflammation is not simply a late consequence of motoneuron degeneration but actively contributes to the balance between neuroprotection and neurotoxicity. The microglial and T cell activation states influence the rate of disease progression; initially microglia and T cells slow disease progression, while later, they contribute to disease acceleration.

Overview of ALS Animal Models

Mutant SOD1

Mutated forms of the human SOD1 gene (mSOD1) have been overexpressed in transgenic mice and rats, which subsequently develop a chronic progressive motoneuron disease that reflect many clinical and pathological features of ALS (Rosen *et al.*, 1993; Gurney *et al.*, 1994). The mechanisms of motoneuron injury are "noncell autonomous;" a phrase that denotes that other cell types are involved in the pathoprogression of disease. Mice chimeric for mSOD1 revealed that wild-type (WT) motoneurons, when surrounded by mSOD1-expressing glia, were injured, while mSOD1-expressing motoneurons surrounded by WT glia appeared normal. The lack or reduction of mSOD1 expression in microglia slowed disease progression and prolonged survival of mSOD1 mice, while disease onset was not altered (Beers *et al.*, 2006; Boillee *et al.*, 2006). While early attempts at overexpressing mSOD1 predominantly in neurons were unsuccessful at inducing motoneuron injury, high homozygous mSOD1^{G93A} overexpression in mice induced a motoneuron disease, although disease was dramatically delayed or absent (Jaarsma *et al.*, 2008).

C9ORF72 Model

Targeted reduction or knockdown of C9ORF72 homologs in mice and zebrafish have so far produced conflicting results, which neither rule out, nor confirm reduced expression of C9ORF72 as a pathogenic mechanism in ALS or frontotemporal dementia (FTD) (Ciura *et al.*, 2013; Suzuki *et al.*, 2013). In transgenic mice, transcription of the mouse C9ORF72 ortholog was most abundant in the neuronal cells that are known to degenerate in ALS and FTD. Although this study suggests that C9ORF72 mutations act predominantly through noncell autonomous mechanisms, the known synthesis and release of dipeptide proteins that could activate a toxic microglial response leading to neuronal injury was not investigated.

In contrast to the mouse model, the zebrafish C9ORF72 ortholog is selectively expressed in the developing nervous system and that the loss of functional transcripts caused both behavioral and cellular deficits related to locomotion without major neuronal morphological abnormalities; overexpression of human C9ORF72 mRNA transcripts rescued these deficits. These results suggest that C9ORF72 haploinsufficiency could be a contributing factor in the spectrum of ALS/FTD neurodegenerative disorders. An alternative interpretation is the possibility that C9ORF72 depletion is not a causative factor in the etiology of the disease but a consequence of toxic cellular processes involved in neurodegeneration, such as the toxic activation of microglia.

When 30 expanded RNA GGGGCC repeats were expressed in the Drosophila eye or motoneurons, they caused an age-dependent disruption of the eye and reduction in locomotion, respectively. These effects were specific to the 30 expanded RNA GGGGCC repeat-expressing flies, suggesting that the observed cell death is a direct result of these repeat RNAs expressed in these cells.

TDP-43 Model

Wild-type TDP-43 and several TDP-43 mutations have been overexpressed in neurons of mice and rats, which resulted in growth retardation, gait abnormalities, degeneration of motoneurons and pyramidal neurons in layer 5 of the frontal cortex, microglial and astroglial activation, cognitive impairments, and premature death; the severity of the phenotype correlated with the levels at which the transgene accumulated in the neuron (Joyce *et al.*, 2011). In addition, abnormal nuclear inclusions composed of TDP-43 and FUS/TLS are found in motoneurons, with substantial accumulations of mitochondria in cytoplasmic inclusions, a lack of mitochondria in axon terminals, and immature neuromuscular junctions. Moderate overexpression of mutant TDP-43 or truncated TDP-43 resulted in up-regulated cytoplasmic and nuclear ubiquitin and aggregates of phosphorylated TDP-43 with enhanced motoneuron degeneration.

Overview of Regulatory T Cells

CD4+ T cells are a major lymphocyte population that plays an important role in governing acquired immune responses to diverse antigens. Many CD4+ T cell subsets have been described, including four distinct subsets [T helper (Th) Th1, Th2, Th17, and regulatory T cells (Tregs)], each of which has specialized functions to control immune responses (Jiang and Dong, 2013). In neurodegenerative diseases, these four T cell subsets fall into two main classes: those that are neuroprotective, Th2 cells and Tregs, and those that are proinflammatory and neurotoxic, Th1 and Th17 cells. Clearly, such a designation is oversimplified and does not fully explain all the relevant immune interactions, but it does provide a way to model the involvement of the immune system in neuroprotection or cytotoxicity. Whether T cells polarized towards a neuroprotective or a cytotoxic phenotype can be influenced by the cytokine milieu, which in turn is dependent on monocytes and dendritic cells (DC) in the periphery and microglia in the CNS; this phenomenon is often referred to as "functional plasticity." DC, monocytes, and microglia can act as antigen-presenting cells (APC) that present cognate antigens on their surface in the context of major histocompatibility complex class II (MHC II) and is recognized by a T lymphocyte through a selective T cell receptor (TCR). Interaction of co-stimulatory molecules on the APC with CD28 on the T cell prompts expansion of the T cells, and secretion from APC of cytokines, which direct the differentiation into effector T cells (Teffs) subtypes. Thus, the specific cytokine milieu created by activated APCs is critical for specifying immune responses.

T cells in general, and Tregs in particular, should not be considered permanently differentiated, but rather phenotypically activated along a continuum with the ability to acquire a Th1, Th2, and Th17 functional states depending on the immune response and cytokine milieu they encounter, and the expression of modifying transcription factors, such as T-bet, IRF4, and STAT3, Bcl-6, respectively. Importantly, Tregs and Teffs that are recruited to the same sites of inflammation generally express similar sets of chemokine receptors, such as CXCR3 for Th1 and CCR6 for Th17 cells. It is therefore likely that, similarly to all T cells, Tregs are able to sense environmental or inflammatory cues, in the particular cytokine milieu, and adaptively differentiate in response to particular inflammatory cues. It is also possible that Tregs are capable of secreting inflammatory cytokines such as interferon gamma (IFN-γ) until they receive strong TCR stimulation, which induces the expression of the forkhead box protein 3 transcription factor (Foxp3 in mice and FOXP3 in humans) and then a potent suppressive function. It is now known that the induction of peripheral immunologic tolerance requires Tregs, which suppress autoimmunity and promote allograft survival. Constitutive expression of Foxp3, in conjunction with the constitutive expression of the high affinity interleukin 2 (IL-2) receptor subunit CD25, is necessary for Tregs to regulate self-tolerance (Kitagawa et al., 2013).

Since the identification of Foxp3, several molecules and in vivo pathways have been found to play a role in the generation and homeostasis of Tregs. These pathways are primarily downstream of T cell activation through TCR stimulation, CD28 co-stimulation, or cytokine receptors, particularly IL-2/IL-2R. During thymocyte development, Foxp3+ Tregs emerge from the pool of double positive cells, and TCR engagement with MHC II and B7/CD28 interactions are crucial for this process. However, subsequent studies suggest that a multistage commitment process may direct the Treg development even at an earlier stage of thymocyte development. However, it is not yet known whether TCR signaling alone is sufficient to drive Treg development or whether other signals can induce Foxp3 expression to initiate Treg differentiation independent of TCR signals.

In addition to expression of Foxp3, Tregs have been described to constitutively express high levels of CD25, with initial reports using high CD25 expression as a surrogate marker for Tregs. Stimulation of T cells with IL-2 leads to the up-regulation of CD25, which, together with the constitutive CD122 (IL-2Rb) and CD132 [common c chain (cc)] subunits, forms a fully functional IL-2R. Signals through IL-2/IL-2R activate signal transducer and activator of transcription 5 (STAT5), which promote cell survival and proliferation. Cytotoxic T-lymphocyte antigen 4 (CTLA-4) is another co-signaling molecule with vital importance to Treg function.

Despite extensive studies on CD4+CD25+ Tregs, current evidence suggests that naturally occurring CD8+CD122+ T cells are also Tregs with the capacity to inhibit T-cell responses and suppress autoimmunity (Dai et al., 2014). CD8+CD122+ T cells are memory-like Tregs that resemble a central memory T cell phenotype. Although the mechanisms underlying CD8+CD122+ Tregs suppressive abilities are still not well understood, they may include the production of IL-10. One study suggests that the programmed death-1 (PD-1) protein expression distinguishes between regulatory and memory CD8+CD122+ T cells and that CD8+CD122+ Tregs undergo faster homeostatic proliferation and are more potent in the suppression of rejection than conventional CD4+CD25+ Tregs.

Foxp3 has been assumed to be a master regulator and a specific molecular marker for Tregs, which include naturally occurring regulatory T cells (nTregs), thymus-derived regulatory T cells (tTregs), peripherally induced regulatory T cells (iTreg), and in vitro induced Tregs (Curotto de Lafaille and Lafaille, 2009). Although a subset of CD4+CD25+ T cells in the thymus develop into nTregs, in peripheral lymphoid tissues, TGF-β induces naive T cells to develop into iTregs. However, nTregs and iTregs have different functional characteristics. Several studies suggest that nTregs are more stable compared to iTregs, and this may be related to the epigenetic regulation of Foxp3. However, there is evidence that Foxp3 expression is not a distinct and reliable marker or a sole regulator of functionally stable Tregs; TCR-stimulated conventional T cells are able to express Foxp3 transiently without suppressive functions (Kitagawa et al., 2013). Furthermore, a fraction of Foxp3+ T cells in a healthy person's blood does not possess suppressive activity but is capable of being proinflammatory. Thus, there are differences between Tregs and Foxp3-transduced conventional T cells, suggesting that Foxp3 expression may not be sufficient for delineating functional Tregs and that there are additional requirements for full Tregs suppressive functions.

DNA methylation and histone modifications are essential for cell differentiation and cell lineage stabilization (Lal and Bromberg, 2009). DNA methylation is important for nTregs because immunological dysregulation would result if Tregs stability is lost along with the ensuing loss of their suppressive functions. Several studies have shown that stable Foxp3 expression correlated with DNA demethylation of Foxp3 conserved noncoding regulatory-T-cell-specific demethylated region (TSDR) (Morikawa and Sakaguchi, 2014). This epigenetic change is acquired through TCR stimulation TSDR, before Foxp3 expression. On TCR stimulation, Foxp3 strongly represses many genes including IL-2. Thus, as was previously discussed with all T cells, functional Tregs can be defined as T cells possessing a Treg-phenotypic epigenome, rather than T cells expressing Foxp3+; a continuum of heterogeneic Tregs with the ability to acquire functional stability and plasticity.

Immunologic Aspects of Microglia and Tregs in ALS

Research linking immunity and neurodegeneration has focused primarily on microglia and innate immunity (Glezer et al., 2007; Henkel et al., 2009). However, infiltrating T cells of the adaptive immune response are also present in areas of CNS motoneuron degeneration. Depending on their phenotype and activation status, T cells can cross-talk with neurons and microglia and either protect or damage neurons from stressful stimuli. In ALS patients' autopsy tissues, neuroinflammation is observed specifically at sites of motoneuron injury, highlighted by the presence of activated/proliferating microglia and infiltrating DC and T cells.

Neuroinflammation is now established as an important factor in the pathogenesis of many neurodegenerative diseases, including ALS (Henkel *et al.*, 2009). At various time points, microglia and T cells are markedly activated, producing either neuroprotective or proinflammatory molecules, which can decrease or increase the rate of primary motoneuron degeneration, respectively. Recent research has shown that this neuroinflammatory component is affected by the peripheral immune system. T cells in particular are able to cross the blood–brain barrier (BBB) into the brain and spinal cord parenchyma, where they interact with resident microglia, inducing them to adopt either an M1 or M2 phenotype, depending on the stage of disease. Classically activated microglia (M1) are cytotoxic due to the secretion of reactive oxygen species (ROS) and proinflammatory cytokines. In contrast, alternatively activated microglia (M2) block proinflammatory responses, and produce high levels of anti-inflammatory cytokines and neurotrophic factors (see Chapters 5 and 6 for further discussion on M1 and M2 polarization). Clearly understanding the changes that occur to allow the interaction between peripheral and central immune responses will be essential in any attempt to manipulate the disease process via neuroinflammatory mechanisms (Fig. 15.1).

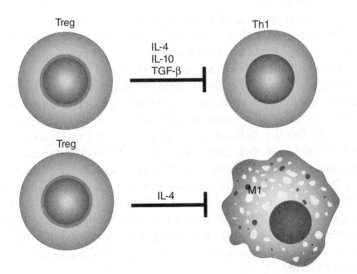

Figure 15.1 Tregs suppress Th1 cells and M1 microglia. Tregs, through the release of IL-10, TGF-β, and IL-4 suppress the proliferation of Th1 cells and inhibit the synthesis of IFN-γ. Tregs are capable of releasing IL-4 and have the potential to inhibit an injurious M1 response and maintain/augment a protective M2 phenotype. Passive transfer of early phase mSOD1 Tregs prolonged the slow phase of disease in mSOD1 mice, augmented M2 markers, and suppressed M1 markers and their proinflammatory cytokines. Patients with ALS with rapidly progressing disease had decreased numbers of Tregs, and the numbers of Tregs were inversely correlated with disease progression rates.

The mSOD1 transgenic mouse model of ALS has been extensively used to study immune/neuron interactions, and although the mechanisms whereby mSOD1 causes disease are unknown, there is compelling evidence suggesting immune system involvement in mSOD1-mediated motoneuron injury. Several studies have demonstrated the presence of activated microglia, T cells, and DC in the spinal cords of mice expressing the G93A form of mSOD1; the presence of DC and their transcripts was elevated in mSOD1 spinal cord beginning at 110 days (Alexianu et al., 2001; Henkel et al., 2004; Henkel et al., 2006; Beers et al., 2008; Henkel et al., 2009). CCL2 mRNA and immunoreactivity were up-regulated in neuronal and glial cells as early as 15 days, before any evidence of microglial activation and correlated with a breakdown in the BBB. In addition, at 39 days of age, before evidence of disease onset, CD68 immunoreactivity, a myeloid-specific LAMP protein expressed by phagocytic cells, was present in lumbar spinal cords of mSOD1 mice. Other studies also indicate an immune activation in mSOD1 mice including activated microglia, increased inducible nitric oxide synthase (iNOS), increased IL-1β, IL-6, and tumor necrosis factor alpha (TNF-α) expression. Although it is not clear if these responses are protective or injurious, there is clear evidence suggestive of an early immune response in mSOD1 mice, as has been shown in patients with ALS.

T Cells and ALS

Several studies have addressed T cell infiltration in post-mortem material from patients with ALS and identified substantial T cells in 38 of 48 spinal cords from patients with ALS (Troost et al., 1989; Kawamata et al., 1992; McGeer and McGeer, 2002). T cells were identified along the vessel walls in the precentral gyrus and extending into the areas of neuronal injury in all eight patients with ALS who were examined. Others have found perivascular and intraparenchymal T cells infiltrates in the corticospinal tracts and ventral horns of 18 of 27 consecutive ALS autopsy cases compared to 1 of 11 control brains, but B cells were not detected (Engelhardt et al., 1993). CD4+ T cells were present in the proximity of degenerating corticospinal tracts, while both CD4+ and CD8+ T cells were demonstrated in ventral horns. Another study reported perivascular infiltration of T cells in the spinal cords of all six patients with ALS studied (Graves et al., 2004).

Of importance is the fact that mSOD1 mice show a similar T cell response that is observed in patients with ALS (Alexianu et al., 2001; Beers et al., 2008). The presence of CD3+ T cells has been demonstrated in the spinal cords of mSOD1 mice at end-stage disease. At early stages of disease, only CD4+ T cells are found in lumbar spinal cords of mSOD1 mice. CD8+ T cells were observed only at end-stage disease, but even at this stage, CD4+ T cells still predominated, accounting for approximately 60% of the total T cell population, while remaining T cells were CD8+. The fact that CD4+ T cells first enter the spinal cords of mSOD1 mice, and that their numbers increase as disease progresses, suggests that they are active participants throughout the course of disease in these mice.

To determine the role for T cells in mSOD1 transgenic mice, mSOD1 mice were bred with RAG-2 knockout mice that lack functional T and B cells. Interestingly, double transgenic mice (mSOD1$^+$/RAG-2$^{-/-}$) had an accelerated disease course, and the mice died earlier than the heterozygous (mSOD1$^+$/RAG-2$^{+/-}$) control mice, indicating that T cells, and possibly B cells, contribute to a neuroprotective environment (Beers et al., 2008); the disease course of

$mSOD1^+/RAG-2^{+/-}$ mice was identical to mSOD1 mice. Similar results were obtained when mSOD1 mice were bred with CD4 knockout mice, indicating that $CD4^+$ T cells contribute to the prolongation of disease duration. These results were confirmed when mSOD1 mice were bred with mice deficient for the TCR β chain; the specific ablation of T cells led to accelerated disease progression and shorter life spans (Chiu *et al.*, 2008). The participation of $CD4^+$ T cells has been further supported by the evidence that the passive transfer of *ex vivo*-activated $CD4^+$ T cells improves neurological function and life span of mSOD1 mice (Banerjee *et al.*, 2008). Taken in its entirety, these results established that the lack of T cell recruitment, through the loss of CCR2 or developmental inhibition, accelerates disease progression and the demise of mSOD1 mice. Therefore, adaptive immune responses mediated by $CD4^+$ T cells serve an important neuroprotective function in the ALS mouse.

Another study demonstrated quantitative and qualitative immune deficits in lymphoid cell and T cell function were seen in mSOD1 mice (Banerjee *et al.*, 2008). Spleens of these animals showed reductions in size, weight, lymphocyte numbers, and morphological deficits at terminal stages of disease compared to their WT littermates. Deficits were readily seen in T cell proliferation coincident with increased annexin-V associated apoptosis and necrosis of lymphocytes. In addition, among $CD4^+$ T cells in patients with ALS, levels of $CD45RA^+$ (naïve) T cells were diminished, while $CD45RO^+$ (memory) T cells were increased compared to age-matched caregivers. In attempts to correct mutant SOD1-associated immune deficits, these investigators reconstituted mSOD1 mice with unfractionated naïve lymphocytes or anti-CD3 activated $CD4^+CD25^+$ Tregs or $CD4^+CD25^-$ Teffs from WT donor mice. While naive lymphocytes failed to enhance survival, both polyclonal-activated Tregs and Teffs subsets delayed loss of motor function and extended survival. However, only Tregs delayed neurological symptom onset, whereas Teffs increased latency between disease onset and entry into late stage.

Tregs and ALS

T cells have been shown to directly communicate with microglia/macrophage, and infiltrating Th cells can be both toxic and protective. As mentioned earlier, although an oversimplification, Th cells can be subdivided into Th1, Th2, Th17, and Treg cells. Prompted by different types of cytokines produced by antigen-presenting monocytes/macrophages/microglia, as well as by DC and other cell sources, undifferentiated Th cells develop into the Th1 or Th2 lineages.

Recent studies have systematically evaluated the dynamic changes that occur in the $CD4^+$ subsets, Th1, Th2, Th17, and Tregs, during progression of disease in mSOD1 mice (Beers *et al.*, 2011). In lumbar spinal cords of mSOD1 mice at early slowly progressing stages, Tregs were increased accompanied by increased levels of IL-4, IL-10, and M2 markers, and then decreased when disease rapidly accelerated. During the rapid stage of disease, there was an increased expression of mRNA for Th1 cells and decreased expression of mRNA for Th2 cells; microglia were predominantly M1. IL-17 expression was not detected at any time in the course of disease, suggesting that Th17 may not be involved in the pathogenesis of ALS in the mouse model.

Th17 cells, an emerging subset of T cells characterized by predominant production of IL-17, are distinct from Th1 or Th2 cells and have been suggested to be crucial in destructive autoimmunity. IL-23 is a proinflammatory cytokine that is produced by macrophages and DC and plays a role in the stimulation and survival of Th17 cells. Serum levels of IL-17 and IL-23 were higher in patients with ALS compared to patients with noninflammatory neurological disorders (Fiala *et al.*, 2010; Rentzos *et al.*, 2010). IL-17 and IL-23 cerebrospinal fluid (CSF) levels were also increased in patients with ALS. However, IL-17 and IL-23 levels were not correlated with disease duration, burden of disease, or clinical subtype of the disease onset in patients with ALS. With the higher expression of IL-17 but lower expression of IL-10 in patients with ALS than controls, the activation of Tregs pathways may be suppressed in patients, suggesting a higher vulnerability of patients with ALS to IL-17-mediated damage. These results suggest that IL-17 and IL-23 may be involved in the pathology of ALS and are potential markers of Th17 cells activation in patients with ALS.

Cytokines and ALS

At early stages of disease in mSOD1 mice, increased expression of IL-4 and IL-10 was noted, suggesting that these cytokines were able to skew microglia toward an M2 phenotype. Although Th2 cells are one of the major sources of IL-4, Th2 are not increased in the lumbar region of ALS mice spinal cords. Tregs are the likely source of IL-4, as our own studies as well as those from other laboratories have documented that Tregs are capable of releasing IL-4 and have the potential to maintain the protective M2 phenotype (Tiemessen *et al.*, 2007; Beers *et al.*, 2011). In addition, as previously discussed, passive transfer of early phase mSOD1 Tregs prolonged the slow phase of disease in mSOD1 mice, augmented M2 markers, and suppressed M1 markers and their proinflammatory cytokines. It was further demonstrated that Tregs, through their secretion of IL-4, can directly suppress the toxic properties of microglia (Zhao *et al.*, 2012). It was previously shown that suppressing the toxic attributes of microglia leads to prolonged survival in this model of ALS. Moreover, M2 cells also have the ability to induce $CD4^+$ Tregs with a strong suppressive function. mSOD1 microglia induced more IL-4-expressing Tregs from mSOD1 mice. Thus, Tregs during the early stages of disease are immunocompetent and actively contribute to neuroprotection through their interactions with microglia. As disease progresses, a transformation occurs from a supportive Tregs/M2 response to an injurious Th1/M1 response. It is known that Th1 cells produce IFN-γ, which promotes M1 microglial activation, and M1 cells can promote proliferation and function of Th1 cells. This vicious cycle is believed to be a significant driving force for acceleration of disease course. Therefore, the dialogue between T cells and microglia modulates their phenotypic profiles and subsequently drives disease progression.

When disease entered the rapidly progressing stage, transplantation of Treg cells could not reverse the acceleration of disease. What causes the transformation and dysfunction of Tregs remains unknown, but cytokines released from activated microglia, astrocytes, and T cells are likely candidates. Both Th1 cells and M1 microglia release TNF-α, which has been recently demonstrated to induce the dysfunction of Tregs by inhibiting phosphorylation of FoxP3 (Nie *et al.*, 2013). IL-1β was required to drive the conversion of Tregs to Th17-producing cells. Moreover, IL-6 has been reported to inhibit the generation of $FoxP3^+$ Tregs (Bettelli *et al.*, 2006). In the mSOD1 mouse model, the transition from protection to toxicity coincided with increased expression of IL-6; IL-6 can be produced by activated microglia, astrocytes, and Th1 cells. Nevertheless, it is unlikely that any single cytokine such as IL-6 is solely responsible for the transformation from neuroprotective Treg/Th2/M2 cells to cytotoxic Th1/M1cells, and it appears much more likely that multiple proinflammatory cytokines mediate the transition.

In vitro, Tregs isolated from mSOD1 mice were found to suppress cytotoxic microglial factors such as NOX2, a subunit of NADPH oxidase found mostly in macrophages/microglia, and iNOS through an IL-4-mediated mechanism, whereas Teffs were only minimally effective; antibodies directed at IL-4 blocked the suppressive response of the Tregs (Zhao *et al.*, 2012). In addition, conditioned media from mSOD1 mice Tregs, or the addition of IL-4, reduced microglial NOX2 expression. During the stable disease phase, as detected using flow cytometry, the total number of Tregs, specifically the numbers of $CD4^+CD25^{high}IL-4^+$, $CD4^+CD25^{high}IL-10^+$, and $CD4^+CD25^{high}TGF-\beta^+$ Tregs, were increased in mSOD1 mice compared to WT mice; Tregs isolated during this phase reduced Teffs proliferation. In contrast, during the rapidly progressing phase, the number of mSOD1 mice Tregs decreased, while the proliferation of mSOD1 mice Teffs increased. The combination of IL-4, IL-10, and TGF-β was required to inhibit the proliferation of mSOD1 mice Teffs by mSOD1 mice Tregs that were isolated during the slow phase, while inhibition of mSOD1 mice Teffs by mSOD1 mice Tregs during the rapid phase, as well as WT mice Teffs, was not dependent on these factors. Thus, mSOD1 mice Tregs at the slow phase suppressed microglial toxicity and mSOD1 mice Teffs proliferation through different mechanisms; microglial activation was suppressed through IL-4, whereas mSOD1 mice Teffs were suppressed by IL-4, IL-10, and TGF-β.

The documented changes in T cell populations that occur in mSOD1 mice were also examined in patients with ALS. Diminished levels of naïve (CD45RA) T cells and increased levels of memory (CD45RO) cells within the $CD4^+$ T cell subset were reported in peripheral blood of patients with ALS. Henkel *et al.* (2013) found that there were T cell alterations present in the peripheral blood and spinal cord tissues of patients with ALS (Henkel *et al.*, 2013). The numbers of $CD4^+CD25^{high}$ Tregs, FoxP3, and CD25 mRNA levels were reduced in patients with ALS with rapidly progressing disease. Similarly, Gata3, TGF-β, and IL-4 mRNA levels were also reduced in rapidly progressing patients. The levels of these Tregs and Th2 markers inversely correlated with the rate of disease progression. Similar results on peripheral Tregs were reported in a recent study (Rentzos *et al.*, 2012). Furthermore, in post-mortem spinal cord tissues of patients with ALS, Tbx21 levels, IFN-γ, and NOX2 levels were up-regulated in rapidly progressing patients, and FoxP3 expression was decreased. These data suggest that decreased Tregs/Th2 and enhanced Th1/M1 cells contribute to rapid disease progression. Most importantly, low FoxP3 mRNA levels early in disease predicted a rapid progression and reduced survival. For the first time, we may be able to predict rapid progression of disease in patients with ALS, and such predictive ability may be of value in stratification for enrollment in clinical trials.

Conclusions

The study and treatment of Lou Gehrig's disease still remains in its infancy even after a century of intense investigation and discovery. The pathways involved in motoneuron death in ALS have been shown to be very complex with diverse cellular and molecular contributions leading to motoneuron injury and eventual neuronal death (Fig. 15.2). Neuroinflammation in ALS has evolved from what was once thought as a secondary effect or consequence of motoneuron injury

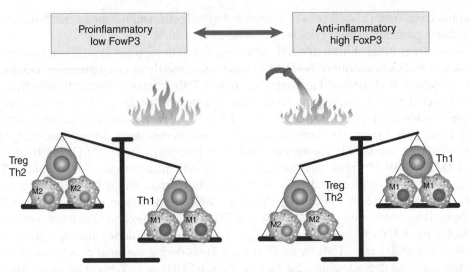

Figure 15.2   The therapeutic goal is to decrease Th1/M1 responses and simultaneously increase Tregs/M2 responses. During the rapidly progressing phase of ALS, the proinflammatory versus anti-inflammatory balance is weighted toward a proinflammatory response and thus fanning the flames of inflammation. However, the possibility of using Tregs cell therapy, either alone or in conjunction with M2 cell therapy, we may be able shift the balance toward an anti-inflammatory response and thus extinguish the flames of inflammation. The dialog between T cells and microglia modulates their phenotypic profiles and subsequently either drives protective of injurious disease progression response.

to a well-accepted concept that it plays a central role in motoneuron pathophysiology and disease propagation. The fact that mutations in different genes can result in common clinical manifestations of ALS as well as the fact that neurons do not die alone suggests that neuroinflammation is the common denominator and necessary to induce neurodegeneration in ALS.

Centrally located as early responders in the disease, resident CNS microglia contribute to the neuroinflammatory response and undergo rapid morphological and functional activation in the presence of signals derived from injured motoneurons. Such neuroinflammation may not initiate neuronal injury but may amplify and propagate injury, initiated by motoneuron "danger signals" such as misfolded proteins, peptide fragments, or dipeptide repeat proteins, and activate microglia. The studies described in this chapter demonstrate a plasticity of microglia on a continuum from a M1 (proinflammatory/neurotoxic) phenotype to a M2 (anti-inflammatory/neuroprotective) phenotype. In the ALS disease course, this continuum is seen with a M2 state early in the disease that transitions to an M1 response during the clinical acceleration and disease progression. A similar transition over the course of disease has been documented in T cells with an early Tregs/Th2 (neuroprotective) response to a Th1/Th17 (neurotoxic) response. This T cell response has the ability to influence the local microglia response in the disease and can even be used as a prediction of rate of disease progression. The converse may also be true; the local microglial milieu may influence the phenotypic response of infiltrating T cells.

Despite many studies defining the multiple intraneuronal pathways compromised in ALS, no therapies have really provided meaningful benefits to patients with ALS. Current data suggests that therapies aimed at affecting and modulating the neuroinflammatory response in ALS might provide these therapeutic benefits. Tregs are especially attractive as a potential therapy, as the passive transfer of Tregs in the mSOD1 mouse model of ALS demonstrated clinical improvement and prolonged survival. Alternative therapies include compounds that can maintain the early microglial M2 phenotype and other compounds that transform the late microglial M1 phenotype into a protective M2 phenotype. Further investigations of the neuroinflammatory responses in ALS will lead to greater understandings about the specific signals involved in the microglial-T cell dialog, and how immunomodulatory therapies may be quickly translated into the clinic to arrest the progressive and devastating nature of this disease, thus providing hope for patients with ALS.

References

Alexianu, M.E., Kozovska, M. & Appel, S.H. (2001) Immune reactivity in a mouse model of familial ALS correlates with disease progression. *Neurology*, **57**, 1282–1289.

Andersen, P.M. & Al-Chalabi, A. (2011) Clinical genetics of amyotrophic lateral sclerosis: What do we really know? *Nature Reviews Neurology*, **7**, 603–615.

Banerjee, R., Mosley, R.L., Reynolds, A.D. *et al.* (2008) Adaptive immune neuroprotection in G93A-SOD1 amyotrophic lateral sclerosis mice. *PLoS One*, **3**, e2740.

Beers, D.R., Henkel, J.S., Zhao, W., Wang, J. & Appel, S.H. (2008) CD4+ T cells support glial neuroprotection, slow disease progression, and modify glial morphology in an animal model of inherited ALS. *Proceedings of the National Academy of Sciences of the United States of America*, **105**, 15558–15563.

Beers, D.R., Henkel, J.S., Zhao, W. *et al.* (2011) Endogenous regulatory T lymphocytes ameliorate amyotrophic lateral sclerosis in mice and correlate with disease progression in patients with amyotrophic lateral sclerosis. *Brain*, **134**, 1293–1314.

Beers, D.R., Henkel, J.S., Xiao, Q. *et al.* (2006) Wild-type microglia extend survival in PU.1 knockout mice with familial amyotrophic lateral sclerosis. *Proceedings of the National Academy of Sciences of the United States of America*, **103**, 16021–16026.

Bettelli, E., Carrier, Y., Gao, W. *et al.* (2006) Reciprocal developmental pathways for the generation of pathogenic effector TH17 and regulatory T cells. *Nature*, **441**, 235–238.

Boillee, S., Yamanaka, K., Lobsiger, C.S. *et al.* (2006) Onset and progression in inherited ALS determined by motor neurons and microglia. *Science*, **312**, 1389–1392.

Chiu, I.M., Chen, A., Zheng, Y. *et al.* (2008) T lymphocytes potentiate endogenous neuroprotective inflammation in a mouse model of ALS. *Proceedings of the National Academy of Sciences of the United States of America*, **105**, 17913–17918.

Ciura, S., Lattante, S., Le Ber, I. *et al.* (2013) Loss of function of C9orf72 causes motor deficits in a zebrafish model of amyotrophic lateral sclerosis. *Annals of Neurology*, **74**, 180–187.

Cronin, S., Hardiman, O. & Traynor, B.J. (2007) Ethnic variation in the incidence of ALS: A systematic review. *Neurology*, **68**, 1002–1007.

Curotto de Lafaille, M.A. & Lafaille, J.J. (2009) Natural and adaptive foxp3+ regulatory T cells: More of the same or a division of labor? *Immunity*, **30**, 626–635.

Dai, Z., Zhang, S., Xie, Q., Wu, S., Su, J., Li, S., Xu, Y. & Li, X.C. (2014) Natural CD8+CD122+ T cells are more potent in suppression of allograft rejection than CD4+CD25+ regulatory T cells. *American Journal of Transplantation*, **14** (1), 39–48.

DeJesus-Hernandez, M. *et al.* (2011) Expanded GGGGCC hexanucleotide repeat in noncoding region of C9ORF72 causes chromosome 9p-linked FTD and ALS. *Neuron*, **72**, 245–256.

Engelhardt, J.I., Tajti, J. & Appel, S.H. (1993) Lymphocytic infiltrates in the spinal cord in amyotrophic lateral sclerosis. *Archives of Neurology*, **50**, 30–36.

Fiala, M., Chattopadhay, M., La Cava, A. *et al.* (2010) IL-17A is increased in the serum and in spinal cord CD8 and mast cells of ALS patients. *Journal of Neuroinflammation*, **7**, 76.

Fischer, L.R., Culver, D.G., Tennant, P. *et al.* (2004) Amyotrophic lateral sclerosis is a distal axonopathy: Evidence in mice and man. *Experimental Neurology*, **185**, 232–240.

Glezer, I., Simard, A.R. & Rivest, S. (2007) Neuroprotective role of the innate immune system by microglia. *Neuroscience*, **147**, 867–883.

Graves, M.C., Fiala, M., Dinglasan, L.A. *et al.* (2004) Inflammation in amyotrophic lateral sclerosis spinal cord and brain is mediated by activated macrophages, mast cells and T cells. *Amyotrophic Lateral Sclerosis and Other Motor Neuron Disorders*, **5**, 213–219.

Gurney, M.E., Pu, H., Chiu, A.Y. *et al.* (1994) Motor neuron degeneration in mice that express a human Cu,Zn superoxide dismutase mutation. *Science*, **264**, 1772–1775.

Henkel, J.S., Beers, D.R., Siklos, L. & Appel, S.H. (2006) The chemokine MCP-1 and the dendritic and myeloid cells it attracts are increased in the mSOD1 mouse model of ALS. *Molecular and Cellular Neurosciences*, **31**, 427–437.

Henkel, J.S., Beers, D.R., Zhao, W. & Appel, S.H. (2009) Microglia in ALS: The good, the bad, and the resting. *Journal of Neuroimmune Pharmacology*, **4**, 389–398.

Henkel, J.S., Engelhardt, J.I., Siklos, L. *et al.* (2004) Presence of dendritic cells, MCP-1, and activated microglia/macrophages in amyotrophic lateral sclerosis spinal cord tissue. *Annals of Neurology*, **55**, 221–235.

Henkel, J.S., Beers, D.R., Wen, S. *et al.* (2013) Regulatory T-lymphocytes mediate amyotrophic lateral sclerosis progression and survival. *EMBO Molecular Medicine*, **5**, 64–79.

Jaarsma, D., Teuling, E., Haasdijk, E.D., De Zeeuw, C.I. & Hoogenraad, C.C. (2008) Neuron-specific expression of mutant superoxide dismutase is sufficient to induce amyotrophic lateral sclerosis in transgenic mice. *Journal of Neuroscience*, **28**, 2075–2088.

Jiang, S. & Dong, C. (2013) A complex issue on CD4(+) T-cell subsets. *Immunological Reviews*, **252**, 5–11.

Joyce, P.I., Fratta, P., Fisher, E.M. & Acevedo-Arozena, A. (2011) SOD1 and TDP-43 animal models of amyotrophic lateral sclerosis: Recent advances in understanding disease toward the development of clinical treatments. *Mammalian Genome*, **22**, 420–448.

Kawamata, T., Akiyama, H., Yamada, T. & McGeer, P.L. (1992) Immunologic reactions in amyotrophic lateral sclerosis brain and spinal cord tissue. *American Journal of Pathology*, **140**, 691–707.

Kitagawa, Y., Ohkura, N. & Sakaguchi, S. (2013) Molecular determinants of regulatory T cell development: The essential roles of epigenetic changes. *Frontiers in Immunology*, **4**, 106.

Lal, G. & Bromberg, J.S. (2009) Epigenetic mechanisms of regulation of Foxp3 expression. *Blood*, **114**, 3727–3735.

McGeer, P.L. & McGeer, E.G. (2002) Inflammatory processes in amyotrophic lateral sclerosis. *Muscle & Nerve*, **26**, 459–470.

Morikawa, H. & Sakaguchi, S. (2014) Genetic and epigenetic basis of Treg cell development and function: From a FoxP3-centered view to an epigenome-defined view of natural Treg cells. *Immunological Reviews*, **259**, 192–205.

Neumann, M., Sampathu, D.M., Kwong, L.K. *et al.* (2006) Ubiquitinated TDP-43 in frontotemporal lobar degeneration and amyotrophic lateral sclerosis. *Science*, **314**, 130–133.

Nie, H., Zheng, Y., Li, R. *et al.* (2013) Phosphorylation of FOXP3 controls regulatory T cell function and is inhibited by TNF-alpha in rheumatoid arthritis. *Nature Medicine*, **19**, 322–328.

Renton, A.E. *et al.* (2011) A hexanucleotide repeat expansion in C9ORF72 is the cause of chromosome 9p21-linked ALS-FTD. *Neuron*, **72**, 257–268.

Rentzos, M., Evangelopoulos, E., Sereti, E. *et al.* (2012) Alterations of T cell subsets in ALS: A systemic immune activation? *Acta Neurologica Scandinavica*, **125**, 260–264.

Rentzos, M., Rombos, A., Nikolaou, C. *et al.* (2010) Interleukin-17 and interleukin-23 are elevated in serum and cerebrospinal fluid of patients with ALS: A reflection of Th17 cells activation? *Acta Neurologica Scandinavica*, **122**, 425–429.

Rosen, D.R., Siddique, T., Patterson, D. *et al.* (1993) Mutations in Cu/Zn superoxide dismutase gene are associated with familial amyotrophic lateral sclerosis. *Nature*, **362**, 59–62.

Rowland, L.P. (2001) How amyotrophic lateral sclerosis got its name: The clinical-pathologic genius of Jean-Martin Charcot. *Archives of Neurology*, **58**, 512–515.

Suzuki, N., Maroof, A.M., Merkle, F.T. *et al.* (2013) The mouse C9ORF72 ortholog is enriched in neurons known to degenerate in ALS and FTD. *Nature Neuroscience*, **16**, 1725–1727.

Tiemessen, M.M., Jagger, A.L., Evans, H.G., van Herwijnen, M.J., John, S. & Taams, L.S. (2007) CD4+CD25+Foxp3+ regulatory T cells induce alternative activation of human monocytes/macrophages. *Proceedings of the National Academy of Sciences of the United States of America*, **104**, 19446–19451.

Traub, R., Mitsumoto, H. & Rowland, L.P. (2011) Research advances in amyotrophic lateral sclerosis, 2009 to 2010. *Current Neurology and Neuroscience Reports*, **11**, 67–77.

Troost, D., van den Oord, J.J., de Jong, J.M. & Swaab, D.F. (1989) Lymphocytic infiltration in the spinal cord of patients with amyotrophic lateral sclerosis. *Clinical Neuropathology*, **8**, 289–294.

Worms, P.M. (2001) The epidemiology of motor neuron diseases: A review of recent studies. *Journal of the Neurological Sciences*, **191**, 3–9.

Zhao, W., Beers, D.R., Liao, B., Henkel, J.S. & Appel, S.H. (2012) Regulatory T lymphocytes from ALS mice suppress microglia and effector T lymphocytes through different cytokine-mediated mechanisms. *Neurobiology of Disease*, **48**, 418–428.

16 An Adaptive Role for TNFα in Synaptic Plasticity and Neuronal Function

Renu Heir and David Stellwagen

Department of Neurology and Neurosurgery, Centre for Research in Neuroscience, The Research Institute of the McGill University Health Center, Montreal, Quebec, Canada

Introduction

The central nervous system (CNS) was originally thought of as an immune-privileged site, kept separate from the peripheral immune system and immune signaling molecules by the blood–brain barrier (Barker and Billingham, 1977). This was proposed in part because of the lack of conventional lymphatic vessels as well as the extended survival of foreign tissue grafts in the brain, suggesting that it was not capable of normal immune responses. However, it was later found that under certain pathological conditions such as neuroinflammation, cytokines are produced in the brain (Hopkins and Rothwell, 1995). It is becoming evident that many immune molecules are present in the nervous system even under nonpathological conditions, and also play a role in regulating synaptic function (Vitkovic *et al.*, 2000). This chapter focuses on the function of the proinflammatory cytokine tumor necrosis factor alpha (TNFα) in the nervous system.

TNFα is a cytokine with well-defined roles in the inflammatory response, cell survival, and organogenesis. The role of TNFα during neuroinflammation is complex: it can contribute to both neuronal cell death and survival (Hsu *et al.*, 1995). Importantly, TNFα mRNA is also basally present in the brain (Vitkovic *et al.*, 2000), suggesting that it could be playing a role under healthy, noninflammatory conditions. Recent evidence in systems ranging from dissociated cell culture to more intact *in vivo* models has demonstrated that TNFα can play an important modulatory role in the brain, particularly at the synapse.

TNFα is translated as a single-pass transmembrane protein, which then assembles into stable homotrimers (Smith and Baglioni, 1987). This membrane-bound TNFα can signal directly in its membrane-bound form (Grell *et al.*, 1995) but is more often cleaved by the matrix metalloprotease ADAM17 (otherwise known as TNFα-converting enzyme, TACE) to release soluble and biologically active TNFα (Black *et al.*, 1997).

Neuroinflammation: New Insights into Beneficial and Detrimental Functions, First Edition. Edited by Samuel David.
© 2015 John Wiley & Sons, Inc. Published 2015 by John Wiley & Sons, Inc.

TNFα signaling occurs through two receptors: TNFR1 and TNFR2 (MacEwan, 2002). TNFR1 expression is ubiquitous, but TNFR2 expression is generally restricted to endothelial and immune cells (Wajant et al., 2003). While the mechanism of receptor specificity is not yet fully understood, TNFR2 can only be maximally activated by membrane-bound TNFα, while TNFR1 is activated by both membrane and soluble TNFα (Grell et al., 1995). TNFR1 and TNFR2 also differ in their downstream signaling pathways: TNFR1 signaling is diverse, and can result in proliferation, activation, and apoptosis, while TNFR2 signaling generally results in proinflammatory and pro-survival processes (Wajant et al., 2003).

Developmental Roles of TNFα

TNFα has a broad range of effects beyond its classical regulation of cell survival and appears to modulate the maturation and function of central synapses. At this time, it is unclear if TNFα can directly regulate synapse formation or indirectly affects connectivity. In *Xenopus* tadpoles, chronic administration of TNFα leads to increased neuronal connectivity (Lee et al., 2010), suggesting an increase in synapse formation, although this effect could also be due to a lack of refinement through decreased synapse elimination. TNFα also appears to regulate neuronal morphology in the hippocampus (Golan et al., 2004), although this, too, could be indirectly due to altered synaptic maturation.

TNFα in Presynaptic Function

There is also some evidence that TNFα regulates presynaptic function by modulating neurotransmitter release probability. Miniature excitatory postsynaptic currents (mEPSCs) are the postsynaptic response to unitary release of neurotransmitter, and the frequency of these events is thought to be proportional to the probability of neurotransmitter release during an action potential. TNFα treatment causes a transient increase in mEPSC frequency (Grassi et al., 1994; Beattie et al., 2002) consistent with an increase in the probability for excitatory neurotransmitter release, although this effect could be indirect due to potentiating factors released from glia (Santello et al., 2011). TNFα treatment also causes a decrease in miniature inhibitory postsynaptic current (mIPSC) frequency (Pribiag and Stellwagen, 2013), suggesting that changes in release probability is not restricted to excitatory synapses.

TNFα Effects on Postsynaptic Receptor Trafficking

The majority of work, however, has focused on the postsynapse, where TNFα has a much clearer role in regulating the trafficking of neurotransmitter receptors. Excitatory synaptic transmission occurs primarily through the signaling of α-amino-3-hydroxy-5-methyl-4-isoxazolepropionic acid-type glutamate receptors (AMPARs), with the number of receptors largely determining the size of the synaptic response (Malinow and Malenka, 2002). The dynamics of AMPAR trafficking to the cell surface, therefore, determine synaptic strength and can be modulated under certain circumstances to result in plasticity of synapses (Malinow and Malenka, 2002; Shepherd and Huganir, 2007). Numerous studies have been conducted to assess the effect of exogenous application of TNFα to cultured neurons in terms of AMPAR surface levels. One of the first showed through immunocytochemistry that application of TNFα to dissociated hippocampal cultures results in trafficking of AMPARs to the neuronal cell surface (Beattie *et al.*, 2002). These additional receptors colocalize with synaptic markers, indicating that they are well-positioned to modify synaptic strength. Furthermore, exocytosis of receptors occurs on a time scale of just 10 min and results in more than double the number of surface receptors, underscoring the potential of TNFα-mediated AMPAR trafficking to make important adjustments to synaptic strength. Interestingly, TNFα signaling was also shown, through the use of function-blocking antibodies to TNFR1, to play a role not only in the trafficking of AMPAR in response to exogenous TNFα, but also in maintaining basal levels of surface expression through this receptor in culture. This suggests a constitutive role for TNFα in the nervous system, and that the TNFα that is released originates with resident cells of the brain rather than immune cells that have infiltrated under pathological conditions.

Changes in synaptic strength in response to TNFα application have also been assayed using electrophysiological methods to corroborate findings by immunocytochemistry. The amplitude of mEPSCs can be used as a measure of the strength of individual synapses. Consistent with immunocytochemical data, TNFα increases mEPSC amplitude in response to TNFα application in cultured hippocampal cells, as well as in the more biologically intact system of acute hippocampal slices (Stellwagen *et al.*, 2005). These studies also revealed that trafficking of receptors is dependent on phosphatidylinositol-4,5-bisphosphate 3-kinase (PI3K) signaling through TNFR1.

It is important to note that the newly inserted AMPA receptors are also of a particular subunit composition. AMPARs are tetramers composed of the subunits GluA1-A4 (Wisden and Seeburg, 1993) and are most often found in one of two combinations: GluA1/GluA2 or GluA2/GluA3 heteromers, although a minority of receptor complexes are GluA1 homomers (Wenthold *et al.*, 1996; Shi *et al.*, 2001). The GluA2 subunit is of particular importance, as it confers calcium ion impermeability to the heteromeric complex (Burnashev *et al.*, 1992). Receptors lacking this subunit are permeable to calcium, which has implications in terms of the calcium-dependent processes of synaptic plasticity as well as excitotoxic cell death and is thought to be important during several disease states (Dong *et al.*, 2009). Several reports have shown that TNFα induces the exocytosis of GluA2-lacking receptors (Ogoshi *et al.*, 2005; Stellwagen *et al.*, 2005), although this does not exclude the exocytosis of GluA2-containing receptor as well. Furthermore, GluA2-lacking receptors may be replaced with GluA2-containing receptors over time, due to the constitutive cycling of AMPARs.

In contrast to AMPARs, TNFα application has no clear effect on the trafficking of other glutamate receptor subtypes. There is no change in synaptic localization of *N*-methyl D-aspartate-type glutamate receptors (NMDARs) despite changes in synaptic AMPAR localization in hippocampal neurons (Beattie *et al.*, 2002), nor are there changes in NMDAR-mediated whole cell currents on cortical neurons (He *et al.*, 2012). Long-term treatment with TNFα may decrease NMDAR currents in the hippocampus (Furukawa and Mattson, 1998), although in the spinal cord, TNFα has been reported to increase NMDAR function (Kawasaki *et al.*, 2008; Han and Whelan, 2010). To date, there have been no reports of TNFα regulating kainate-type glutamate receptors.

Table 16.1 The synaptic effects of TNFα treatment

Preparation	TNFα treatment	Result	Reference
Xenopus tectal neurons	30 nM, 10–12 d	↑ Connectivity	Lee *et al.*, 2010
Rat hippocampal cultures	10 nM, 2–5 min	↑ Glutamate release probability	Grassi *et al.*, 1994
	0.6–60 nM, 15 min	↑ Glutamate release probability ↑ Surface AMPARs	Beattie *et al.*, 2002
	6 nM, 45 min	↓ GABA release probability ↓ Surface GABARs ↓ GABAR current	Pribiag and Stellwagen, 2013
	60 nM, 15–20 min	↑ Surface AMPARs ↑ AMPAR current ↓ Surface GABARs ↓ GABAR current	Stellwagen *et al.*, 2005
Mouse acute hippocampal slices	6 nM, 15 min	↑ surface AMPARs	Ogoshi *et al.*, 2005
Rat acute hippocampal slices	600 nM, 2–3 h	↑ AMPAR current ↓ GABAR current	Stellwagen *et al.*, 2005

In addition to glutamate receptors, γ-aminobutyric acid receptors (GABARs) are also regulated by TNFα. GABARs are the principal receptors responsible for fast inhibitory transmission in the brain (Jacob *et al.*, 2008) and therefore are critical to maintaining the balance of excitatory to inhibitory signaling. Exogenous TNFα increases surface AMPAR, as previously discussed, and simultaneously decreases surface GABARs, as observed by both immunocytochemistry and measurement of mIPSC amplitudes in neuronal culture (Stellwagen *et al.*, 2005). Detailed mechanistic examination of this process has revealed that the down-regulation of GABARs requires the sequential activation of p38 mitogen-activated protein kinase (MAPK), PI3K, and protein phosphatase 1 (PP1), leading to the dephosphorylation of the GABARs (Pribiag and Stellwagen, 2013). Similar effects of TNFα on GABARs were also found in acute hippocampal slices. It is important to note that this study also demonstrated that GABAR endocytosis is followed by down-regulation of the scaffolding protein, gephyrin, indicating that TNFα is capable of regulation of not only the receptor content of GABAergic synapses, but also their structural components. Taken together, these data regarding the results of TNFα application emphasize its potential for wide-reaching regulation of nervous system dynamics (Table 16.1). By modulating both the major excitatory and inhibitory neurotransmitter receptors, TNFα is aptly positioned to function as a critical regulator of circuit excitability (Fig. 16.1).

The potential source of TNFα in this type of synaptic modulation is also of great interest. To this end, studies have shown that treatment of neurons with glial-conditioned medium phenocopies administration of TNFα alone in terms of increasing surface AMPARs, indicating that the source of TNFα allowing for the modulation of synapses is glial cells (Beattie *et al.*, 2002). This is further supported by the fact that addition of soluble TNFR1, which blocks normal TNFα signaling, abolishes this effect of glial-conditioned medium on neuronal cultures.

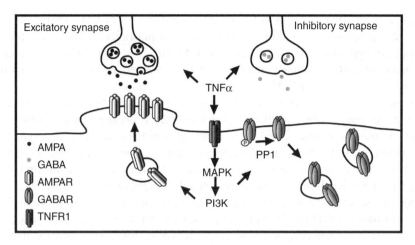

Figure 16.1   The role of TNFα at excitatory and inhibitory synapses. TNFα exerts its effects on postsynaptic trafficking through the activation of TNFR1. Common signaling downstream of TNFR1 diverges between excitatory and inhibitory synapses at the level of PI3K. At excitatory synapses, this leads to exocytosis of AMPARs and increased synaptic strength. At inhibitory synapses, PP1 is activated, which goes on to dephosphorylate GABARs and results in their endocytic removal from the synapse. At the presynapse, TNFα also increases glutamate release probability while decreasing GABA release probability. All of these effects together result in a higher excitatory–inhibitory balance, and increased neuronal activity.

TNFα and Synaptic Plasticity

While examination of the effects of exogenous application of TNFα has yielded a wealth of information in terms of the potential effects of TNFα on neurotransmission, to understand the endogenous role of TNFα in nervous system function, it is vital to consider under which conditions TNFα may be released and therefore under which conditions these effects are biologically relevant. Neuronal circuits are dynamically regulated in the healthy brain, primarily through the modulation of neurotransmitter receptor levels during the process of synaptic plasticity. This is critical to the activity of neural circuits, as they depend on the combined effects of the strengths of the individual synaptic connections within them. Circuits are subject to modification by both Hebbian and non-Hebbian forms of synaptic plasticity. Hebbian forms, such as long-term potentiation (LTP) and long-term depression (LTD), rapidly adjust the strength of individual synapses in response to synchronous synaptic activity (Malinow and Malenka, 2002) and are thought to be necessary for information storage and refinement of connections during development. Non-Hebbian forms are thought to provide stability to neuronal circuits, allowing them to adapt to changing conditions (Turrigiano and Nelson, 2004).

TNFα has an ambiguous role in Hebbian forms of plasticity. There are reports that TNFα pretreatment blocks LTP induction in the dentate gyrus (Cunningham *et al.*, 1996; Wang *et al.*, 2005), and in CA1 of the hippocampus (Tancredi *et al.*, 1992). However, normal LTP and LTD in the CA1 can be elicited following TNFα treatment, despite a change in synaptic function (Stellwagen and Malenka, 2006). Although LTD was reported to be absent in TNFR knockout (KO) mice according to one report (Albensi and Mattson, 2000), other evidence demonstrates normal LTP and LTD in TNFα KO and TNFR1/TNFR2 double KO mice (Stellwagen and Malenka, 2006).

Overall, this suggests that TNFα is not required for either LTP or LTD, though it may have a modulatory influence on the induction of these forms of plasticity. In particular, the change in basal synaptic strength induced by TNFα may alter the threshold for induction and thus represent a form of meta-plasticity (Abraham and Bear, 1996). However, TNFα is clearly not part of the core machinery responsible for Hebbian plasticity.

Hebbian plasticity of course is not the only type of synaptic plasticity. Because both forms of Hebbian plasticity function in a positive feedback manner, it is necessary to counter these types of plasticity in order to prevent either runaway strengthening or weakening of synapses, which could have deleterious effects on neural circuit function. A homeostatic process termed synaptic scaling negatively regulates these mechanisms by uniformly adjusting the strength of all of the synapses on a given cell in response to prolonged changes in overall firing rates (Turrigiano et al., 1998). This serves to keep activity levels within the optimal range for transmission without losing the information conferred by LTP and LTD, as differences in relative synaptic strengths are preserved. TNFα has been implicated in the process of scaling up excitatory synaptic strength in response to activity blockade (Stellwagen and Malenka, 2006). Forty-eight hour treatment of dissociated hippocampal cultures with tetrodotoxin (TTX), which blocks Na^+ channels thus preventing the generation of action potentials, leads to an increase in surface AMPARs, an increase in mEPSC amplitudes, a decrease in surface GABARs, and a decrease in mIPSC amplitudes. This leads to an overall increase in circuit strength, and is accompanied by an increase in TNFα concentration in the culture medium that can be blocked by treatment with soluble TNFR1, which prevents TNFα signaling. Together, this is strong evidence that TNFα-mediated receptor trafficking through TNFR1 signaling is an important cellular response to prolonged activity deprivation.

The relevant AMPAR subunit that is trafficked in this type of plasticity was not exhaustively tested in that study, but increases in surface GluA1 staining were observed following activity deprivation. Together with previous data that TNFα application results in exocytosis of GluA2-lacking AMPARs (Stellwagen et al., 2005), this suggests that GluA1 homomers are increased at the cell surface after TTX treatment. Other reports of homeostatic plasticity support this suggestion, showing an increase in GluA2-lacking receptors after activity deprivation (Thiagarajan et al., 2005; Sutton et al., 2006; Aoto et al., 2008; Hou et al., 2008; Garcia-Bereguiain et al., 2013), although there has been one report showing a requirement for GluA2 in synaptic scaling using knockdown studies (Gainey et al., 2009). However, there is also data using neuronal cultures from animals with genetic deletions of GluA1, GluA2, and GluA3, demonstrating that there is no subunit requirement for synaptic scaling (Altimimi and Stellwagen, 2013), which may be a result of compensation by other AMPARs to the absence of particular AMPAR subunits.

Glial Release of TNFα During Plasticity

Another important question in the examination of TNFα in synaptic scaling is its source. While previous studies indicated that glia produce TNFα basally in culture, and that this TNFα is capable of driving surface expression of AMPARs in neuronal cultures treated with glial-conditioned medium (Beattie et al., 2002), it was unclear if this held true for synaptic scaling. Banker-style cultures where neurons are grown physically separated from a feeder layer of glial cells allow for the detailed examination of the relative contribution of each cell type to synaptic scaling. In this system, it was shown that TNFα −/− glia are unable to support synaptic scaling in WT neurons (Stellwagen and Malenka, 2006), suggesting that the relevant source for TNFα in the context of synaptic scaling is glia.

This is an important finding, as it establishes TNFα as not only a neuromodulatory factor, but also as a gliotransmitter. It was a long-held belief that glial cells merely provided physical and trophic support for neurons, but it has recently come to light that they are capable of modulating neurotransmission through the secretion of factors, termed gliotransmitters, that act upon neurons (Haydon, 2001; Volterra and Meldolesi, 2005; Perea et al., 2009). In this way, synapses are thought to have not just a pre- and postsynaptic component, but also a glial element, resulting in their characterization as tripartite structures. The role of TNFα in synaptic scaling reinforces this idea of the tripartite synapse, where glial cells are able to actively participate in setting synaptic properties.

While a role for TNFα in receptor trafficking during synaptic plasticity is clear, there is evidence that it may also play other more complex roles in the regulation of synapses. In addition to its function as a gliotransmitter itself, there is evidence supporting a role in regulating other gliotransmitters, namely glutamate (Santello et al., 2011). It has been shown that glutamate can be released from astrocytes in the dentate gyrus in response to stimulation of their P2Y1 purinergic receptors by neuronal activity, resulting in an increase in synaptic neurotransmitter release through modulation of NMDARs (Jourdain et al., 2007). Santello et al. show that this P2Y1-dependent increase in glutamate release from astrocytes and subsequent synaptic strengthening is dependent on the presence of TNFα. In this case, TNFα would act to increase vesicle fusion, a function that could be analogous to the increase in release probability reported at excitatory synapses.

It is important to note that the concept of gliotransmission is a highly controversial one. While there exists a large body of literature demonstrating roles for gliotransmitters such as glutamate in the regulation of synaptic transmission (Araque et al., 2014), numerous reports also question the ability of astrocytes to exocytose the purported gliotransmitters, as well question their ability to exert effects on synaptic transmission (Agulhon et al., 2010). Overall, these data suggest that an important part of the role of TNFα in neural cultures is a homeostatic function in responding to long-lasting changes in activity levels. It is therefore of interest to consider whether this idea may hold true in more intact systems that approximate similar circumstances. This idea has been investigated in one such system: denervation of entorhino-hippocampal slice cultures. The entorhinal cortex is the major input and output structure for the hippocampus. Projections from the entorhinal cortex to the dentate gyrus, termed the perforant path, have long been studied in terms of both structure (Witter, 2007) and plasticity (Bliss and Lomo, 1973; Douglas and Goddard, 1975). In entorhino-hippocampal slice cultures, these projections can be preserved so that the effects of subsequent denervation of the cultures can be assessed. Recently, data have shown that entorhinal denervation results in a homeostatic scaling up of mEPSC amplitudes in the dentate gyrus reaching a peak 3–4 days after lesion (Vlachos et al., 2012; Vlachos et al., 2013), and that this scaling was not additive with increases in synaptic strength observed after prolonged TTX treatment. This suggests a common mechanism for the homeostatic response to the two methods of decreasing activity. This system, therefore, bears remarkable similarity to the dissociated cell culture system in terms of responses to long-lasting decreases in overall activity.

Indeed, TNFα is also required for this form of plasticity: slice cultures either made from TNFα KO animals, or treated with soluble TNFR to block TNFα signaling lack the late-stage (3–4 day) component of increased mEPSC amplitude (Becker *et al.*, 2013). Further similarities to synaptic scaling in culture lie with the source of TNFα. A combination of *in situ* hybridization for TNFα and immunofluorescent labeling of the astrocytic marker glial fibrillary acidic protein (GFAP) revealed the presence of TNFα mRNA in astrocytes in the denervated area of the dentate gyrus. Although this does not exclude alternate sources of TNFα such as microglia or neurons, the presence of TNFα mRNA in astrocytes highlights the possibility that they are capable of supplying the TNFα required for this form of plasticity.

TNFα-Mediated Homeostatic Plasticity *in Vivo*

The visual system has offered insight into TNFα-dependent plasticity processes *in vivo*. The visual cortex is particularly plastic during a time in early development termed the critical period (Hubel and Wiesel, 1970). During this time, monocular deprivation by suturing one eye closed results in a shift in the responses detected in the visual cortex. Initially, there is a decrease in responses to stimulation of the closed eye, followed by increased responses following stimulation of the open eye (Frenkel and Bear, 2004). Experiments in animals lacking TNFα have revealed that TNFα is necessary for potentiation of open-eye responses, but not for decreases in closed-eye responses (Kaneko *et al.*, 2008). Interestingly, open-eye responses can also potentiate following monocular deprivation in the adult animal (outside of the critical period), albeit to a lesser extent (Sawtell *et al.*, 2003), and this is not dependent on TNFα (Ranson *et al.*, 2012). The requirement of TNFα for some forms of visual system plasticity is an important finding, as it represents an example of TNFα-dependent plasticity in an intact animal, highlighting the biological relevance of TNFα in modulating synaptic function.

TNFα-Mediated Plasticity in the Striatum

Taken together, all of the previously discussed data highlight the ability of TNFα to modulate synaptic transmission in the excitatory cells of the hippocampus and cortex. From systems of neuronal culture, to acute slices, to slice culture and finally *in vivo*, the data suggest that TNFα has an overall function to homeostatically regulate synaptic strength. However, whether TNFα carries out similar functions in other brain areas or in other cell types remains largely unexplored. Furthermore, the role of TNFα under inflammatory conditions is uncertain. Traditionally, inflammation during pathology has been viewed as largely deleterious, but given the role of TNFα in homeostatic plasticity, it may serve at least initially to help stabilize circuit function in the face of disruption. In this context, TNFα-mediated synaptic changes could in fact be beneficial. Recently, the striatum was investigated in terms of TNFα and synaptic plasticity during pathological conditions.

The striatum is a key center for processing information in the basal ganglia: it receives cortical, thalamic, and brainstem inputs and serves to integrate sensorimotor, cognitive, and motivational information. It is composed primarily of GABAergic medium spiny neurons (MSNs), which constitute its only output (Gerfen and Wilson, 1996). Recently, TNFα was implicated in determining

AMPAR content at corticostriatal synapses (Lewitus *et al.*, 2014). In contrast with results in pyramidal neurons, experiments where acute striatal slices are treated with exogenous TNFα resulted in decreased excitatory synaptic strength. In addition, both biochemical methods (cell surface biotinylation) and electrophysiological analysis suggest that this decrease in synaptic function is due to an endocytosis of GluA2-lacking AMPARs, the same subtype that is exocytosed in pyramidal neurons in response to TNFα treatment.

In this study, TNFα was also implicated *in vivo* as a limiting factor for synaptic strength in the corticostriatal circuit. Removal of TNFα from the system, whether it be by using TNFα −/− animals, or by administration of a dominant negative form of TNFα to wild-type animals, resulted in an increase in AMPA/NMDA ratios and therefore corticostriatal synaptic strength. This is strong evidence that under basal conditions, TNFα functions to down-regulate surface AMPARs *in vivo*. Furthermore, TNFα was also implicated in the modulation of striatal-dependent behavior. Chronic blockade of D_2 dopamine receptors by drugs such as haloperidol results in elevated striatal TNFα levels, increased AMPA binding, as well as the development of involuntary movements of the face (tardive dyskinesia), suggesting that there is a dysfunction in the striatal circuit responsible for movement under these conditions (Schmitt *et al.*, 2003; Bishnoi *et al.*, 2008). Lewitus *et al.* show that decreasing TNFα by dominant negative TNFα treatment results in more frequent involuntary movements, suggesting that TNFα serves to limit the adverse effects of chronic haloperidol administration on the corticostriatal circuit, and that this is through the endocytosis of calcium-permeable AMPARs. Furthermore, restoring TNFα signaling normalized the behavior, suggesting that TNFα is acting in an ongoing manner to reduce the severity of the circuit perturbation.

While these results showing that TNFα mediates endocytosis of AMPARs in the striatum initially appear to contradict data showing that TNFα mediates exocytosis of AMPARs in pyramidal neurons, it is important to note that the MSNs of the striatum are inhibitory, in contrast to excitatory pyramidal cells. Both decreasing inhibition and increasing excitation would have the ultimate result of increasing the activity of neural circuits, so TNFα would be exerting the same overall effect in both of these cases. There is also a precedent for differential effects of activity deprivation on AMPAR trafficking in excitatory versus inhibitory cells in hippocampal cultures, with AMPARs being decreased on inhibitory parvalbumin-expressing interneurons (Chang *et al.*, 2010). Similar signaling mechanisms inverting the AMPAR response in inhibitory cells could be functioning in the case of the effect of TNFα on striatal MSNs. Thus, data from the hippocampus, cortex, and striatum suggest that TNFα may have a general role in homeostatic regulation of neuronal circuits, regardless of brain area or cell type.

Implications of TNFα-Mediated Synaptic Regulation

There is now a wealth of evidence for a neuromodulatory role for TNFα at the synapse outside of the context of neuroinflammation. Overall, these data suggest that TNFα acts to homeostatically regulate circuit function by inducing appropriate alterations in synaptic strength, and slight elevation of TNFα during neuronal pathologies such as dyskinesia may be an adaptive response to circuit disruption. While the importance of these experiments in understanding brain function is clear, they may also give valuable insight into the mechanisms at play during pathological conditions where there is inflammation and infiltration of cytokine-secreting immune cells.

The inflammatory response to injury or prolonged CNS disease results in the chronic production of high levels of proinflammatory cytokines, which could be contributing to the synaptic dysfunction observed in many disease states (Allan and Rothwell, 2001; Leonoudakis et al., 2004). For example, cytokines, including TNFα, are prime candidates for the induction and maintenance of chronic pain states, which result at least in part from increased excitatory and decreased inhibitory drive on central pain pathways (Kawasaki et al., 2008) and is consistent with receptor trafficking induced by TNFα (Stellwagen et al., 2005). Furthermore, the fact that TNFα treatment of pyramidal neurons results in the trafficking of AMPARs that are permeable to calcium would result in a higher intracellular calcium concentration after neuronal activity. This is an important consideration because excitotoxic cell death has been attributed to elevated intracellular calcium leading to the inappropriate activation of enzymes such as phospholipases, endonucleases, and proteases (Sattler and Tymianski, 2000). Indeed, it has been shown that TNFα-induced delivery of calcium-permeable AMPARs makes neurons more susceptible to the excitotoxic insult of kainate treatment (Leonoudakis et al., 2008), and to spinal cord injury (Ferguson et al., 2008). Similarly, elevated GluA1 levels and decreased GluA2 levels in mouse models of amyotropic lateral sclerosis (ALS) (Zhao et al., 2008) may result in increased calcium-permeable AMPARs at the synapse and increased excitotoxic motor neuron death. Conversely, several studies have observed a neuroprotective role for TNFα and other cytokines to excitotoxic insults, (Carlson et al., 1998, 1999; Liu et al., 1999), although it is unclear if this is related to the effect of TNFα on synapses.

TNFα can also broadly regulate nervous system function. Acute elevation of cytokines, including TNFα, results in "sickness behavior," characterized by decreased motor activity and food intake, social withdrawal, and increased slow wave sleep (Dantzer et al., 2008). This response is thought to be adaptive and is likely due to regulation of circuit function of hypothalamic nuclei, but the details are unknown at this time. TNFα also generally increases excitability in the brain, potentially increasing seizure susceptibility (Galic et al., 2012), and acute exposure to cytokines during development can have lasting impact on endocrine responses and metabolism (Spencer et al., 2011). This suggests that TNFα-mediated changes in circuit function can have a lasting impact on nervous system function.

In conclusion, TNFα modulates far more in the nervous system than neuronal cell survival and cell death. It is used by the healthy nervous system to homeostatically regulate circuit function, and a neuroinflammatory response may at times be an adaptive response to circuit disruption. In other circumstances, particularly during high levels or chronic elevation, TNFα may be contributing to pathology through a dysregulation of synaptic function.

References

Abraham, W.C. & Bear, M.F. (1996) Metaplasticity: The plasticity of synaptic plasticity. Trends in Neurosciences, 19, 126–130.

Agulhon, C., Fiacco, T.A. & McCarthy, K.D. (2010) Hippocampal short- and long-term plasticity are not modulated by astrocyte Ca2+ signaling. Science, 327, 1250–1254.

Albensi, B.C. & Mattson, M.P. (2000) Evidence for the involvement of TNF and NF-kappaB in hippocampal synaptic plasticity. Synapse, 35, 151–159.

Allan, S.M. & Rothwell, N.J. (2001) Cytokines and acute neurodegeneration. *Nature reviews Neuroscience*, **2**, 734–744.

Altimimi, H.F. & Stellwagen, D. (2013) Persistent synaptic scaling independent of AMPA receptor subunit composition. *Journal of Neuroscience*, **33**, 11763–11767.

Aoto, J., Nam, C.I., Poon, M.M., Ting, P. & Chen, L. (2008) Synaptic signaling by all-trans retinoic acid in homeostatic synaptic plasticity. *Neuron*, **60**, 308–320.

Araque, A., Carmignoto, G., Haydon, P.G., Oliet, S.H., Robitaille, R. & Volterra, A. (2014) Gliotransmitters travel in time and space. *Neuron*, **81**, 728–739.

Barker, C.F. & Billingham, R.E. (1977) Immunologically privileged sites. *Advances in Immunology*, **25**, 1–54.

Beattie, E.C., Stellwagen, D., Morishita, W. *et al.* (2002) Control of synaptic strength by glial TNFalpha. *Science*, **295**, 2282–2285.

Becker, D., Zahn, N., Deller, T. & Vlachos, A. (2013) Tumor necrosis factor alpha maintains denervation-induced homeostatic synaptic plasticity of mouse dentate granule cells. *Frontiers in Cellular Neuroscience*, **7**, 257.

Bishnoi, M., Chopra, K. & Kulkarni, S.K. (2008) Differential striatal levels of TNF-alpha, NFkappaB p65 subunit and dopamine with chronic typical and atypical neuroleptic treatment: Role in orofacial dyskinesia. *Progress in Neuro-Psychopharmacology & Biological Psychiatry*, **32**, 1473–1478.

Black, R.A., Rauch, C.T., Kozlosky, C.J. *et al.* (1997) A metalloproteinase disintegrin that releases tumour-necrosis factor-alpha from cells. *Nature*, **385**, 729–733.

Bliss, T.V. & Lomo, T. (1973) Long-lasting potentiation of synaptic transmission in the dentate area of the anaesthetized rabbit following stimulation of the perforant path. *Journal of Physiology*, **232**, 331–356.

Burnashev, N., Monyer, H., Seeburg, P.H. & Sakmann, B. (1992) Divalent ion permeability of AMPA receptor channels is dominated by the edited form of a single subunit. *Neuron*, **8**, 189–198.

Carlson, N.G., Bacchi, A., Rogers, S.W. & Gahring, L.C. (1998) Nicotine blocks TNF-alpha-mediated neuroprotection to NMDA by an alpha-bungarotoxin-sensitive pathway. *Journal of Neurobiology*, **35**, 29–36.

Carlson, N.G., Wieggel, W.A., Chen, J., Bacchi, A., Rogers, S.W. & Gahring, L.C. (1999) Inflammatory cytokines IL-1 alpha, IL-1 beta, IL-6, and TNF-alpha impart neuroprotection to an excitotoxin through distinct pathways. *Journal of Immunology*, **163**, 3963–3968.

Chang, M.C., Park, J.M., Pelkey, K.A. *et al.* (2010) Narp regulates homeostatic scaling of excitatory synapses on parvalbumin-expressing interneurons. *Nature Neuroscience*, **13**, 1090–1097.

Cunningham, A.J., Murray, C.A., O'Neill, L.A., Lynch, M.A. & O'Connor, J.J. (1996) Interleukin-1 beta (IL-1 beta) and tumour necrosis factor (TNF) inhibit long-term potentiation in the rat dentate gyrus in vitro. *Neuroscience Letters*, **203**, 17–20.

Dantzer, R., O'Connor, J.C., Freund, G.G., Johnson, R.W. & Kelley, K.W. (2008) From inflammation to sickness and depression: When the immune system subjugates the brain. *Nature Reviews Neuroscience*, **9**, 46–56.

Dong, X.X., Wang, Y. & Qin, Z.H. (2009) Molecular mechanisms of excitotoxicity and their relevance to pathogenesis of neurodegenerative diseases. *Acta Pharmacologica Sinica*, **30**, 379–387.

Douglas, R.M. & Goddard, G.V. (1975) Long-term potentiation of the perforant path-granule cell synapse in the rat hippocampus. *Brain Research*, **86**, 205–215.

Ferguson, A.R., Christensen, R.N., Gensel, J.C. *et al.* (2008) Cell death after spinal cord injury is exacerbated by rapid TNF alpha-induced trafficking of GluR2-lacking AMPARs to the plasma membrane. *Journal of Neuroscience*, **28**, 11391–11400.

Frenkel, M.Y. & Bear, M.F. (2004) How monocular deprivation shifts ocular dominance in visual cortex of young mice. *Neuron*, **44**, 917–923.

Furukawa, K. & Mattson, M.P. (1998) The transcription factor NF-kappaB mediates increases in calcium currents and decreases in NMDA- and AMPA/kainate-induced currents induced by tumor necrosis factor-alpha in hippocampal neurons. *Journal of Neurochemistry*, **70**, 1876–1886.

Gainey, M.A., Hurvitz-Wolff, J.R., Lambo, M.E. & Turrigiano, G.G. (2009) Synaptic scaling requires the GluR2 subunit of the AMPA receptor. *Journal of Neuroscience*, **29**, 6479–6489.

Galic, M.A., Riazi, K. & Pittman, Q.J. (2012) Cytokines and brain excitability. *Frontiers in Neuroendocrinology*, **33**, 116–125.

Garcia-Bereguiain, M.A., Gonzalez-Islas, C., Lindsly, C., Butler, E., Hill, A.W. & Wenner, P. (2013) In vivo synaptic scaling is mediated by GluA2-lacking AMPA receptors in the embryonic spinal cord. *Journal of Neuroscience*, **33**, 6791–6799.

Gerfen, C. & Wilson, C. (1996) The basal ganglia. In: Björklund, A., Hökfelt, T. & Swanson, L.M. (eds), *Handbook of Chemical Neuroanatomy. Integrated Systems of the CNS. Part III*. Elsevier, Amsterdam, The Netherlands, pp. 371–468.

Golan, H., Levav, T., Mendelsohn, A. & Huleihel, M. (2004) Involvement of tumor necrosis factor alpha in hippocampal development and function. *Cerebral Cortex*, **14**, 97–105.

Grassi, F., Mileo, A.M., Monaco, L., Punturieri, A., Santoni, A. & Eusebi, F. (1994) TNF-alpha increases the frequency of spontaneous miniature synaptic currents in cultured rat hippocampal neurons. *Brain Research*, **659**, 226–230.

Grell, M., Douni, E., Wajant, H. *et al.* (1995) The transmembrane form of tumor necrosis factor is the prime activating ligand of the 80 kDa tumor necrosis factor receptor. *Cell*, **83**, 793–802.

Han, P. & Whelan, P.J. (2010) Tumor necrosis factor alpha enhances glutamatergic transmission onto spinal motoneurons. *Journal of Neurotrauma*, **27**, 287–292.

Haydon, P.G. (2001) GLIA: Listening and talking to the synapse. *Nature Reviews Neuroscience*, **2**, 185–193.

He, P., Liu, Q., Wu, J. & Shen, Y. (2012) Genetic deletion of TNF receptor suppresses excitatory synaptic transmission via reducing AMPA receptor synaptic localization in cortical neurons. *FASEB Journal*, **26**, 334–345.

Hopkins, S.J. & Rothwell, N.J. (1995) Cytokines and the nervous system. I: Expression and recognition. *Trends in neurosciences*, **18**, 83–88.

Hou, Q., Zhang, D., Jarzylo, L., Huganir, R.L. & Man, H.Y. (2008) Homeostatic regulation of AMPA receptor expression at single hippocampal synapses. *Proceedings of the National Academy of Sciences of the United States of America*, **105**, 775–780.

Hsu, H., Xiong, J. & Goeddel, D.V. (1995) The TNF receptor 1-associated protein TRADD signals cell death and NF-kappa B activation. *Cell*, **81**, 495–504.

Hubel, D.H. & Wiesel, T.N. (1970) The period of susceptibility to the physiological effects of unilateral eye closure in kittens. *Journal of Physiology*, **206**, 419–436.

Jacob, T.C., Moss, S.J. & Jurd, R. (2008) GABA(A) receptor trafficking and its role in the dynamic modulation of neuronal inhibition. *Nature Reviews Neuroscience*, **9**, 331–343.

Jourdain, P., Bergersen, L.H., Bhaukaurally, K. *et al.* (2007) Glutamate exocytosis from astrocytes controls synaptic strength. *Nature Neuroscience*, **10**, 331–339.

Kaneko, M., Stellwagen, D., Malenka, R.C. & Stryker, M.P. (2008) Tumor necrosis factor-alpha mediates one component of competitive, experience-dependent plasticity in developing visual cortex. *Neuron*, **58**, 673–680.

Kawasaki, Y., Zhang, L., Cheng, J.K. & Ji, R.R. (2008) Cytokine mechanisms of central sensitization: Distinct and overlapping role of interleukin-1beta, interleukin-6, and tumor necrosis factor-alpha in regulating synaptic and neuronal activity in the superficial spinal cord. *The Journal of Neuroscience*, **28**, 5189–5194.

Lee, R.H., Mills, E.A., Schwartz, N. *et al.* (2010) Neurodevelopmental effects of chronic exposure to elevated levels of pro-inflammatory cytokines in a developing visual system. *Neural development*, **5**, 2.

Leonoudakis, D., Zhao, P. & Beattie, E.C. (2008) Rapid tumor necrosis factor alpha-induced exocytosis of glutamate receptor 2-lacking AMPA receptors to extrasynaptic plasma membrane potentiates excitotoxicity. *Journal of Neuroscience*, **28**, 2119–2130.

Leonoudakis, D., Braithwaite, S.P., Beattie, M.S. & Beattie, E.C. (2004) TNFalpha-induced AMPA-receptor trafficking in CNS neurons; relevance to excitotoxicity? *Neuron Glia Biology*, **1**, 263–273.

Lewitus, G.M., Pribiag, H., Duseja, R., St-Hilaire, M. & Stellwagen, D. (2014) An adaptive role of TNFalpha in the regulation of striatal synapses. *Journal of Neuroscience*, **34**, 6146–6155.

Liu, X.H., Xu, H. & Barks, J.D. (1999) Tumor necrosis factor-a attenuates N-methyl-D-aspartate-mediated neurotoxicity in neonatal rat hippocampus. *Brain Research*, **851**, 94–104.

MacEwan, D.J. (2002) TNF receptor subtype signalling: Differences and cellular consequences. *Cellular Signalling*, **14**, 477–492.

Malinow, R. & Malenka, R.C. (2002) AMPA receptor trafficking and synaptic plasticity. *Annual Review of Neuroscience*, **25**, 103–126.

Ogoshi, F., Yin, H.Z., Kuppumbatti, Y., Song, B., Amindari, S. & Weiss, J.H. (2005) Tumor necrosis-factor-alpha (TNF-alpha) induces rapid insertion of Ca2+-permeable alpha-amino-3-hydroxyl-5-methyl-4-isoxazole-propionate (AMPA)/kainate (Ca-A/K) channels in a subset of hippocampal pyramidal neurons. *Experimental Neurology*, **193**, 384–393.

Perea, G., Navarrete, M. & Araque, A. (2009) Tripartite synapses: Astrocytes process and control synaptic information. *Trends in Neurosciences*, **32**, 421–431.

Pribiag, H. & Stellwagen, D. (2013) TNF-alpha downregulates inhibitory neurotransmission through protein phosphatase 1-dependent trafficking of GABA(A) receptors. *Journal of Neuroscience*, **33**, 15879–15893.

Ranson, A., Cheetham, C.E., Fox, K. & Sengpiel, F. (2012) Homeostatic plasticity mechanisms are required for juvenile, but not adult, ocular dominance plasticity. *Proceedings of the National Academy of Sciences of the United States of America*, **109**, 1311–1316.

Santello, M., Bezzi, P. & Volterra, A. (2011) TNFalpha controls glutamatergic gliotransmission in the hippocampal dentate gyrus. *Neuron*, **69**, 988–1001.

Sattler, R. & Tymianski, M. (2000) Molecular mechanisms of calcium-dependent excitotoxicity. *Journal of Molecular Medicine*, **78**, 3–13.

Sawtell, N.B., Frenkel, M.Y., Philpot, B.D., Nakazawa, K., Tonegawa, S. & Bear, M.F. (2003) NMDA receptor-dependent ocular dominance plasticity in adult visual cortex. *Neuron*, **38**, 977–985.

Schmitt, A., May, B., Muller, B. *et al.* (2003) Effects of chronic haloperidol and clozapine treatment on AMPA and kainate receptor binding in rat brain. *Pharmacopsychiatry*, **36**, 292–296.

Shepherd, J.D. & Huganir, R.L. (2007) The cell biology of synaptic plasticity: AMPA receptor trafficking. *Annual Review of Cell and Developmental Biology*, **23**, 613–643.

Shi, S., Hayashi, Y., Esteban, J.A. & Malinow, R. (2001) Subunit-specific rules governing AMPA receptor trafficking to synapses in hippocampal pyramidal neurons. *Cell*, **105**, 331–343.

Smith, R.A. & Baglioni, C. (1987) The active form of tumor necrosis factor is a trimer. *Journal of Biological Chemistry*, **262**, 6951–6954.

Spencer, S.J., Galic, M.A. & Pittman, Q.J. (2011) Neonatal programming of innate immune function. *American Journal of Physiology Endocrinology and Metabolism*, **300**, E11–18.

Stellwagen, D. & Malenka, R.C. (2006) Synaptic scaling mediated by glial TNF-alpha. *Nature*, **440**, 1054–1059.

Stellwagen, D., Beattie, E.C., Seo, J.Y. & Malenka, R.C. (2005) Differential regulation of AMPA receptor and GABA receptor trafficking by tumor necrosis factor-alpha. *Journal of Neuroscience*, **25**, 3219–3228.

Sutton, M.A., Ito, H.T., Cressy, P., Kempf, C., Woo, J.C. & Schuman, E.M. (2006) Miniature neurotransmission stabilizes synaptic function via tonic suppression of local dendritic protein synthesis. *Cell*, **125**, 785–799.

Tancredi, V., D'Arcangelo, G., Grassi, F. *et al.* (1992) Tumor necrosis factor alters synaptic transmission in rat hippocampal slices. *Neuroscience Letters*, **146**, 176–178.

Thiagarajan, T.C., Lindskog, M. & Tsien, R.W. (2005) Adaptation to synaptic inactivity in hippocampal neurons. *Neuron*, **47**, 725–737.

Turrigiano, G.G. & Nelson, S.B. (2004) Homeostatic plasticity in the developing nervous system. *Nature Reviews Neuroscience*, **5**, 97–107.

Turrigiano, G.G., Leslie, K.R., Desai, N.S., Rutherford, L.C. & Nelson, S.B. (1998) Activity-dependent scaling of quantal amplitude in neocortical neurons. *Nature*, **391**, 892–896.

Vitkovic, L., Bockaert, J. & Jacque, C. (2000) "Inflammatory" cytokines: Neuromodulators in normal brain? *Journal of Neurochemistry*, **74**, 457–471.

Vlachos, A., Becker, D., Jedlicka, P., Winkels, R., Roeper, J. & Deller, T. (2012) Entorhinal denervation induces homeostatic synaptic scaling of excitatory postsynapses of dentate granule cells in mouse organotypic slice cultures. *PLoS One*, **7**, e32883.

Vlachos, A., Ikenberg, B., Lenz, M. *et al.* (2013) Synaptopodin regulates denervation-induced homeostatic synaptic plasticity. *Proceedings of the National Academy of Sciences of the United States of America*, **110**, 8242–8247.

Volterra, A. & Meldolesi, J. (2005) Astrocytes, from brain glue to communication elements: The revolution continues. *Nature Reviews Neuroscience*, **6**, 626–640.

Wajant, H., Pfizenmaier, K. & Scheurich, P. (2003) Tumor necrosis factor signaling. *Cell Death and Differentiation*, **10**, 45–65.

Wang, Q., Wu, J., Rowan, M.J. & Anwyl, R. (2005) Beta-amyloid inhibition of long-term potentiation is mediated via tumor necrosis factor. *European Journal of Neuroscience*, **22**, 2827–2832.

Wenthold, R.J., Petralia, R.S., Blahos, J. II & Niedzielski, A.S. (1996) Evidence for multiple AMPA receptor complexes in hippocampal CA1/CA2 neurons. *Journal of Neuroscience*, **16**, 1982–1989.

Wisden, W. & Seeburg, P.H. (1993) Mammalian ionotropic glutamate receptors. *Current Opinion in Neurobiology*, **3**, 291–298.

Witter, M.P. (2007) The perforant path: Projections from the entorhinal cortex to the dentate gyrus. *Progress in Brain Research*, **163**, 43–61.

Zhao, P., Ignacio, S., Beattie, E.C. & Abood, M.E. (2008) Altered presymptomatic AMPA and cannabinoid receptor trafficking in motor neurons of ALS model mice: Implications for excitotoxicity. *European Journal of Neuroscience*, **27**, 572–579.

17 Resolution of Inflammation in the Lesioned Central Nervous System

Jan M. Schwab,[1,2,3,4]* Harald Prüss,[1,5]* and Charles N Serhan[6]

[1]*Department of Neurology and Experimental Neurology, Clinical and Experimental Spinal Cord Injury Research (Neuroparaplegiology), Charite – Universitatsmedizin Berlin, Berlin, Germany*
[2]*Spinal Cord Injury Center, Trauma Hospital Berlin, Berlin, Germany*
[3]*Department of Neurology & Center for Brain and Spinal Cord Repair, The Ohio State University Medical Center, Columbus, OH, USA*
[4]*Department of Neuroscience, The Ohio State University Medical Center, Columbus, OH, USA*
[5]*German Center for Neurodegenerative Diseases (DZNE), Berlin, Germany*
[6]*Center for Experimental Therapeutics and Reperfusion Injury, Department of Anesthesiology, Perioperative and Pain Medicine, Harvard Institutes of Medicine, Brigham and Women's Hospital and Harvard Medical School, Boston, MA, USA*

Introduction

Acute inflammation is a highly regulated process characterized by adhesion molecule upregulation, vasoactive mediator expression, leukocyte diapedesis, phagocytosis, and release of chemical mediators such as eicosanoids, prostaglandins, and complement components. As acute inflammation could perpetuate and result in spreading, chronicity, and tissue injury, a complete resolution is required (Serhan, 2014; Buckley *et al.*, 2014). While there is ample information available about the recruitment of leukocyte entry into the central nervous system (CNS), little is known about their exposure time to the lesioned CNS parenchyma and their exit. Likewise, resolution is also a finely orchestrated, active process, which is distinct from anti-inflammation as local inflammatory stimuli do not simply fizzle out (Serhan *et al.*, 2007; Serhan 2014; Buckley *et al.*, 2014). Resolution is already encoded at the onset of the acute inflammatory response and includes limiting further leukocyte influx and clearance of inflammatory cells, reduction of proinflammatory factors, and release of pro-resolving factors (Serhan and Savill 2005; Serhan 2014; Buckley *et al.*, 2014). Complete resolution should eventually lead to restoration of tissue homeostasis (Gilroy *et al.*, 2004, Serhan *et al.*, 2007). Pioneering efforts were antedated by the discovery of mediators

---

*These authors contributed equally.

Neuroinflammation: New Insights into Beneficial and Detrimental Functions, First Edition. Edited by Samuel David.
© 2015 John Wiley & Sons, Inc. Published 2015 by John Wiley & Sons, Inc.

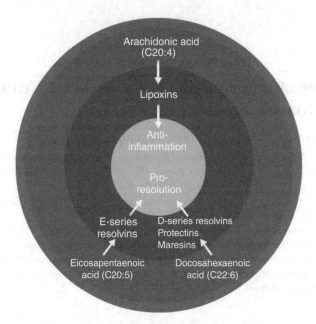

Figure 17.1   Resolution phase lipid mediators of inflammation: agonists of resolution. The specialized pro-resolving mediators (SPM): The three polyunsaturated fatty acids arachidonic acid, eicosapentaenoic acid (EPA), and docosahexaenoic acid (DHA) are substrates for the formation of lipid mediators, which regulate the endogenous termination of inflammation via anti-inflammatory and pro-resolution actions. Lipoxins are formed from arachidonic acid, E-series resolvins are formed from EPA, and D-series resolvins, protectins and maresins are formed from DHA.

with a dual anti-inflammatory and pro-resolutive function such as Lipoxin A_4 as the first member of its class (Serhan *et al.*, 1986). Subsequently, an intense and exciting discovery unraveled consecutive families of novel mediators including resolvins, protectins, and maresins together referred to as specialized pro-resolving mediators (SPMs) (Fig. 17.1; Serhan, 2014; Buckley *et al.*, 2014).

A simple and relatively easy way to quantify resolution of inflammation is by estimating the number of particular immune cell populations in tissue sections or possibly by fluorescence-activated cell sorting (FACS) analysis. The main events in resolution can be quantified by resolution indices consisting of the resolution interval (Ri) and the resolution plateau (Rp) as complementary objective measures of resolution capacity in different organ systems (Fig. 17.2; Prüss *et al.*, 2011). It is likely that cell recruitment and resolution vary substantially between different organs and lesion etiologies (Navarro Xavier *et al.*, 2010). In this chapter, we provide evidence for defective cellular and molecular resolution program in inflammatory CNS lesions with direct implications for a perpetuated immunopathology. We emphasize the predisposition of the CNS as an immune-privileged organ unprepared to deal with exacerbated inflammation and in turn being disabled to accomplish its complete resolution (Figs. 17.2a and 17.2b).

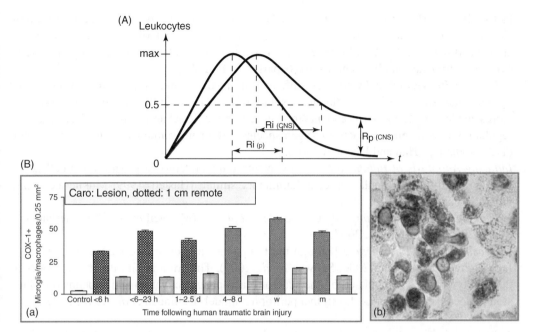

Figure 17.2 Modeling neuroinflammatory resolution phenotypes *in vivo*: Objective measures. (A) Based on cell trafficking into and away from inflammatory lesions, integrative indices were established to quantitatively determine the main events of resolution. These include the Resolution index (Ri) as the time between the maximum and the point when cells numbers are reduced by 50%. In case of a nonresolving CNS acute inflammation, a model of a resolution deficit with respect to the resolution plateau (Rp) can be determined. The black line illustrates the course of an self-limiting inflammatory response (e.g., peritonitis). The blue line illustrates the inflammatory response in CNS lesions as being delayed, sustained and non-self-limiting. (B) Impaired resolution of inflammation is also evident in CNS lesions of noninflammatory origin such as stroke or traumatic brain injury. Following traumatic brain injury, COX-1+ microglia/macrophage numbers remain signficantly elevated at the lesion site (orange colored caro bars) for up to months (m) compared to neuropathological unaltered controls (white bar) and remote areas (dotted bars) (Schwab *et al.*, 2002) (a). The nonresolving CNS lesion milieu is dominated by CD68+ lipid-laden microglia/macrophages (>80%) (brown) coexpressing proinflammatory enzymes such as COX-1 (blue) in areas of ongoing neuronal degeneration (Schwab *et al.*, 2000a) (b). *Source*: Part (b) is from Schwab *et al.* (2013), with permission from Springer. (*See insert for color representation of this figure.*)

Mechanisms of Resolution

Resolution is already encoded at the onset of inflammation, involving at least six principal mechanisms:

1. *Limiting Further Leukocyte Migration.* Parenchymal cells within the inflamed tissue (e.g., fibroblasts but also astrocytes) can determine the duration of leukocyte infiltration by normalizing of chemokine gradients, withdrawal of survival signals or induction of leukocyte apoptosis (Filer *et al.*, 2006, Buckley *et al.*, 2001, Kim *et al.*, 2014).
2. *Reducing the Release of Proinflammatory Factors.* During the course of inflammation prostaglandin derivatives increasingly suppress inflammatory pathways, for example, nuclear

factor κB (NF-κB), activating protein-1 (AP1), signal transducer and activator of transcription (STAT), inducible nitric oxide synthase (iNOS), interleukin (IL)-1β, tumor necrosis factor alpha (TNF-α), and IL-12 (Gilroy *et al.*, 2004) while several anti-inflammatory cytokines are expressed, for example, IL-4 and IL-10 (Iribarren *et al.*, 2003).

3. *Release of Pro-resolving Factors.* A shift in lipid-mediator biosynthesis to pro-resolution lipid mediators (i.e., SPMs) accelerates resolution (Levy *et al.*, 2001, Serhan *et al.*, 2000) by increasing leukocyte apoptosis and macrophage clearance (Rajakariar *et al.*, 2007), and down-regulation of extracellular reactive oxygen species and innate immunity via toll-like receptor (TLR) signaling (Han and Ulevitch 2005).

4. *Inducing Apoptosis of Inflammatory Cells.* Neutrophils undergoing programmed cell death lose the ability to degranulate after inflammatory stimuli (Haslett, 1999; Mukherjee *et al.*, 2004; Serhan *et al.*, 2008).

5. *Promoting Clearance of Apoptotic Cells by Macrophages* (Mitchell *et al.*, 2002; Serhan and Savill, 2005; Schwab *et al.*, 2007).

6. *Increasing Exit of Phagocytes.* Through the lymphatics and clearance via the mucosal surface (Schwab and Serhan 2006; Schwab *et al.*, 2007). The emigration rate of macrophages through lymphatics is regulated by the state of macrophage activation and depends on adhesion molecule expression as shown in a peritonitis model (Bellingan *et al.*, 1996, 2002).

Although initiation of inflammation and resolution are separate processes, they share similar features and signaling pathways that are spatially and temporally distinct. Context-specific functionality is achieved by a lipid-mediator class shift, which dampens inflammation and fosters resolution with progressing time after onset of inflammation (Levy *et al.*, 2001). This shift involves a change of arachidonic acid (AA) derived from the proinflammatory lipids such as Leukotriene B4 (LTB$_4$) to the pro-resolution lipid class of Lipoxin A$_4$ (Levy *et al.*, 2001).

"Nonphlogistic" inflammation is the hallmark of the resolution phase and consists of the influx of inflammatory cells without inducing the proinflammatory signaling cascade or tissue damage. The prototypic "nonphlogistic" inflammation occurs only during CNS development when organogenesis requires continuous remodeling, and removal of apoptotic cells is a prerequisite for the maintenance of normal function [for review, see Henson and Hume (2006)]. Uptake and digestion of apoptotic cells in murine brain during development occur within 1–2 h (Coles *et al.*, 1993; Gohlke *et al.*, 2004), which is remarkable as up to 50% of cells is deleted during development in the mammalian brain (Lossi and Merighi, 2003; de la Rosa and de Pablo, 2000). Cell removal itself prevents further tissue damage by causing noninflammatory and nonimmunogenic *in situ* digestion of dying cells (Henson and Hume, 2006).

Resolution Deficit Following CNS Lesions

The resolution phase at a histological level is defined as the interval from maximum leukocyte infiltration to the point when they are cleared from the tissue (Serhan *et al.*, 2007). However, in CNS injury and disease, resolution of inflammation is not complete, and blood-borne cells survive in the tissue at the lesion site for prolonged periods. For example, lipid-laden macrophages appear to constitute a smoldering, nonresolving inflammatory milieu up to years in human CNS ischemic lesions (Schwab *et al.*, 2000a) or traumatic brain injury (Fig. 17.2; Schwab *et al.*, 2002). In multiple sclerosis (MS) lesions, the density of leukocyte infiltrates remains significantly higher in the "normal-appearing white matter" (NAWM) compared to that in the white matter of age-matched controls (Kutzelnigg *et al.*, 2005). This represents a reactive, immunologically "loaded" milieu consistent with the idea of a nonresolving activation of the innate immune system even in areas away from the lesions. Moreover, it appears that immune cells are apparently trapped in the lesioned brain while the blood–brain barrier partially repairs. Thus, the immune privilege of the CNS may constitute a bidirectional shield in which inflammation proceeds behind the blood–brain barrier and to become compartmentalized as discussed for the progressive stage of MS (Lassmann, 2008; Lassmann *et al.*, 2012).

Given that accumulation and persistence of leukocytes is a hallmark of chronic inflammation, the parenchymal "inflammatory residuum" is fully armed with components required to propagate (i) early neuronal injury, (ii) neurodegeneration and gliopathy, (iii) aberrant neuronal function such as blockade of saltatory nerve conduction and pain, and also the development of (iv) autoimmunity. This potency to propagate injury and dysfunction of spared circuitry is aggravated by an impaired endogenous regenerative capacity of the CNS. Unresolved inflammation might therefore lead to dysfunctional recovery associated with fibrotic scarring, late degeneration ("tertiary injury"), and blunted regeneration (Prüss *et al.*, 2012; Shechter and Schwartz, 2013). The resolution deficit inherent to CNS lesions requires a more detailed view of the immunobiology of CNS lesions.

Immunobiology of Resolution in CNS Lesions – Impaired Resolution Contributes to Neuropathology

Most basic mechanisms of resolution also apply to inflammation in the CNS, although some special features exist. At the lesion site, the immune-privilege collapses, resulting in blood–brain barrier breakdown, local cytokine effects, facilitation of antigen drainage to the periphery, appearance of dendritic cells (DCs), and establishment of tertiary lymphoid tissue in the meninges and even in the CNS parenchyma (Ankeny *et al.*, 2009). Clearance of leukocytes from the tissue is generally possible through returning to the systemic circulation via lymphatic drainage (Bellingan *et al.*, 1996, 2002) or death by apoptosis and subsequent phagocytosis (Fig. 17.3).

Clearance by recirculation has been shown for microglia and bone-marrow-derived DCs that can leave the CNS via the blood stream and home to mesenteric lymph nodes and spleen (Hochmeister *et al.*, 2008). In contrast, the route of "lymphatic drainage" of the CNS is strikingly different compared to that of most organs of the human body and is represented by the perivascular spaces of capillaries and arteries, which are in continuity with the subarachnoid space (Ransohoff and Engelhardt, 2012; Weller *et al.*, 2008). However, the cellular efflux is very limited via the perivascular route, and cellular drainage from the brain parenchyma to cervical lymph nodes is absent (Carare *et al.*, 2008) even if cells from cerebrospinal fluid (CSF) appear in the cervical lymphoid tissue (Hatterer *et al.*, 2006; Carare *et al.*, 2008).

The noninflammatory removal of leukocytes by apoptosis in the brain consists of further peculiarities. All CNS cells express fasL, which results in apoptosis of incoming fas-positive T cells, irrespective of their antigen specificity (Bauer *et al.*, 1998; Bechmann *et al.*, 1999). Besides

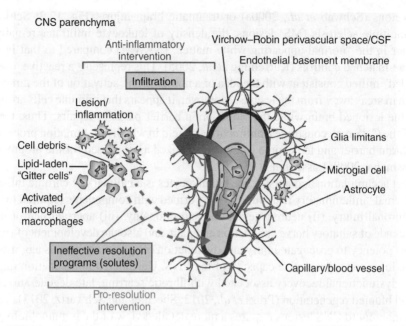

Figure 17.3 Infiltration and exit routes of inflammatory traffic in the immune-privileged CNS: Targets for anti-inflammatory versus pro-resolution intervention. Traditional anti-inflammatory treatments focussing mostly on leukocyte infiltration (left upper part) are likely to be insufficient if impaired resolution of inflammation is part of the underlying CNS pathophysiology (left lower part). This is supported by the lack of efficacy of classical anti-inflammatory approaches in chronic inflammatory CNS disease such as progressive MS. Published experimental and human neuropathological and neuroimmunological evidence suggests a CNS lesion environment, which blocks effective resolution of inflammation. Given that the acute inflammatory response in CNS lesions is delayed or non-self-limiting, SPMs qualify as good candidates with robust bioactivity to shape a maladaptive immune response. Reducing the exposure time of vulnerable neurons, oligodendrocytes and other neuropil to the hostile milieu of chronic inflammation by treatment with SPMs can be expected to attenuate inflammation-mediated pain and neurodegeneration. (*See insert for color representation of this figure.*)

professional phagocytes, microglia can induce T cell apoptosis (Ford *et al.*, 1996) and release anti-inflammatory cytokines (Aloisi 2001; Kreutzberg 1996) and phagocytose apoptotic cells in the brain (Magnus *et al.*, 2001). The contribution is essential, as myelin clearance by microglia and macrophages is necessary for remyelination of damaged axons (See Chapter 13 for more details).

On the cellular level, there are signatures of inflammatory episodes remaining visible in the CNS lesion site long after its occurance and representing the inability to return to the preinjury state. This inability to erase "inflammatory signatures" well illustrates, the low and inefficient resolution capacity of the CNS. After CNS injury, microglia, the resident macrophages of the CNS, are at the center stage during this process, as there is virtually no pathology without their participation (Kreutzberg, 1996; David and Kroner, 2011). On becoming activated, they may not always return to a resting state and become "primed." Primed microglia/macrophages are characterized by a dysfunctionally exaggerated inflammatory response and constitute a well-documented pathoimmunological part during aging, neurodegeneration, and pain (Perry and Holmes, 2014). In chronic MS, as the disease turns into the progressive stage, chronically activated microglia/macrophages at the extending lesion margin were found to be dysfunctional and proposed to contribute to "frustrated phagocytosis," a cellular hallmark of impaired resolution (Prineas *et al.*, 2001). This implies that inflammatory neuropathology progresses in the absence of florid perivascular cell infiltration or other histological signs of proinflammatory events (Prineas *et al.*, 2001). A similar observation stems from chronic lesions of noninflammatory origin such as stroke (Schwab *et al.*, 2000a), spinal cord injury (SCI; Schwab *et al.*, 2000b; Fleming *et al.*, 2006), or traumatic brain injury (TBI; Fig. 17.2b; Schwab *et al.*, 2002; Beschorner *et al.*, 2002). Subsequent to CNS injury, elevated numbers of lipid-laden microglia/macrophages were detected at the lesion margin constituting a smoldering, nonresolving inflammatory milieu lasting years, resulting in an elevated resolution plateau. It should be emphasized that this refers to CNS injury, not inflammatory disease. Thus, a continuation of the initial inflammatory disease process as the underlying reason is unlikely and suggests an impaired resolution capacity at the CNS lesion site irrespective of its origin. Noteworthy, after acute human CNS lesions, perivascular spaces get cleared of microglia/macrophages months after injury, whereas in the lesion parenchyma, microglia/macrophages fail to return to control levels (Beschorner *et al.*, 2002). A compensatory and sustained induction of resolution active proteins such as heme oxygenase 1 (HO-1) synthesis concomitant to persistent accumulation of inflammatory cells at the lesion site (Beschorner *et al.*, 2000) implies the inability of lesioned CNS tissue to mount an effective, counter-regulatory response to clear inflammatory cells. In rodent models, evidence for a microglia/macrophages program to turn them into an anti-inflammatory phenotype shortly after phagocytic activity is observed to be effective *in vitro* but appears to be blocked *in vivo*, due to resolution inhibiting factors in the CNS inflammatory milieu (Kroner *et al.*, 2014). Thus, published experimental and human neuropathological and neuroimmunological evidence suggests a lesion environment in the CNS, which blocks effective resolution of inflammation. This may relate to tightly regulated signaling of cell-intrinsic and cell-extrinsic factors known to regulate leukocyte migration in nonlymphoid organs (Weninger *et al.*, 2014). In addition to the presence of active resolution blocking molecules, a lack of resolution promoting factors also needs to be considered. Molecular determinants impairing CNS-specific resolution are not known.

Late Degeneration/"Tertiary" Injury and Autoimmunity as a Consequence of Failed Resolution of Inflammation in CNS Lesions?

Neurodegeneration

Once inflammation has become chronic, the spared neuronal tissue becomes more vulnerable to several coinciding pathological conditions. One explanation is the "priming" of microglia, which increases expression of immune receptors on the cell surface after clearing of apoptotic cells. In this way, microglia show an augmented response to inflammation somewhere in the body, which could result in neuronal damage due to restimulation of the existing CNS lesions (Perry and Holmes, 2014). This hypothesis is supported by findings in patients with MS that there is an association between systemic infection and MS relapses (Buljevac *et al.*, 2002). Also, after experimental stroke, systemic application of endotoxins mimicking aspects of infections re-inflames residual, nonresolved inflammatory foci and exacerbates neurodegeneration (Cunningham *et al.*, 2005). Thus, residual inflammatory signatures are triggers for propagated neuronal death that can be set-off even long after injury. Similar results were obtained in humans in Alzheimer's disease (AD), unravelling an association between dementia and infection (Holmes *et al.*, 2009).

Other examples for the progressive damage after CNS injury coincidental with prolonged inflammation at the lesion site are the structural changes after TBI or SCI. Progressive atrophy of both grey and white matter continues after TBI and ongoing cell death of neurons, and oligodendrocytes, demyelination of intact fiber tracts, retrograde axonal degeneration, and progressive conduction failure are observed after chronic SCI (Bramlett and Dietrich 2007; James *et al.*, 2011). The putative relevance of a sustained Rp is further supported by the finding that stimulation of macrophages with lipopolysaccharide (LPS) is sufficient to induce demyelinating lesions (Felts *et al.*, 2005). Thus, unresolved inflammation is likely to be involved in delayed ongoing demyelination and subsequent neuronal degeneration after SCI (Arvanian *et al.*, 2009; Bramlett and Dietrich, 2007). Given that the Rp relates to incomplete resolution of inflammation, additional work is needed to determine (i) whether a higher resolution plateau containing persisting blood-borne cells leads to worse clinical outcome and histopathological damage and (ii) what effects do resolution agonists have in modifying Rp behind the blood–brain barrier?

Autoimmunity

Besides propagation of neurodegeneration, the chronic inflammation milieu may trigger autoimmune disease *de novo*. Some examples have arisen in the last few years that resolution failure can facilitate chronic autoimmune disease. Impaired clearance of apoptotic cells has, for example, been linked to the pathogenesis of systemic lupus erythematodes (SLE) (Muñoz *et al.*, 2010). In the CNS, accumulating evidence demonstrates that acute CNS lesions of noninflammatory, traumatic, or hypoxic origin subsequently acquire hallmarks of chronic autoimmune disease. This involves T- and B-lymphocytes (Jones, 2014). Among T lymphocytes, a subgroup of CD8+ cells impairs saltatory nerve conduction and propagates neuronal cell death (Lassmann, 2008; Yarom *et al.*, 1983). Acute CNS injury triggers the formation of ectopic lymphoid follicles composed of B cells synthesizing autoantibodies that bind CNS proteins (Ankeny *et al.*, 2009). Also, after ischemic brain injury, 25% of patients with stroke displayed CSF-specific immunoglobulin synthesis, suggesting development of autoimmunity (Prüss *et al.*, 2012). The factors that determine if a patient develops CSF antibody synthesis are still not known.

Moreover, persistent chronic inflammation is not only capable of generating *de novo* autoimmunity but can also exacerbate the neuropathology driven by existing autoimmunity such as MS. A clinical example supporting this view is the slow expansion of demyelinated plaques in secondary progressive MS (Kutzelnigg *et al.*, 2005) with low-grade inflammation and microglia activation at plaque borders (Prineas *et al.*, 2001). Inflammatory CNS lesions provide a B-cell fostering environment through a chemokine pattern for plasma cell survival, including the B-cell survival factor BAFF (Meinl *et al.*, 2008). As a result, 40% of patients with secondary progressive MS have B-cell follicles in their meninges (Serafini *et al.*, 2004; Magliozzi *et al.*, 2007). This compartmentalization behind the blood–brain barrier does not require another infiltration episode and is largely dependent on the nonresolving inflammatory mileu. This may explain why early phase relapsing-remitting MS turns into relapse-free progressive MS, in which classic anti-inflammatory interventions become ineffective and fail to wipe-out residual parenchymal inflammatory cells (Ransohoff, 2012). The CNS appears unable to resolve inflammation effectively due to anatomical constraints but also due to its inability to generate an effective pro-resolution permissive milieu. A sustained inflammatory response can contribute to fibrotic scar formation, demyelination, chronic neurodegeneration, development of neuropathic pain, and decline of neurological function.

Evidence for the Effectiveness of Pro-resolution Mediators in CNS Lesions

Treatment with resolution agonists is effective to treat conditions of impaired resolution (Gilroy *et al.*, 2004). A systems approach to investigate self-limited (self-resolving) inflammatory models in mice and elucidation of the molecular structure of these reagents uncovered novel endogenous resolution phase mediators that stimulate resolution mechanisms *in vivo*. The resolving inflammatory milieu utilizes docosahexaenoic acid (DHA) and another omega-3 (ω-3) eicosapentaenoic acid (EPA) to produce three structurally distinct families of potent di- and trihydroxy-containing products, with several stereospecific potent mediators in each family. New classes of small, local, and stereoselectively active endogenous autacoids, namely, the lipoxins, D and E series resolvins, (neuro) protectins, and maresins, have been identified to be bioeffective in picogram concentrations. These SPMs prevent excessive inflammation and promote removal of microbes and apoptotic cells, thereby expediting resolution and return to tissue homeostasis (Fig. 17.1). As part of their molecular mechanism, SPMs exert their potent actions via activating specific G-protein coupled receptors [for recent review on SPM biosynthesis see Serhan (2014)].

The best-investigated SPM bioactivity in the neuropathology is their effect on neuropathic pain. Postlesional neuropathic pain is propagated by aberrant neuronal function and enduring gliopathy, which is described as a remnant of the inflammatory response linked to failed resolution of inflammation (Hulsebosch, 2008). Indeed, the anti-inflammatory and pro-resolution lipoxins and aspirin-triggered Lipoxins (ATL) attenuate inflammation-induced pain implicated in spinal nociceptive processing (Svensson *et al.*, 2007; Wang *et al.*, 2014a, 2014b; Li *et al.*, 2013). Moreover, DHA-derived Resolvin D1 (RvD1) and EPA-derived Resolvin E1 (RvE1) also attenuate inflammatory pain [for review see Ji *et al.* (2011)] after binding to their receptors on immune cells and neurons to normalize exaggerated pain via regulation of inflammatory mediators, transient receptor potential (TRP) ion channels, and spinal cord synaptic transmission.

Another solid body of evidence identifies neuroprotection as a neurobiological effect of SPMs and their substrate the Omega-3 (ω-3) polyunsaturated fatty acids (PUFA), which comprise both EPA and DHA. In particular, the DHA-derived neuroprotectin D1 (NPD1) exerts potent neuroprotective effects on the CNS (Bazan *et al.*, 2012; Mukherjee *et al.*, 2004; Marcheselli *et al.*, 2003). In case of the ω-3 EPA and the ω-6 arachidonic acid (AA), only the SPMs reveal potent neuroprotection, whereas their substrate is less effective. Of note, also a robust neuroprotective effect of the AA-derived Lipoxin A_4 has been replicated in experimental stroke (Sobrado *et al.*, 2009; Ye *et al.*, 2010; Wu *et al.*, 2012; Hawkins *et al.*, 2014). Evidence for the neuroprotective and immune modulatory effects of the SPM substrates themselves after acute CNS lesions was reported earlier by applying ω-3 PUFA (King *et al.*, 2006; Michael-Titus and Priestley, 2014). This was confirmed in transgenic *FAT-1* mice, which are able to synthesize ω-3 PUFA (Lim *et al.*, 2013). These mice reveal substantial neuroprotection after spinal cord injury (Lim *et al.*, 2013). However, only DHA was found to have neuroprotective effects, not EPA (Hall *et al.*, 2012; Orr *et al.*, 2013). DHA-derived SPMs likely account for the major part of these effects.

Lastly, chronic, nonresolving inflammation propagates CNS neurodegeneration and represents a major target for neurodegenerative diseases (Glass *et al.*, 2010). There is good evidence demonstrating that sustained inflammation will result in impaired cognitive function (Hein *et al.*, 2010). Although DHA exerts a protective effect and prevents cognitive decline, the underlying molecular effector mechanisms remained unclear. In 2005, the first investigations confirmed that DHA-derived NPD1 is reduced in the hippocampus in AD. Supplying NPD-1 resulted in anti-apoptotic gene expression and reduced Aβ42-induced neurotoxicity (Lukiw *et al.*, 2005). Further investigations also showed that LXA_4 is reduced in the AD brain paralleled by downregulation of potent resolving proteins known to act downstream of SPMs such as HO-1 and PPAR-γ (Wang *et al.*, 2014a, 2014b). Together, these human data point to an impaired resolution of inflammation in neurodegenerative disease, possibly due to poorly sustained resolution programs, which is associated with disease progression (Wang *et al.*, 2014a, 2014b). Additional proof that SPMs counteract inflammation-triggered neuronal dysfunction was substantiated by the evidence that AT-RvD1 prevents memory loss in a model of surgery-induced cognitive decline (Terrando *et al.*, 2013). Surgery-induced cognitive decline is a prevalent challenge in aged patients. The elevated level of constitutive microglia activation in the aged brain suggests a defective counter-regulatory resolution program. This impaired resolution in the primed aged CNS becomes superaggravated by surgery-induced responses to sedative anesthetica and bacterial load. Nonexhaustive or possibly "delayed" resolution pathways may suggest a defective resolution program also present in patients with highly active MS, thereby contributing to neurodegeneration (Prüss *et al.*, 2013).

The evidence surveyed previously identifies several types of CNS lesions to be responsive to SPM treatment. Modifying inflammatory phenotypes after acute and chronic CNS lesions by SPMs is therefore feasible and improves neuropathological and functional outcome in experimental models. SPMs and their receptors offer new reagents and targets, respectively, and comprise an excellent group of therapeutics to promote active resolution of inflammation, as opposed to the conventionally used enzyme inhibitors and receptor antagonists. This approach may offer new targets for drug design suitable for treating inflammation-related CNS diseases, for the new terrain of resolution pharmacology.

Conclusion

Defective clearance of acute inflammatory cells is an underlying mechanism of the neuropathology after CNS injury and disease and contributes to the maladaptive neuroimmunological response. Late and not self-limiting CNS inflammation may be due in part to a "reverse effect" of the blood–brain barrier, in that immune cells are not able to exit the lesion site. Orthodox anti-inflammatory treatments are likely to be ineffective if impaired resolution of inflammation is part of the underlying CNS pathophysiology. This is supported by the lack of efficacy of classical anti-inflammatory approaches in chronic inflammatory CNS disease such as in the progressive phase of MS. Published experimental and human neuropathological and neuroim-munological evidence suggests a CNS lesion environment, which blocks effective resolution of inflammation. Similarly to unknown molecular factors blocking remyelination in the adult CNS milieu, resolution antagonist contributing to the resolution impermissive milieu have yet to be defined. The understanding of resolution of inflammation has not yet reached neurology or neuropathology textbooks. SPMs constitute a group of drug targets already validated in numerous non-CNS inflammatory disease models (Serhan 2014; Buckley *et al.*, 2014), which have been shown to have robust effects in some experimental models of CNS neuropathology. Further research is warranted to pave the way for clinical applications of resolution agonists in CNS. Specifically, to what extent diseases of the CNS require different pro-resolution molecules and effective treatment time frames as compared to other peripheral organs.

Acknowledgment

We thank Dr. Sam David for critically reading the manuscript and helpful comments. This work was supported by the Else–Kröner–Fresenius Foundation, Wings for Life Spinal Cord Research Foundation (Grant No. WfL-DE-006/1) (to J.M.S.), US National Institutes of Health (R01GM038765 and P01GM095467) and the Mérieux Foundation (France) (to CNS).

References

Aloisi, F. (2001) Immune function of microglia. *Glia*, **36**, 165–179.

Ankeny, D.P., Guan, Z. & Popovich, P.G. (2009) B cells produce pathogenic antibodies and impair recovery after spinal cord injury in mice. *Journal of Clinical Investigation*, **119**, 2990–2999.

Arvanian, V.L., Schnell, L., Lou, L. *et al.* (2009) Chronic spinal hemisection in rats induces a progressive decline in transmission in uninjured fibers to motoneurons. *Experimental Neurology*, **216**, 471–480.

Bauer, J., Bradl, M., Hickley, W.F. *et al.* (1998) T-cell apoptosis in inflammatory brain lesions: Destruction of T cells does not depend on antigen recognition. *American Journal of Pathology*, **153**, 715–724.

Bechmann, I., Mor, G., Nilsen, J., Eliza, M., Nitsch, R. & Naftolin, F. (1999) FasL (CD95L, ApoIL) is expressed in the normal rat and human brain: Evidence for the existence of an immunological brain barrier. *Glia*, **27**, 62–74.

Bellingan, G.J., Xu, P., Cooksley, H. *et al.* (2002) Adhesion molecule-dependent mechanisms regulate the rate of macrophage clearance during the resolution of peritoneal inflammation. *Journal of Experimental Medicine*, **196**, 1515–1521.

Bellingan, G.J., Caldwell, H., Howie, S.E., Dransfield, I. & Haslett, C. (1996) In vivo fate of the inflammatory macrophage during the resolution of inflammation: Inflammatory macrophages do not die locally, but emigrate to the draining lymph nodes. *Journal of Immunology*, **157**, 2577–2585.

Bazan, N.G., Eady, T.N., Khoutorova, L. *et al.* (2012) Novel aspirin-triggered neuroprotectin D1 attenuates cerebral ischemic injury after experimental stroke. *Experimental Neurology*, **236**, 122–130.

Beschorner, R., Adjodah, D., Schwab, J.M. *et al.* (2000) Long-term expression of heme oxygenase-1 (HO-1, HSP-32) following focal cerebral infarctions and traumatic brain injury in humans. *Acta Neuropathologica*, **100**, 377–384.

Beschorner, R., Nguyen, T.D., Gözalan, F. *et al.* (2002) CD14 expression by activated parenchymal microglia/macrophages and infiltrating monocytes following human traumatic brain injury. *Acta Neuropathologica*, **103**, 541–549.

Bramlett, H.M. & Dietrich, W.D. (2007) Progressive damage after brain and spinal cord injury: Pathomechanisms and treatment strategies. *Progress in Brain Research*, **161**, 125–141.

Buckley, C.D., Pilling, D., Lord, J.M., Akbar, A.N., Scheel-Toellner, D. & Salmon, M. (2001) Fibroblasts regulate the switch from acute resolving to chronic persistent inflammation. *Trends in Immunology*, **22**, 199–204.

Buckley, C.D., Gilroy, D.W. & Serhan, C.N. (2014) Proresolving lipid mediators and mechanisms in the resolution of acute inflammation. *Immunity*, **40**, 315–327.

Buljevac, D., Flach, H.Z., Hop, W.C. *et al.* (2002) Prospective study on the relationship between infections and multiple sclerosis exacerbations. *Brain*, **125**, 952–960.

Carare, R.O., Bernardes-Silva, M., Newman, T.A. *et al.* (2008) Solutes, but not cells, drain from the brain parenchyma along basement membranes of capillaries and arteries: Significance for cerebral amyloid angiopathy and neuroimmunology. *Neuropathology and Applied Neurobiology*, **34**, 131–144.

Coles, H.S., Burne, J.F. & Raff, M.C. (1993) Large-scale normal cell death in the developing rat kidney and its reduction by epidermal growth factor. *Development*, **118**, 777–784.

Cunningham, C., Wilcockson, D.C., Campion, S., Lunnon, K. & Perry, V.H. (2005) Central and systemic endotoxin challenges exacerbate the local inflammatory response and increase neuronal death during chronic neurodegeneration. *Journal of Neuroscience*, **25**, 9275–9284.

David, S. & Kroner, A. (2011) Repertoire of microglial and macrophage responses after spinal cord injury. *Nature Reviews Neuroscience*, **12**, 388–399.

de la Rosa, E.J. & de Pablo, F. (2000) Cell death in early neural development: Beyond the neurotrophic theory. *Trends in Neurosciences*, **23**, 454–458.

Felts, P.A., Woolston, A.M., Fernando, H.B. *et al.* (2005) Inflammation and primary demyelination induced by the intraspinal injection of lipopolysaccharide. *Brain*, **128**, 1649–1666.

Filer, A., Pitzalis, C. & Buckley, C.D. (2006) Targeting the stromal microenvironment in chronic inflammation. *Current Opinion in Pharmacology*, **6**, 393–400.

Fleming, J.C., Norenberg, M.D., Ramsay, D.A. *et al.* (2006) The cellular inflammatory response in human spinal cords after injury. *Brain*, **129**, 3249–3269.

Ford, A.L., Foulcher, E., Lemckert, F.A. & Sedgwick, J.D. (1996) Microglia induce CD4 T lymphocyte final effector function and death. *Journal of Experimental Medicine*, **184**, 1737–1745.

Gilroy, D.W., Lawrence, T., Perretti, M. & Rossi, A.G. (2004) Inflammatory resolution: New opportunities for drug discovery. *Nature Review Drug Discovery*, **3**, 401–416.

Glass, C.K., Saijo, K., Winner, B., Marchetto, M.C. & Gage, F.H. (2010) Mechanisms underlying inflammation in neurodegeneration. *Cell*, **140**, 918–934.

Gohlke, J.M., Griffith, W.C. & Faustman, E.M. (2004) The role of cell death during neocortical neurogenesis and synaptogenesis: Implications from a computational model for the rat and mouse. *Brain Research. Developmental Brain Research*, **151**, 43–54.

Hall, J.C., Priestley, J.V., Perry, V.H. & Michael-Titus, A.T. (2012) Docosahexaenoic acid, but not eicosapentaenoic acid, reduces the early inflammatory response following compression spinal cord injury in the rat. *Journal of Neurochemistry*, **121**, 738–750.

Han, J. & Ulevitch, R.J. (2005) Limiting inflammatory responses during activation of innate immunity. *Nature Immunology*, **6**, 1198–1205.

Haslett, C. (1999) Granulocyte apoptosis and its role in the resolution and control of lung inflammation. *American Journal of Respiratory and Critical Care Medicine*, **160**, S5–S11.

Hatterer, E., Davoust, N., Didier-Bazes, M. *et al.* (2006) How to drain without lymphatics? Dendritic cells migrate from the cerebrospinal fluid to the B-cell follicles of cervical lymph nodes. *Blood*, **107**, 806–812.

Hawkins, K.E., DeMars, K.M., Singh, J. *et al.* (2014) Neurovascular protection by post-ischemic intravenous injections of the lipoxin A4 receptor agonist, BML-111, in a rat model of ischemic stroke. *Journal of Neurochemistry*, **129**, 130–142.

Hein, A.M., Stasko, M.R., Matousek, S.B. *et al.* (2010) Sustained hippocampal IL-1beta overexpression impairs contextual and spatial memory in transgenic mice. *Brain, Behavior, and Immunity*, **24**, 243–253.

Henson, P.M. & Hume, D.A. (2006) Apoptotic cell removal in development and tissue homeostasis. *Trends in Immunology*, **27**, 244–250.

Hochmeister, S., Zeitelhofer, M., Bauer, J. *et al.* (2008) After injection into the striatum, in vitro-differentiated microglia- and bone marrow-derived dendritic cells can leave the central nervous system via the blood stream. *American Journal of Pathology*, **173**, 1669–1681.

Holmes, C., Cunningham, C., Zotova, E. *et al.* (2009) Systemic inflammation and disease progression in Alzheimer disease. *Neurology*, **73**, 768–774.

Hulsebosch, C.E. (2008) Gliopathy ensures persistent inflammation and chronic pain after spinal cord injury. *Experimental Neurology*, **214**, 6–9.

Iribarren, P., Cui, Y.H., Le, Y. *et al.* (2003) IL-4 down-regulates lipopolysaccharide-induced formyl peptide receptor 2 in murine microglial cells by inhibiting the activation of mitogen-activated protein kinases. *Journal of Immunology*, **171**, 5482–5488.

James, N.D., Bartus, K., Grist, J., Bennetts, D.L., McMahon, S.B. & Bradbury, E.J. (2011) Conduction failure following spinal cord injury: Functional and anatomical changes from acute to chronic stages. *Journal of Neuroscience*, **31**, 18543–18555.

Ji, R.R., Xu, Z.Z., Strichartz, G. & Serhan, C.N. (2011) Emerging roles of resolvins in the resolution of inflammation and pain. *Trends in Neurosciences*, **34**, 599–609.

Jones, T.B. (2014) Lymphocytes and autoimmunity after spinal cord injury. *Experimental Neurology*, **258C**, 78–90.

Kim, R.Y., Hoffman, A.S., Itoh, N. *et al.* (2014) Astrocyte CCL2 sustains immune cell infiltration in chronic experimental autoimmune encephalomyelitis. *Journal of Neuroimmunology*, **274**, 53–61.

King, V.R., Huang, W.L., Dyall, S.C., Curran, O.E., Priestley, J.V. & Michael-Titus, A.T. (2006) Omega-3 fatty acids improve recovery, whereas omega-6 fatty acids worsen outcome, after spinal cord injury in the adult rat. *Journal of Neuroscience*, **26**, 4672–4680.

Kreutzberg, G.W. (1996) Microglia: A sensor for pathological events in the CNS. *Trends in Neurosciences*, **19**, 312–318.

Kroner, A., Greenhalgh, A.D., Zarruk, J.G., Passos Dos Santos, R., Gaestel, M. & David, S. (2014) TNF and increased intracellular iron alter macrophage polarization to a detrimental M1 phenotype in the injured spinal cord. *Neuron*, **83**, 1098–1116.

Kutzelnigg, A., Lucchinetti, C.F., Stadelmann, C. *et al.* (2005) Cortical demyelination and diffuse white matter injury in multiple sclerosis. *Brain*, **128**, 2705–12.

Lassmann, H. (2008) Mechanisms of inflammation induced tissue injury in multiple sclerosis. *Journal of the Neurological Sciences*, **74**, 45–47.

Lassmann, H., van Horssen, J. & Mahad, D. (2012) Progressive multiple sclerosis: Pathology and pathogenesis. *Nature Reviews Neurology*, **8**, 647–656.

Levy, B.D., Clish, C.B., Schmidt, B., Gronert, K. & Serhan, C.N. (2001) Lipid mediator class switching during acute inflammation: Signals in resolution. *Nature Immunology*, **2**, 612–619.

Li, Q., Tian, Y., Wang, Z.F. *et al.* (2013) Involvement of the spinal NALP1 inflammasome in neuropathic pain and aspirin-triggered-15-epi-lipoxin A4 induced analgesia. *Neuroscience*, **254**, 230–240.

Lim, S.N., Gladman, S.J., Dyall, S.C. *et al.* (2013) Transgenic mice with high endogenous omega-3 fatty acids are protected from spinal cord injury. *Neurobiology of Disease*, **51**, 104–112.

Lossi, L. & Merighi, A. (2003) In vivo cellular and molecular mechanisms of neuronal apoptosis in the mammalian CNS. *Progress in Neurobiology*, **69**, 287–312.

Lukiw, W.J., Cui, J.G., Marcheselli, V.L. *et al.* (2005) A role for docosahexaenoic acid-derived neuroprotectin D1 in neural cell survival and Alzheimer disease. *Journal of Clinical Investigation*, **115**, 2774–2783.

Magliozzi, R., Howell, O., Vora, A. *et al.* (2007) Meningeal B-cell follicles in secondary progressive multiple sclerosis associate with early onset of disease and severe cortical pathology. *Brain*, **130**, 1089–1104.

Magnus, T., Chan, A., Grauer, O., Toyka, K.V. & Gold, R. (2001) Microglial phagocytosis of apoptotic inflammatory T cells leads to down-regulation of microglial immune activation. *Journal of Immunology*, **167**, 5004–5010.

Meinl, E., Krumbholz, M., Derfuss, T., Junker, A. & Hohlfeld, R. (2008) Compartmentalization of inflammation in the CNS: A major mechanism driving progressive multiple sclerosis. *Journal of Neurological Sciences*, **274**, 42–44.

Marcheselli, V.L., Hong, S., Lukiw, W.J. *et al.* (2003) Novel docosanoids inhibit brain ischemia-reperfusion-mediated leukocyte infiltration and pro-inflammatory gene expression. *Journal of Biological Chemistry*, **278**, 43807–43817.

Michael-Titus, A.T. & Priestley, J.V. (2014) Omega-3 fatty acids and traumatic neurological injury: From neuroprotection to neuroplasticity? *Trends in Neurosciences*, **37**, 30–38.

Mitchell, S., Thomas, G., Harvey, K. *et al.* (2002) Lipoxins, aspirin-triggered epi-lipoxins, lipoxin stable analogues, and the resolution of inflammation: Stimulation of macrophage phagocytosis of apoptotic neutrophils in vivo. *Journal of the American Society of Nephrology*, **13**, 2497–2507.

Mukherjee, P.K., Marcheselli, V.L., Serhan, C.N. & Bazan, N.G. (2004) Neuroprotectin D1: A docosahexaenoic acid-derived docosatriene protects human retinal pigment epithelial cells from oxidative stress. *Proceedings of the National Academy of Sciences of the United States of America*, **101**, 8491–8496.

Muñoz, L.E., Lauber, K., Schiller, M., Manfredi, A.A. & Herrmann, M. (2010) The role of defective clearance of apoptotic cells in systemic autoimmunity. *Nature Reviews. Rheumatology*, **6**, 280–289.

Navarro-Xavier, R.A., Newson, J., Silveira, V.L., Farrow, S.N., Gilroy, D.W. & Bystrom, J. (2010) A new strategy for the identification of novel molecules with targeted proresolution of inflammation properties. *Journal of Immunology*, **184**, 1516–1525.

Orr, S.K., Palumbo, S., Bosetti, F. *et al.* (2013) Unesterified docosahexaenoic acid is protective in neuroinflammation. *Journal of Neurochemistry*, **127**, 378–393.

Perry, V.H. & Holmes, C. (2014) Microglial priming in neurodegenerative disease. *Nature Reviews Neurology*, **10**, 217–24.

Prineas, J.W., Kwon, E.E., Cho, E.S. *et al.* (2001) Immunopathology of secondary-progressive multiple sclerosis. *Annals of Neurology*, **50**, 646–657.

Prüss, H., Rosche, B., Sullivan, A.B. *et al.* (2013) Proresolution lipid mediators in multiple sclerosis – Differential, disease severity-dependent synthesis – A clinical pilot trial. *PLoS One*, **8**, e55859.

Prüss, H., Iggena, D., Baldinger, T. *et al.* (2012) Evidence of intrathecal immunoglobulin synthesis in stroke: A cohort study. *Archives of Neurology*, **69**, 714–717.

Prüss, H., Kopp, M.A., Brommer, B. *et al.* (2011) Non-resolving aspects of acute inflammation after spinal cord injury (SCI): Indices and resolution plateau. *Brain Pathology*, **21**, 652–660.

Rajakariar, R., Hilliard, M., Lawrence, T. *et al.* (2007) Hematopoietic prostaglandin D2 synthase controls the onset and resolution of acute inflammation through PGD2 and 15-deoxyDelta12 14 PGJ2. *Proceedings of the National Academy of Sciences of the United States of America*, **104**, 20979–20984.

Ransohoff, R.M. (2012) Animal models of multiple sclerosis: The good, the bad and the bottom line. *Nature Neuroscience*, **15**, 1074–1077.

Ransohoff, R.M. & Engelhardt, B. (2012) The anatomical and cellular basis of immune surveillance in the central nervous system. *Nature Reviews Immunology*, **12**, 623–635.

Schwab, J.M., Chiang, N., Arita, M. & Serhan, C.N. (2007) Resolvin E1 and protectin D1 activate inflammation-resolution programmes. *Nature*, **447**, 869–874.

Schwab, J.M. & Serhan, C.N. (2006) Lipoxins and new lipid mediators in the resolution of inflammation. *Current Opinion in Pharmacology*, **6**, 414–420.

Schwab, J.M., Beschorner, R., Meyermann, R., Gözalan, F. & Schluesener, H.J. (2002) Persistent accumulation of cyclooxygenase-1-expressing microglial cells and macrophages and transient upregulation by endothelium in human brain injury. *Journal of Neurosurgery*, **96**, 892–899.

Schwab, J.M., Nguyen, T.D., Postler, E., Meyermann, R. & Schluesener, H.J. (2000a) Selective accumulation of cyclooxygenase-1-expressing microglial cells/macrophages in lesions of human focal cerebral ischemia. *Acta Neuropathologica*, **99**, 609–614.

Schwab, J.M., Brechtel, K., Nguyen, T.D. & Schluesener, H.J. (2000b) Persistent accumulation of cyclooxygenase-1 (COX-1) expressing microglia/macrophages and upregulation by endothelium following spinal cord injury. *Journal of Neuroimmunology*, **111**, 122–130.

Serafini, B., Rosicarelli, B., Magliozzi, R., Stigliano, E. & Aloisi, F. (2004) Detection of ectopic B-cell follicles with germinal centers in the meninges of patients with secondary progressive multiple sclerosis. *Brain Pathology*, **14**, 164–167.

Serhan, C.N. (2014) Pro-resolving lipid mediators are leads for resolution physiology. *Nature*, **510**, 92–101.

Serhan, C.N., Chiang, N. & Van Dyke, T.E. (2008) Resolving inflammation: Dual anti-inflammatory and pro-resolution lipid mediators. *Nature Reviews Immunology*, **8**, 349–361.

Serhan, C.N., Brain, S.D., Buckley, C.D. *et al.* (2007) Resolution of inflammation: State of the art, definitions and terms. *FASEB Journal*, **21**, 325–332.

Serhan, C.N. & Savill, J. (2005) Resolution of inflammation: The beginning programs the end. *Nature Immunology*, **6**, 1191–1197.

Serhan, C.N., Clish, C.B., Brannon, J., Colgan, S.P., Chiang, N. & Gronert, K. (2000) Novel functional sets of lipid-derived mediators with antiinflammatory actions generated from omega-3 fatty acids via cyclooxygenase 2-nonsteroidal antiinflammatory drugs and transcellular processing. *Journal of Experimental Medicine*, **192**, 1197–1204.

Serhan, C.N., Nicolaou, K.C., Webber, S.E. *et al.* (1986) Lipoxin A. Stereochemistry and biosynthesis. *Journal of Biological Chemistry*, **261**, 16340–16345.

Shechter, R. & Schwartz, M. (2013) CNS sterile injury: Just another wound healing? *Trends in Molecular Medicine*, **19**, 135–143.

Sobrado, M., Pereira, M.P., Ballesteros, I. *et al.* (2009) Synthesis of lipoxin A4 by 5-lipoxygenase mediates PPARgamma-dependent, neuroprotective effects of rosiglitazone in experimental stroke. *Journal of Neuroscience*, **29**, 3875–3884.

Svensson, C.I., Zattoni, M. & Serhan, C.N. (2007) Lipoxins and aspirin-triggered lipoxin inhibit inflammatory pain processing. *Journal of Experimental Medicine*, **204**, 245–252.

Terrando, N., Gómez-Galán, M., Yang, T. *et al.* (2013) Aspirin-triggered resolvin D1 prevents surgery-induced cognitive decline. *FASEB Journal*, **27**, 3564–3571.

Wang, X., Zhu, M., Hjorth, E. *et al.* (2014a) Resolution of inflammation is altered in Alzheimer's disease. *Alzheimer's and Dementia*. Feb 12, 2014. Doi: 10.1016/j.jalz.2013.12.024. (Epub ahead of print).

Wang, Z.F., Li, Q., Liu, S.B. *et al.* (2014b) Aspirin-triggered Lipoxin A4 attenuates mechanical allodynia in association with inhibiting spinal JAK2/STAT3 signaling in neuropathic pain in rats. *Neuroscience*, **273**, 65–78.

Weller, R.O., Subash, M., Preston, S.D., Mazanti, I. & Carare, R.O. (2008) Perivascular drainage of amyloid-beta peptides from the brain and its failure in cerebral amyloid angiopathy and Alzheimer's disease. *Brain Pathology*, **18**, 253–266.

Weninger, W., Biro, M. & Jain, R. (2014) Leukocyte migration in the interstitial space of non-lymphoid organs. *Nature Reviews Immunology*, **14**, 232–246.

Wu, Y., Wang, Y.P., Guo, P. *et al.* (2012) A lipoxin A4 analog ameliorates blood-brain barrier dysfunction and reduces MMP-9 expression in a rat model of focal cerebral ischemia-reperfusion injury. *Journal of Molecular Neuroscience*, **46**, 483–491.

Yarom, Y., Naparstek, Y., Lev-Ram, V., Holoshitz, J., Ben-Nun, A. & Cohen, I.R. (1983) Immunospecific inhibition of nerve conduction by T lymphocytes reactive to basic protein of myelin. *Nature*, **5914**, 246–247.

Ye, X.H., Wu, Y., Guo, P.P. *et al.* (2010) Lipoxin A4 analogue protects brain and reduces inflammation in a rat model of focal cerebral ischemia reperfusion. *Brain Research*, **1323**, 174–183.

Index

Neuroinflammation: New Insights into Beneficial and Detrimental Functions, First Edition. Edited by Samuel David.
© 2015 John Wiley & Sons, Inc. Published 2015 by John Wiley & Sons, Inc.